Radiography Procedure and Competency Manual

Radiography Procedure and Competency Manual

■ ■ ■

ANITA BIEDRZYCKI, BS, RT(R)
Larchmont Imaging Associates, L.L.C.
Burlington County, New Jersey

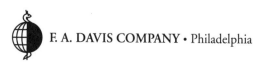
F. A. DAVIS COMPANY • Philadelphia

...3

...A. Davis Company

...s by F.A. Davis Company. All rights reserved. This book is protected by copyright. No part of it
...oduced, stored in a retrieval system, or transmitted in any form or by any means, electronic, mechan-
ical, photocopying, recording, or otherwise, without written permission from the publisher.

Chapter opening art used with permission from Scanlon, V, and Saunders, T, *Essentials of Anatomy and Physiology*,
ed. 3. F.A. Davis, Philadelphia, 1999.

Printed in the United States of America

Last digit indicates print number: 10 9 8 7 6 5 4 3 2

Acquisitions Editor: Christa A Fratantoro
Development and Production Services: Dovetail Content Solutions
Cover Designer: Elizabeth DiFebo

As new scientific information becomes available through basic and clinical research, recommended treatments
and drug therapies undergo changes. The author and publisher have done everything possible to make this book
accurate, up to date, and in accord with accepted standards at the time of publication. The authors, editors, and
publisher are not responsible for errors or omissions or for consequences from application of the book, and make
no warranty, expressed or implied, in regard to the contents of the book. Any practice described in this book
should be applied by the reader in accordance with professional standards of care used in regard to the unique
circumstances that may apply in each situation. The reader is advised always to check product information (pack-
age inserts) for changes and new information regarding dose and contraindications before administering any
drug. Caution is especially urged when using new or infrequently ordered drugs.

Library of Congress Cataloging in Publication Data

Biedrzycki, Anita.
  Radiography procedure and competency manual / Anita Biedrzycki. —2nd ed.
      p. ; cm.
  Rev. ed. of: The radiography procedure & competency manual / Anita Biedrzycki. 2000.
  Includes bibliographical references and index.
  ISBN-13: 978-0-8036-1874-9
  1. Radiology, Medical—Handbooks, manuals, etc. 2. Radiologic technologists—Handbooks,
manuals, etc. I. Biedrzycki, Anita. Radiography procedure & competency manual. II. Title.
  [DNLM: 1. Radiography—methods—Examination Questions. WN 18.2 B586r 2008]
  RC78.B48 2008
  616.07'57–dc22
                                                                                                    2007046907

Dedication

To MOM

Mother, You filled my days with rainbow lights,
Fairytales and sweet dream nights,
A kiss to wipe away my tears,
Gingerbread to ease my fears.
You gave the gift of life to me,
And then in love, you set me free.
I thank you for your tender care,
For deep warm hugs and being there.
I hope that when you think of me,
A part of you, you'll always see.

~Author Unknown~

Preface

Radiography Procedure and Competency Manual is designed to aid students in achieving their goal of becoming competent, meticulous, conscientious, confident, and professional radiologic technologists. I'm sure that other radiography educators have experienced frustrations similar to my own in trying to find a comprehensive, organized, and practical method to teach and track performance and competency. I hope this text will fill that void.

Balancing the many components of producing high-quality radiographs is a daunting task. This manual introduces students to new material, provides a foundation from which to expand, and provides students and instructors with an easy-to-follow, comprehensive text that explains intricacies on a comprehensible level. It is a progressive text based on clinical theories that are the foundations for mastering all clinical applications and skills, and it bridges the gap between theory and performance. Because this manual is very detailed, students can use it as a reference to practice and learn from their mistakes. When students are familiar with the format of the manual, they acquire habits that allow them to perform systematically, without leaving out important details.

The Joint Review Committee on Education in Radiologic Technology (JRCERT) requires critical-thinking and problem solving-skills in the curriculum of radiography programs to further enhance students' competence. As of January 1, 2002, the American Registry of Radiologic Technologists (ARRT) required documentation of mandatory and elective student competency performances. This book addresses both the JRCERT and the ARRT requirements. It also includes additional examinations that are not required by the ARRT, to broaden the scope of practice and not to limit exams to the "norms," mainly because the routine protocols are not always achievable.

All program directors are required to sign documentation verifying that each student has met competency requirements as identified by the ARRT before the student is eligible to take the national certification examination. This text was written so that ARRT standards and student progression toward meeting the requirements can easily be accomplished and monitored. Also required by the ARRT is documentation of general patient care, including cardiopulmonary resuscitation, vital signs, sterile and aseptic technique, venipuncture, transfer of patients, and care of patient medical equipment. A section documenting each of the required components is included in the Radiography Procedure and Competency Table of Contents and Grade Record.

I genuinely hope that this text will contribute to the knowledge, confidence, and expertise of students and their future careers as radiologic technologists, and ultimately to the enhancement of quality patient care.

Acknowledgments

Carley, Christopher, and Zeke ~ Just thinking of you all inspires, motivates, and brightens each day! May your innocence be recognized, your youth be respected, your lives be cherished, and your growth be infamously untouchable!

Paula "Wubby" and Chris "Doc" ~ You both are always so supportive and such GREAT friends!

And of course, thanks to **Frank** for always finding your "puddles," leaving me time to concentrate, and "making life easy." ☺ Also for supporting me in everything I do (or dream to do someday) ~ just for being you!!!

Radiography Procedure and Competency
Table of Contents and Grade Record

Student Name:_____

Expected Year of Graduation:_____

Requirements
M – ARRT Mandatory (36)
E – ARRT Elective (15 of 30)
PE – Program Elective

P – Performed on Patient
S – Simulated (up to 8 mandatory procedures may be simulated)
Circle One (P/S)

PAGE				PROCEDURE EVALUATION		REPEAT EVALUATION		COMPETENCY EVALUATION	
				GRADE	DATE	GRADE	DATE	GRADE	DATE
1	**CHAPTER 1 ■ Clinical Equipment**								
3	Radiology Equipment								
5	**CHAPTER 2 ■ Abdomen**								
7	Supine Abdomen	**M**	**P/S**						
	Abdomen – Upright or Decubitis:	**M**							
11	Erect Abdomen	PE	**P/S**						
15	Decubitus Abdomen	PE	**P/S**						
19	Dorsal Decubitus Abdomen	PE	**P/S**						
23	Obstruction Series	PE	**P/S**						
27	Lateral Abdomen	PE	**P/S**						
31	Pediatric Abdomen (Age 6 or Younger)	**E**	**P/S**						
35	**CHAPTER 3 ■ Chest**								
37	Routine Chest	**M**	**P/S**						
41	Lordotic Chest	PE	**P/S**						
45	Bilateral Decubitus Chest	**E**	**P/S**						
49	Bilateral Oblique Chest	PE	**P/S**						
	AP Chest – Wheelchair or Stretcher:	**M**							
53	Wheelchair Chest	PE	**P/S**						
57	Stretcher Chest	PE	**P/S**						
61	Pediatric Chest (Age 6 or Younger)	**M**	**P/S**						
65	**CHAPTER 4 ■ Upper Extremities**								
67	Finger/Thumb	**M**	**P/S**						
71	Hand	**M**	**P/S**						

Note: * *Each Program has the right to alter the grading system to fit their needs. At the discretion of each Program, specific criteria performed incorrectly, necessitating a repeat exposure or when criteria are erroneously omitted may result in an automatic failing grade. For example: failure to assess the patient's possibility of pregnancy, document the date of the patient's last menstrual period, have the patient sign a pregnancy consent form, shield (when appropriate), and/or obtain a full and accurate history is unacceptable and automatically results in a failing grade; no exceptions.*

GENERAL PATIENT CARE ~ All six of the following general patient care competencies are *mandatory* per ARRT guidelines prior to graduation.

- CPR certification competence verified and documentation filed with program by:

  Program Personnel Name: _____ Date: _____

- Vital signs (blood pressure, pulse, respiration and temperature) competence verified and documentation filed with program by:

  Program Personnel Name: _____ Date: _____

- Sterile and aseptic technique competence verified and documentation filed with program by:

  Program Personnel Name: _____ Date: _____

- Venipuncture competence verified and documentation filed with program by:

  Program Personnel Name: _____ Date: _____

- Transfer of patient competence verified and documentation filed with program by:

  Program Personnel Name: _____ Date: _____

- Care of medical equipment (e.g. oxygen tank, IV tubing) competence verified and documentation filed with program by:

  Program Personnel Name: _____ Date: _____

Note to Educators

The complexities of positioning patients for radiographic examinations must be introduced systematically and without confusion. Learning each detail is often overwhelming, but to ensure that the patient is never compromised, no facet can ever be overlooked. This text is very detailed to encourage students to acquire the exemplary behaviors that are basic habits of experienced technologists.

Radiography Procedure and Competency Manual is intended to serve as a record of a student's entire clinical education. It is organized by anatomical sections, beginning with the most basic of exams and ending with the most comprehensive. Each section is broken down by required tasks for the instructor or evaluator's use in the lab and in the clinical setting.

Although some projections are the same as others in different examinations, the manual is written so that each evaluation is a complete and individual exam. As an example, a complete abdomen examination requires an AP projection only, while a complete obstruction series examination requires two AP projections: an AP erect abdomen and an AP supine abdomen, and often a PA chest. Since both examinations require an AP projection, both evaluations list the AP separately. The manual is detailed and thorough without being needlessly repetitive.

Designed to be user friendly, the manual is presented in such a way that the instructor, after evaluating the student, can easily check "Yes," the student accomplished the objective, or "No," the student did not accomplish the objective. The manual's organization allows the instructor to compare the Procedural (Lab) Evaluation and the Competency Evaluation simultaneously because both evaluations are side by side on the same page. Repetitious weak points can easily be distinguished and addressed before the student acquires bad habits.

In this second edition, based on educator requests, columns have been moved to the right side of the requirements and a third column has been added to allow for the possible need to repeat procedures or competencies. Also, the second edition recognizes that many institutions have acquired state-of-the-art equipment, technology and software. The digital arena is a growing aspect in healthcare, so new technologies are noted throughout the text but they do not replace conventional systems universally. There are still many facilities with conventional technology, CR, DR, or a combination of newer technology.

The manual is a comprehensive text that complements radiographic procedures texts. Additionally, because it bridges the gap between theory and performance, the manual is a valuable teaching and testing tool for both the instructor and the student. For the instructor, it provides a complete, detailed, convenient, and organized tool to compare, track, and evaluate student performance, progression, and competency according to mandatory ARRT standards. Because all requirements are listed in detail, students acquire habits that allow them to function systematically without forgetting or leaving out important details. Students may overlook many important details that are required to perform an exam appropriately if they are not required to perform them more than once. Because the students remembered all the details when performing a hand radiograph does not mean the educator should assume the student will remember to perform all the same required details when performing a wrist radiograph (within the same chapter) or a skull series (in a different chapter) 2 days later or even a barium enema 8 months later. Close attention should consistently and repeatedly be paid to all the details of each exam until the student is able to perform all required tasks autonomously.

Because all requirements are outlined, this text provides the program with a method for achieving higher efficiency and more consistency among multiple instructors and evaluators. All evaluators are required to complete the same objectives, ask the same anatomy questions, and so forth (unless the anatomy is not visible —see Modifications). Because of its systematic approach, this text also provides new and inexperienced instructors with an integral tool to guide them into fair and consistent evaluating habits.

ARRT Clinical Competency Requirements

As of January 1, 2005, the American Registry of Radiologic Technologists updated requirements that each student must demonstrate competency in specific clinical radiological procedures. All program directors sign documentation verifying that these requirements have been met before the student will be eligible to take the national certification examination.

According to the new ARRT requirements, students must demonstrate competency in all 36 mandatory radiological procedures. At least 28 of the 36 mandatory radiological procedure competencies must be demonstrated on patients (not phantoms or simulations). Students must demonstrate competency in at least 15 of the 30 elective radiological procedures. Electives may be demonstrated on patients, on phantoms, or as simulations. In addition to the radiological procedure competencies, the six General Patient Care competencies are mandatory. These competencies may be simulated. Reviewing the text's Grade Record is an easy way to assess a student's progress in meeting and documenting these requirements.

All standard ARRT mandatory and elective requirements are included in this text, as are additional examinations that may be used as program electives. Mandatory ARRT requirements are identified by "M" and elective requirements by "E" on the Radiologic Technology Procedure and Competency Table of Contents and Grade Record at the beginning of the text. Program electives are identified as "PE" on the Grade Record. Program electives can be used to broaden the scope of practice so as not to limit exams to the "norms" mainly because the routine protocols are not always achievable. Institutional protocol determines the positions or projections used for each procedure. Demonstration of competence required by the ARRT and included in this text includes requisition evaluation, patient assessment, room preparation, patient management, equipment operation, technique selection, positioning skills, radiation safety, imaging processing and image evaluation. Competency activities should be varied in patient characteristics (e.g. age, gender, medical condition etc.).

The core requirements mandated by the ARRT are the **minimum** clinical competencies necessary to establish eligibility for participation in the certification examination. The ARRT encourages education and experience beyond these requirements.

Using Each Section Task by Task

This book can be customized to meet the needs of individual programs. Each program decides whether to use the Procedural Evaluations with or without the Radiographic Image Quality and Anatomy sections, which is why they are shaded. Each program can also omit specific requirements that may not apply to their institution or to an individual exam.

The text lists a Procedural Evaluation and a Competency Evaluation for each exam. The Procedural Evaluation should be used as the lab exercise. Following a demonstration lecture/lab, students should have the opportunity to practice exams with fellow classmates on their own. Using the Procedural Evaluation as a dry run, instructors can evaluate students in a lab setting. After the student passes the Procedural Evaluation, he/she is able to perform these exams on patients with **direct supervision** while simultaneously requesting a Competency Evaluation. Once the student passes the Competency Evaluation, he/she is considered fully competent and can perform these exams on patients with **indirect supervision.**

Technicalities are broken down into specific sections: Facility Preparation, Patient Preparation, Tasks (in later chapters), Patient Positioning, Important Details, Radiographic Image Quality, and exam specific Anatomy. In a consistent, thorough, and easy-to-follow fashion, each section addresses pertinent aspects of performing each exam that cannot be neglected. The section labeled Facility Preparation itemizes the student's responsibilities before the patient is involved. Once interactions between the patient and the student occur, the Patient Preparation section continues the evaluation. Subsequently, the examination is conducted and is contained in the Patient Positioning segment, which describes each projection for each exam individually, consistently, and thoroughly.

The section labeled Tasks is not introduced until the exams become more interactive, such as in fluoroscopy, which has responsibilities that are much more involved than the responsibilities during a chest x-ray.

Before an exposure is taken, significant details including markers, collimation, technique, and so forth are listed in the Important Details segment.

Because a Procedural Evaluation is a simulation, a resulting radiograph usually does not exist (unless performed on phantoms). The requirements of Radiographic Image Quality and/or Anatomy can be used at an individual program's discretion. These sections can be disregarded if a program chooses not to include them in its lab setting. Programs may choose to incorporate these sections in their lab settings by using teaching images or discarded images. The Yes/No components of the Procedure Evaluation that may not be required by all programs are shaded to help the instructor simplify calculations when determining a final grade.

The Image Quality and Anatomy sections are standard requirements and must be required during each Competency Evaluation. Both the Image Quality and Anatomy sections conclude a Competency Evaluation. Radiographic Image Quality requires the student to evaluate his/her radiographs as to whether they possess proper density, good detail, scale of contrast, and so forth. It is important to mention that this section requires the instructor to ask the student to verbally critique his/her radiographs. The student should describe each component as it relates to the specific radiographs that are being analyzed. For example, the instructor should ask the student what scale of contrast the image possesses (requirement number six). The student should provide the specific response of long scale of contrast or short scale of contrast. The student might reply that a image is a low contrast image, but the question refers to its scale; therefore, the student's response should be long scale.

The student is also required to analyze the same radiographs and identify pertinent anatomical structures (not listed in any particular order) listed in the Anatomy section. Poor positioning yields inferior radiographs (those that do not display required anatomy). The Anatomy section can be used to identify anatomical landmarks and to reinforce proper positioning (during the Radiographic Image Quality section, requirement number three).

If a specific anatomical structure is not visible for any reason, that particular landmark requirement should be omitted from the evaluation and not counted during calculation of the student's grade (see Grading Evaluations: Modifications 2a).

Modifications

Radiography Procedure and Competency Manual can be customized to meet the needs of individual programs. Each program decides how to use the Procedural Evaluation: with or without the Radiographic Image Quality and Anatomy sections. Each program can also omit specific requirements that may not apply to its institution or to an individual exam. If a specific projection is not required by your institution, all the requirements for that projection can be omitted. For example, if your institution does not require a supine abdomen for a double contrast barium enema, you can skip the supine requirement. Be sure to keep in mind that you do not count the four requirements of this projection when determining a grade. This is also true for the requirement of asking female patients the date of their last menstrual cycle and possibility of pregnancy (Patient Preparation section, requirement number four) for male patients. Obviously, the student would not be required to ask male patients these questions (see Grading Evaluations: Modifications 2b).

During the more interactive exams, the students have the opportunity to jot down notes (those specific to their institution). For example, in the Facility Preparation section in Chapter 9, there is extra space left in number two so the student can list additional supplies such as types and amounts of contrast, routine protocols, and so forth.

Following the entire evaluation, a section entitled Patient Information is available to use as references, future classroom assignments, and/or student projects. A Comments section follows, and the evaluation is concluded with the signature of the evaluator.

Grading Evaluations

Taking into account educator time restraints, this edition has modified each evaluation so that the total number of requirements is obvious at the conclusion of each procedure performed. If for some reason a requirement is omitted, the educator should subtract one from the total.

The following example refers to the routine chest evaluation where a student did not perform (or poorly performed) 5 various objectives:

I. Facility Preparation	1–5 requirements
II. Patient Preparation	6–11 requirements
III. Patient Positioning	12–16 & 17–21 requirements
IV. Important Details	22–34 requirements
V. Radiographic Image Quality	35–40 requirements
VI. Anatomy	41–58 requirements

58 Total requirements
–5 Requirements marked "No"

53 Correct requirements (requirements met)

$$53/58 = .9137 \times 100 = \textbf{91 Final Grade}$$

If the patient were male, then Section II, number 9 would be omitted; therefore, the total number of requirements would be 57.

I. Facility Preparation	1–5 requirements
II. Patient Preparation	6–11 requirements — #9 omitted (-1)
III. Patient Positioning	12–16 & 17–21 requirements
IV. Important Details	22–34 requirements
V. Radiographic Image Quality	35–40 requirements
VI. Anatomy	41–58 requirements

58 Total requirements
-1 (#9 omitted)

57 Total requirements
-5 Requirements marked "No"

52 Correct requirements (requirements met)

$$52/57 = .91222 \times 100 = \textbf{91 Final Grade}$$

- NOTE – Unless the program evaluates the student on anatomy during a procedural evaluation, the Image Evaluation and the Anatomy requirements will also have to be deducted before the Procedural evaluation grade is computed.

I. Facility Preparation	1–5 requirements	
II. Patient Preparation	6–11 requirements — #9 omitted (-1)	
III. Patient Positioning	12–16 & 17–21 requirements	
IV. Important Details	22–34 requirements	
V. Radiographic Image Quality	~~35–40 requirements~~ — all omitted (-6)	
VI. Anatomy	~~41–58 requirements~~ — all omitted (-18)	

33 Total requirements
−5 Requirements marked "No"

28 Correct requirements (requirements met)

$28/33 = .845 \times 100 = $ **84.5 Final Grade** or rounded up = 85

Just as in the first edition, there may be reason for modifications of grading.

Grading Evaluations: Modifications

1. If a student needs a subtle reminder to perform a **necessary** task, I often give the student a chance to rectify an error before the exposure is taken. For example, if a student is ready to take the exposure, I'll say, "What are you forgetting?" Without delay, the student realizes he or she did not collimate and will make the correction **before the exposure is taken.** The student did not perform this requirement totally on his or her own, though I did not blatantly tell the student of the error, nor did I correct it. The student made the correction with a subtle reminder; therefore, I give the student **half credit** for that task (and will circle both the Yes and the No).

Referring to a fresh chest evaluation and in addition to not performing 5 various objectives, 3 other objectives were "half" performed (-1.5), Section IV, Important Details:

	Procedure Yes	No	Repeat Yes	No	Competency Yes	No
24. Provides radiation protection (shield) for the patient, self and others (closes doors).	☐	☐	☐	☐	Ⓨ	ⓃO
25. Applies proper collimation and make adjustments as necessary.	☐	☐	☐	☐	☐	☐
26. Properly measures the patient along the course of the central ray *for each projection*.	☐	☐	☐	☐	Ⓨ	ⓃO
27. Sets the proper exposure technique...	☐	☐	☐	☐	☐	☐
28. Exposes the cassette/receptor after telling the patient to hold still and after giving him or her proper breathing instructions (inspiration) *for each projection*.	☐	☐	☐	☐	Ⓨ	ⓃO

I. Facility Preparation	1–5 requirements	
II. Patient Preparation	6–11 requirements	
III. Patient Positioning	12–16 & 17–21 requirements	
IV. Important Details	22–34 requirements (-1.5 since 3 objectives were "half" performed)	
V. Radiographic Image Quality	35–40 requirements	
VI. Anatomy	41–58 requirements	

58 Total requirements
−6.5 Requirements (5 marked "No" **and** 3 marked "Yes and No")

51.5 Correct requirements (requirements met)

$51.5/58 = .8879 \times 100 = $ **88.7 Final Grade** or rounded up = 89

2. (a) If a student is not required to perform a certain task or point out certain anatomy (as sometimes certain anatomy may not be visible on all radiographs), that task may be omitted. For example, while reviewing anatomy, if a clear view of the sternoclavicular joints is not visible, simply omit it; do not ask it and remember this when calculating the grade (scratch off both the Yes and the No boxes).

Adding to the same examples as above, section VI. Chest Anatomy:

	Procedure		*Repeat*		*Competency*	
	Yes	*No*	*Yes*	*No*	*Yes*	*No*
50. Clavicles	▪	▪	▪	▪	☐	☐
51. Sternoclavicular joints.	▪	▪	▪	▪	⊟	⊟
52. Acromioclavicular joints	▪	▪	▪	▪	☐	☐

I. Facility Preparation	1–5 requirements
II. Patient Preparation	6–11 requirements
III. Patient Positioning	12–16 & 17–21 requirements
IV. Important Details	22–34 requirements — (-1.5 since 3 objectives were "half" performed)
V. Radiographic Image Quality	35–40 requirements
VI. Anatomy	41–58 requirements — #51 omitted (-1)

57 Total requirements
–6.5 Requirements (5 marked "No" **and** 3 marked "Yes and No")
50.5 Correct requirements (requirements met)

$$50.5/57 = .8859 \times 100 = \textbf{88.5 Final Grade} \text{ or rounded up} = 89$$

2. (b) Another good example of this is when performing an exam on a male patient (as mentioned above).

The student would not be required to ask about the patient's last menstrual period or the possibility of pregnancy. That task may be omitted (scratch off both the Yes and No). Adding to the same examples as above except in section II, Patient Preparation:

	Procedure		*Repeat*		*Competency*	
	Yes	*No*	*Yes*	*No*	*Yes*	*No*
8. Explains the exam in terms the patient fully understands and properly communicates with the patient throughout the exam.	☐	☐	☐	☐	☐	☐
9. Asks female patients of child bearing age the date of her last menstrual period and the possibility of pregnancy (also has patient sign pregnancy consent form).	☐	☐	☐	☐	⊟	⊟
10. Removes all obscuring objects (snaps, zippers, necklaces, etc.) so as *not* to produce radiographs artifacts.	☐	☐	☐	☐	☐	☐

I. Facility Preparation	1–5 requirements
II. Patient Preparation	6–11 requirements — #9 omitted (-1)
III. Patient Positioning	12–16 & 17–21 requirements
IV. Important Details	22–34 requirements
V. Radiographic Image Quality	35–40 requirements
VI. Anatomy	41–58 requirements — #51 omitted

56 Total requirements
–6.5 Requirements (5 marked "No" **and** 3 marked "Yes and No")
49.5 Correct requirements (requirements met)

$$49.5/56 = .8839 \times 100 = \textbf{88.3 Final Grade}$$

Critical Thinking and Problem Solving

The JRCERT requires **critical thinking** and **problem solving** skills as part of the curriculum in order to further enhance student competence. Sections in this manual require the student to use critical thinking as well as problem solving skills. The Tasks, Positioning, and Important Details sections initiate critical thinking skills by requiring the student to complete each and every responsibility step by step and know the consequences of omitting one single step. By evaluating their own radiographs during the Radiographic Image and Anatomy sections, students use their problem solving skills to judge their own positioning talents based on whether or not the proper structures are visible. If the appropriate structures are not visible, students should be expected to explain why. Students should be able to perform repeat radiographs of better quality after making the appropriate adjustments.

At the completion of the student's entire curriculum and following the performance of all the necessary Competency Evaluations, both the student and instructor can easily determine the student's level of competence by reviewing each individual exam if they choose, but more effortlessly by reviewing the chart at the beginning of the manual.

New students often observe an experienced technologist position the most difficult patients and obtain "textbook" images. The student lacks confidence, thinking he/she will never be able to do the same. Knowing proper positioning, how to manipulate equipment, centering, and so forth are only half the battle. Actually performing the exams is the other half. After completing this manual, students will have gained the knowledge, confidence and expertise to perform just as the technologist they observed performed. If students are truly competent, after they pass the ARRT certification examination, then the conversion to technologists should be no more than a transfer of paperwork. Radiology is a rapidly expanding profession. Why not expand our students' education before they join the profession?

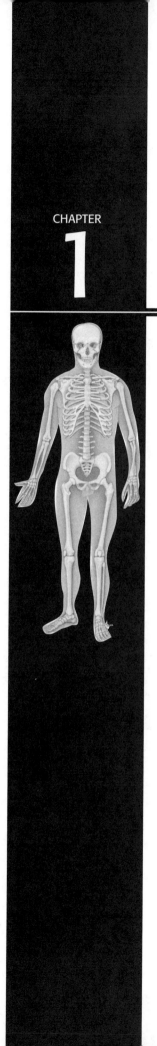

CHAPTER

1

Clinical Equipment

Student Name:_____

RADIOLOGY EQUIPMENT EVALUATION
The student is able to:

Competency

Yes　No

1. Raise and lower the x-ray tube by using the vertical lock. ☐ ☐
2. Move the x-ray tube the length of the table by using the longitudinal lock. ☐ ☐
3. Move the x-ray tube the width of the table by using the transverse lock. ☐ ☐
4. Place 14 × 17, 10 × 12, and 8 × 10 cassettes in the Bucky drawer lengthwise and/or crosswise. ☐ ☐
5. Center the x-ray tube when it is perpendicular to the Bucky drawer. ☐ ☐
6. Use the DETENT button and lock the tube to center it transversely. ☐ ☐
7. Angle the tube cephalad and/or caudad any given degree. ☐ ☐
8. Demonstrate how to rotate the tube head and maintain proper centering of a cassette. ☐ ☐
9. Center the tube when angled to the Bucky drawer. ☐ ☐
10. Demonstrate how to move the Bucky drawer the length of the table and lock it into position. ☐ ☐
11. Employ requested distances to the table or the upright Bucky by using distance markers on the ceiling or behind the x-ray tube (40–44 inches/72 inches). ☐ ☐
12. Center the x-ray tube to the upright Bucky with various cassette sizes lengthwise and/or crosswise. ☐ ☐
13. Demonstrate how to collimate to the appropriate field size. ☐ ☐
14. Demonstrate how to angle to the table (Trendelenburg) by using the table controls as well as the tower controls. ☐ ☐
15. Place the table in the upright position. ☐ ☐
16. Manipulate the tube to place it in the horizontal position for decubitus exposures. ☐ ☐
17. Demonstrate how to lock the fluoroscopic tower over the table so that it does not float back. ☐ ☐
18. Demonstrate how to remove the fluoroscopic tower. ☐ ☐
19. Load and unload spot cassettes in the fluoroscopic tower. ☐ ☐
20. Program the machine for full, split, horizontal, and four-on-one spot images. ☐ ☐
21. Demonstrate how to activate the compression device. ☐ ☐
22. Demonstrate how to lock the tower in place. ☐ ☐
23. Move the tower the length of the table using the motor-driven handle. ☐ ☐
24. Connect the video recording system. ☐ ☐
25. Identify the controls: ☐ ☐

   Conventional systems
   - Generator (on/off, kilovolts peak [kVp], milliamperage [mA], seconds/time, and phototimer, with its cells and density settings)

   or

   CR or DR systems
   - The patient on the work-list (or how to manually type the patient information into the system)

(continued)

- Selection of various body regions, body parts, and views/projections
- Preset parameters:
  —Adult vs. pediatric patients
  ◦ Small, medium, or large
  —Bucky/receptor (upright vs. table) or non-Bucky
  —Automatic exposure control (AEC) vs. fixed
  ◦ If AEC, checks ion chambers
  ◦ Density setting
  —kVp and mA; adjusts if necessary
  —Focal spot/filament size

26. Manipulate the rotor and exposure switch button.   ☐   ☐

Comments:

_____

_____

_____

Competency Evaluator Signature

_____

Date

END RADIOLOGY EQUIPMENT EVALUATION

CHAPTER

2

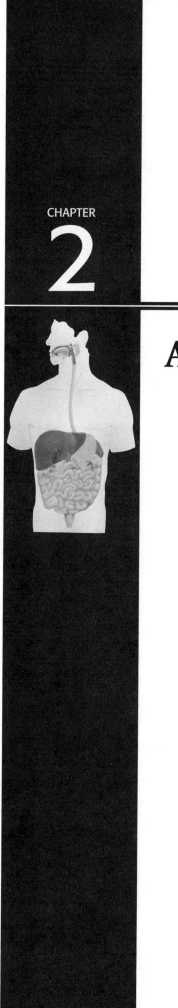

Abdomen

Supine Abdomen

The objective of this evaluation is to determine the student's competency level when performing specific radiographic examinations.

Student Name: _____

Procedure Grade	Repeat Grade	Competency Grade

PATIENT INFORMATION OR SIMULATED PROCEDURE *(circle if simulated)*

	Procedure	Repeat	Competency
Age			
Medical Record No.			
Ability to Cooperate			
Condition/Pathology			
Technical Factors Used			
Exposure Index			

FACILITY PREPARATION
The student:

	Procedure Yes	Procedure No	Repeat Yes	Repeat No	Competency Yes	Competency No
1. Examines the radiographic room and cleans/straightens it before escorting the patient in.	☐	☐	☐	☐	☐	☐
2. Has all equipment and supplies (patient gown, pillow, markers, etc.) readily available before escorting the patient in.	☐	☐	☐	☐	☐	☐
3. Is able to manipulate all radiographic equipment with ease, and centers the central ray to the cassette/receptor.	☐	☐	☐	☐	☐	☐
4. Adjusts the tube to the proper source-to-image receptor distance (SID).	☐	☐	☐	☐	☐	☐
5. Selects a cassette/receptor of the appropriate size.	☐	☐	☐	☐	☐	☐

Comments:

_____

_____

PATIENT PREPARATION
The student:

	Procedure Yes	Procedure No	Repeat Yes	Repeat No	Competency Yes	Competency No
6. Identifies the correct patient and examination according to the requisition while establishing a good rapport with him or her.	☐	☐	☐	☐	☐	☐
7. Obtains and documents the patient's history before the examination.	☐	☐	☐	☐	☐	☐
8. Explains the examination in terms the patient fully understands, and properly communicates with the patient throughout the examination.	☐	☐	☐	☐	☐	☐
9. Asks female patients of childbearing age the date of their last menstrual period and documents this; inquires about the possibility of pregnancy and has them sign pregnancy consent forms.	☐	☐	☐	☐	☐	☐
10. Removes all obscuring objects (snaps, zippers, belt, etc.) so as not to produce radiographic artifacts.	☐	☐	☐	☐	☐	☐

(continued)

	Procedure		Repeat		Competency	
	Yes	No	Yes	No	Yes	No
11. Respects the patient's modesty and provides ample comfort for him or her.	☐	☐	☐	☐	☐	☐

Comments:

_____

_____

PATIENT POSITIONING FOR A SUPINE ABDOMEN (TO INCLUDE THE SYMPHYSIS)

The student:

	Procedure		Repeat		Competency	
	Yes	No	Yes	No	Yes	No
12. Places the patient in the supine position, without rotation on the radiographic table, and with the patient's arms at his or her sides.	☐	☐	☐	☐	☐	☐
13. Selects the appropriate receptor or places the cassette lengthwise. For conventional cassettes, the flash must be at the bottom and away from any anatomy.	☐	☐	☐	☐	☐	☐
14. Centers the central ray to the midsagittal plane of the body.	☐	☐	☐	☐	☐	☐
15. Directs the central ray perpendicularly at the level of the iliac crest.	☐	☐	☐	☐	☐	☐

Comments:

_____

_____

IMPORTANT DETAILS

The student:

	Procedure		Repeat		Competency	
	Yes	No	Yes	No	Yes	No
16. Instills confidence in the patient by exhibiting self-confidence throughout the examination.	☐	☐	☐	☐	☐	☐
17. Places a lead marker in the appropriate area of the cassette/receptor (top/bottom/anteriorly/laterally), where it will be visualized on the finished radiograph, on the proper anatomical side (right/left), and in the appropriate position (face up/face down), depending on the patient's position.	☐	☐	☐	☐	☐	☐
18. Provides radiation protection (shield) for the patient (when appropriate), self, and others (closes doors).	☐	☐	☐	☐	☐	☐
19. Applies proper collimation and makes adjustments as necessary.	☐	☐	☐	☐	☐	☐
20. Properly measures the patient along the course of the central ray.	☐	☐	☐	☐	☐	☐
21. Sets the proper exposure technique:	☐	☐	☐	☐	☐	☐

Conventional systems
- Sets the proper kVp, mA, and time, and makes adjustments as necessary.

or

CR or DR systems
- Identifies the patient on the work-list (or manually types the patient information into the system).
- Selects appropriate body region, specific body part, and accurate view/projection.
- Double-checks preset parameters:
  — Adult vs. pediatric patients
    ◦ Small, medium, or large
  — Bucky/receptor (upright vs. table) or non-Bucky
  — Automatic exposure control (AEC) vs. fixed
    ◦ If AEC, checks ion chambers
    ◦ Density setting

— kVp and mA; adjusts if necessary
— Focal spot/filament size

	Procedure		Repeat		Competency	
	Yes	No	Yes	No	Yes	No
22. Exposes the cassette/receptor after telling the patient to hold still and after giving him or her proper breathing instructions (expiration) for each projection.	☐	☐	☐	☐	☐	☐
23. Provides each radiograph with the proper patient identification (flash) and/or processes each cassette (image) without difficulty (regardless of technology—film, CR, or DR).	▨	▨	▨	▨	☐	☐
24. Properly completes the examination by filling out all necessary paperwork, entering the examination in the computer, having the images checked by the appropriate staff members, and informing the patient that he or she is finished.	▨	▨	▨	▨	☐	
25. Exhibits the ability to adapt to new and difficult situations if and when necessary.	▨	▨	▨	▨	☐	☐
26. Accepts constructive criticism and uses it to his or her advantage.	☐	☐	☐	☐	☐	☐
27. Leaves the radiographic room neat and clean for the next examination.	▨	▨	▨	▨	☐	☐
28. Completes the examination within a reasonable time frame.	☐	☐	☐	☐	☐	☐

Comments:

_____

_____

RADIOGRAPHIC IMAGE QUALITY
The student is able to critique his or her radiographs as to whether they demonstrate:

	Procedure		Repeat		Competency	
	Yes	No	Yes	No	Yes	No
29. Proper technique/optimal density	▨	▨	▨	▨	☐	☐
30. Enhanced detail, without evidence of motion and without any visible artifacts	▨	▨	▨	▨	☐	☐
31. Proper positioning (all anatomy included, evidence of proper centering/ alignment, etc.)	▨	▨	▨	▨	☐	☐
32. Proper marker placement	▨	▨	▨	▨	☐	☐
33. Evidence of proper collimation and radiation protection	▨	▨	▨	▨	☐	☐
34. Long vs. short scale of contrast	▨	▨	▨	▨	☐	☐

Comments:

_____

_____

ABDOMEN ANATOMY
The student is able to identify:

	Procedure		Repeat		Competency	
	Yes	No	Yes	No	Yes	No
35. Kidneys	▨	▨	▨	▨	☐	☐
36. Psoas muscles	▨	▨	▨	▨	☐	☐
37. Bladder	▨	▨	▨	▨	☐	☐
38. Diaphragm	▨	▨	▨	▨	☐	☐
39. Symphysis pubis	▨	▨	▨	▨	☐	☐
40. Iliac crest	▨	▨	▨	▨	☐	☐
41. Hips	▨	▨	▨	▨	☐	☐
42. Stomach	▨	▨	▨	▨	☐	☐
43. Liver	▨	▨	▨	▨	☐	☐

(continued)

	Procedure		Repeat		Competency	
	Yes	No	Yes	No	Yes	No
44. Bowel gas	☐	☐	☐	☐	☐	☐
45. Obvious pathology	☐	☐	☐	☐	☐	☐

Comments:

_____

_____

_____   _____   _____
Procedure Evaluator Signature   Repeat Evaluator Signature   Competency Evaluator Signature

_____   _____   _____
Date   Date   Date

END SUPINE ABDOMEN EVALUATION

Erect Abdomen

The objective of this evaluation is to determine the student's competency level when performing specific radiographic examinations.

Student Name:_____

Procedure Grade	Repeat Grade	Competency Grade

PATIENT INFORMATION OR SIMULATED PROCEDURE *(circle if simulated)*

	Procedure	Repeat	Competency
Age			
Medical Record No.			
Ability to Cooperate			
Condition/Pathology			
Technical Factors Used			
Exposure Index			

FACILITY PREPARATION
The student:

	Procedure Yes	No	Repeat Yes	No	Competency Yes	No
1. Examines the radiographic room and cleans/straightens it before escorting the patient in.	☐	☐	☐	☐	☐	☐
2. Has all equipment and supplies (patient gown, pillow, markers, etc.) readily available before escorting the patient in.	☐	☐	☐	☐	☐	☐
3. Is able to manipulate all radiographic equipment with ease, and centers the central ray to the cassette/receptor.	☐	☐	☐	☐	☐	☐
4. Adjusts the tube to the proper SID.	☐	☐	☐	☐	☐	☐
5. Selects a cassette/receptor of the appropriate size.	☐	☐	☐	☐	☐	☐

Comments:

_____

_____

PATIENT PREPARATION
The student:

	Procedure Yes	No	Repeat Yes	No	Competency Yes	No
6. Identifies the correct patient and examination according to the requisition while establishing a good rapport with him or her.	☐	☐	☐	☐	☐	☐
7. Obtains and documents the patient's history before the examination.	▨	▨	▨	▨	☐	☐
8. Explains the examination in terms the patient fully understands, and properly communicates with the patient throughout the examination.	☐	☐	☐	☐	☐	☐
9. Asks female patients of childbearing age the date of their last menstrual period and documents this; inquires about the possibility of pregnancy and has them sign pregnancy consent forms.	☐	☐	☐	☐	☐	☐
10. Removes all obscuring objects (snaps, zippers, belt, etc.) so as *not* to produce radiographic artifacts.	☐	☐	☐	☐	☐	☐

(continued)

	Procedure		Repeat		Competency	
	Yes	No	Yes	No	Yes	No
11. Respects the patient's modesty and provides ample comfort for him or her.	☐	☐	☐	☐	☐	☐

Comments:

_____

_____

PATIENT POSITIONING FOR AN ERECT ABDOMEN (TO INCLUDE DIAPHRAGMS)

The student:

	Procedure		Repeat		Competency	
	Yes	No	Yes	No	Yes	No
12. Places the patient in the erect position, with his or her back against the upright Bucky/receptor, without rotation, and with the patient's arms at his or her sides.	☐	☐	☐	☐	☐	☐
13. Selects the appropriate receptor or places the cassette lengthwise. For conventional cassettes, the flash must be at the bottom and away from any anatomy.	☐	☐	☐	☐	☐	☐
14. Centers the central ray to the midsagittal plane of the body.	☐	☐	☐	☐	☐	☐
15. Directs the central ray perpendicularly, at a level 1–3 inches above the iliac crest.	☐	☐	☐	☐	☐	☐

Comments:

_____

_____

IMPORTANT DETAILS

The student:

	Procedure		Repeat		Competency	
	Yes	No	Yes	No	Yes	No
16. Instills confidence in the patient by exhibiting self-confidence throughout the examination.	☐	☐	☐	☐	☐	☐
17. Places a lead marker in the appropriate area of the cassette/receptor (top/bottom/anteriorly/laterally), where it will be visualized on the finished radiograph, on the proper anatomical side (right/left), and in the appropriate position (face up/face down), depending on the patient's position.	☐	☐	☐	☐	☐	☐
18. Provides radiation protection (shield) for the patient (when appropriate), self, and others (closes doors).	☐	☐	☐	☐	☐	☐
19. Applies proper collimation and makes adjustments as necessary.	☐	☐	☐	☐	☐	☐
20. Properly measures the patient along the course of the central ray.	☐	☐	☐	☐	☐	☐
21. Sets the proper exposure technique:	☐	☐	☐	☐	☐	☐

Conventional systems
- Sets the proper kVp, mA, and time, and makes adjustments as necessary.

or

CR or DR systems
- Identifies the patient on the work-list (or manually types the patient information into the system).
- Selects appropriate body region, specific body part, and accurate view/projection.
- Double-checks preset parameters:
  —Adult vs. pediatric patients
    ○ Small, medium, or large
  —Bucky/receptor (upright vs. table) or non-Bucky
  —AEC vs. fixed
    ○ If AEC, checks ion chambers
    ○ Density setting

	Procedure		Repeat		Competency	
	Yes	No	Yes	No	Yes	No

—kVp and mA; adjusts if necessary
—Focal spot/filament size

22. Exposes the cassette/receptor after telling the patient to hold still and after giving the patient proper breathing instructions (expiration) *for each projection.*	☐	☐	☐	☐	☐	☐
23. Provides each radiograph with the proper identification (flash) and/or processes each cassette (image) without difficulty (regardless of technology—film, CR, or DR).	☒	☒	☒	☒	☐	☐
24. Properly completes the examination by filling out all necessary paperwork, entering the examination in the computer, having the images checked by the appropriate staff members, and informing the patient that he or she is finished.	☒	☒	☒	☒	☐	☐
25. Exhibits the ability to adapt to new and difficult situations if and when necessary.	☒	☒	☒	☒	☐	☐
26. Accepts constructive criticism and uses it to his or her advantage.	☐	☐	☐	☐	☐	☐
27. Leaves the radiographic room neat and clean for the next examination.	☒	☒	☒	☒	☐	☐
28. Completes the examination within a reasonable time frame.	☐	☐	☐	☐	☐	☐

Comments:

_____

_____

RADIOGRAPHIC IMAGE QUALITY
The student is able to critique his or her radiographs as to whether they demonstrate:

	Procedure		Repeat		Competency	
	Yes	No	Yes	No	Yes	No
29. Proper technique/optimal density	☒	☒	☒	☒	☐	☐
30. Enhanced detail, without evidence of motion and without any visible artifacts	☒	☒	☒	☒	☐	☐
31. Proper positioning (all anatomy included, evidence of proper centering/alignment, etc.)	☒	☒	☒	☒	☐	☐
32. Proper marker placement	☒	☒	☒	☒	☐	☐
33. Evidence of proper collimation and radiation protection	☒	☒	☒	☒	☐	☐
34. Long vs. short scale of contrast	☐	☐	☐	☐	☐	☐

Comments:

_____

_____

ABDOMEN ANATOMY
The student is able to identify:

	Procedure		Repeat		Competency	
	Yes	No	Yes	No	Yes	No
35. Kidneys	☒	☒	☒	☒	☐	☐
36. Psoas muscles	☒	☒	☒	☒	☐	☐
37. Bladder	☒	☒	☒	☒	☐	☐
38. Diaphragm	☒	☒	☒	☒	☐	☐
39. Symphysis pubis	☒	☒	☒	☒	☐	☐
40. Iliac crest	☒	☒	☒	☒	☐	☐
41. Hips	☒	☒	☒	☒	☐	☐

(continued)

	Procedure		Repeat		Competency	
	Yes	No	Yes	No	Yes	No
42. Stomach	☐	☐	☐	☐	☐	☐
43. Liver	☐	☐	☐	☐	☐	☐
44. Bowel gas	☐	☐	☐	☐	☐	☐
45. Obvious pathology	☐	☐	☐	☐	☐	☐

Comments:

_____

_____

_____   _____   _____
Procedure Evaluator Signature   Repeat Evaluator Signature   Competency Evaluator Signature

_____   _____   _____
Date   Date   Date

END ERECT ABDOMEN EVALUATION

Student Name:_____

Procedure Grade	Repeat Grade	Competency Grade

PATIENT INFORMATION OR SIMULATED PROCEDURE *(circle if simulated)*

	Procedure	Repeat	Competency
Age			
Medical Record No.			
Ability to Cooperate			
Condition/Pathology			
Technical Factors Used			
Exposure Index			

FACILITY PREPARATION
The student:

	Procedure Yes No	Repeat Yes No	Competency Yes No
1. Examines the radiographic room and cleans/straightens it before escorting the patient in.	☐ ☐	☐ ☐	☐ ☐
2. Has all equipment and supplies (patient gown, pillow, markers, etc.) readily available before escorting the patient in.	☐ ☐	☐ ☐	☐ ☐
3. Is able to manipulate all radiographic equipment with ease, and centers the central ray to the cassette/receptor *for both projections.*	☐ ☐	☐ ☐	☐ ☐
4. Adjusts the tube to the proper SID *for each projection.*	☐ ☐	☐ ☐	☐ ☐
5. Selects a cassette/receptor of the appropriate size for each projection.	☐ ☐	☐ ☐	☐ ☐

Comments:

_____

_____

PATIENT PREPARATION
The student:

	Procedure Yes No	Repeat Yes No	Competency Yes No
6. Identifies the correct patient and examination according to the requisition while establishing a good rapport with him or her.	☐ ☐	☐ ☐	☐ ☐
7. Obtains and documents the patient's history before the examination.	▦ ▦	▦ ▦	☐ ☐
8. Explains the examination in terms the patient fully understands, and properly communicates with the patient throughout the examination.	☐ ☐	☐ ☐	☐ ☐
9. Asks female patients of childbearing age the date of their last menstrual period and documents this; inquires about the possibility of pregnancy and has them sign pregnancy consent forms.	☐ ☐	☐ ☐	☐ ☐
10. Removes all obscuring objects (snaps, zippers, belt, etc.) so as *not* to produce radiographic artifacts.	☐ ☐	☐ ☐	☐ ☐

(continued)

	Procedure		Repeat		Competency	
	Yes	No	Yes	No	Yes	No
11. Respects the patient's modesty and provides ample comfort for him or her.	☐	☐	☐	☐	☐	☐

Comments:

_____

_____

PATIENT POSITIONING FOR A LEFT OR RIGHT LATERAL DECUBITUS
The student:

	Procedure		Repeat		Competency	
	Yes	No	Yes	No	Yes	No
12. Places the patient in the left or right lateral recumbent position, without rotation and with the patient "built up" to adequately demonstrate the left/right side.	☐	☐	☐	☐	☐	☐
13. Selects the appropriate receptor or places the grid/cassette lengthwise, as close to the patient as possible. For conventional cassettes, the flash must be at the bottom and away from any anatomy.	☐	☐	☐	☐	☐	☐
14. Instructs the patient to raise his or her arms above the area of the abdomen, and adjusts the thorax to a true lateral position, making sure there is no rotation.	☐	☐	☐	☐	☐	☐
15. Using a horizontal beam, centers the central ray to the midsagittal plane.	☐	☐	☐	☐	☐	☐
16. Directs the central ray perpendicularly at the level of the iliac crest.	☐	☐	☐	☐	☐	☐

Comments:

_____

_____

IMPORTANT DETAILS
The student:

	Procedure		Repeat		Competency	
	Yes	No	Yes	No	Yes	No
17. Instills confidence in the patient by exhibiting self-confidence throughout the examination.	☐	☐	☐	☐	☐	☐
18. Places a lead marker in the appropriate area of the cassette/receptor (top/bottom/anteriorly/laterally), where it will be visualized on the finished radiograph, on the proper anatomical side (right/left), and in the appropriate position (face up/face down), depending on the patient's position.	☐	☐	☐	☐	☐	☐
19. Provides radiation protection (shield) for the patient (when appropriate), self, and others (closes doors).	☐	☐	☐	☐	☐	☐
20. Applies proper collimation and makes adjustments as necessary.	☐	☐	☐	☐	☐	☐
21. Properly measures the patient along the course of the central ray *for each projection.*	☐	☐	☐	☐	☐	☐
22. Sets the proper exposure technique:	☐	☐	☐	☐	☐	☐

Conventional systems
• Sets the proper kVp, mA, and time, and makes adjustments as necessary.

or

CR or DR systems
• Identifies the patient on the work-list (or manually types the patient information into the system).
• Selects appropriate body region, specific body part, and accurate view/ projection.
• Double-checks preset parameters:
  —Adult vs. pediatric patients

	Procedure		Repeat		Competency	
	Yes	No	Yes	No	Yes	No

○ Small, medium, or large
—Bucky/receptor (upright vs. table) or non-Bucky
—AEC vs. fixed
  ○ If AEC, checks ion chambers
  ○ Density setting
—kVp and mA; adjusts if necessary
—Focal spot/filament size

	Procedure		Repeat		Competency	
	Yes	No	Yes	No	Yes	No
23. Exposes the cassette/receptor after telling the patient to hold still and after giving the patient proper breathing instructions (expiration) *for each projection.*	☐	☐	☐	☐	☐	☐
24. Provides each radiograph with the proper identification (flash) and/or processes each cassette (image) without difficulty (regardless of technology—film, CR, or DR).	▣	▣	▣	▣	☐	☐
25. Properly completes the examination by filling out all necessary paperwork, entering the examination in the computer, having the images checked by the appropriate staff members, and informing the patient that he or she is finished.	▣	▣	▣	▣	☐	☐
26. Exhibits the ability to adapt to new and difficult situations if and when necessary.	▣	▣	▣	▣	☐	☐
27. Accepts constructive criticism and uses it to his or her advantage.	☐	☐	☐	☐	☐	☐
28. Leaves the radiographic room neat and clean for the next examination.	▣	▣	▣	▣	☐	☐
29. Completes the examination within a reasonable time frame.	☐	☐	☐	☐	☐	☐

Comments:

_____

_____

RADIOGRAPHIC IMAGE QUALITY
The student is able to critique his or her radiographs as to whether they demonstrate:

	Procedure		Repeat		Competency	
	Yes	No	Yes	No	Yes	No
30. Proper technique/optimal density	▣	▣	▣	▣	☐	☐
31. Enhanced detail, without evidence of motion and without any visible artifacts	▣	▣	▣	▣	☐	☐
32. Proper positioning (all anatomy included, evidence of proper centering/ alignment, etc.)	▣	▣	▣	▣	☐	☐
33. Proper marker placement	▣	▣	▣	▣	☐	☐
34. Evidence of proper collimation and radiation protection	▣	▣	▣	▣	☐	☐
35. Long vs. short scale of contrast	▣	▣	▣	▣	☐	☐

Comments:

_____

_____

ABDOMEN ANATOMY
The student is able to identify:

	Procedure		Repeat		Competency	
	Yes	No	Yes	No	Yes	No
36. Kidneys	▣	▣	▣	▣	☐	☐
37. Bladder	▣	▣	▣	▣	☐	☐
38. Diaphragm	▣	▣	▣	▣	☐	☐
39. Symphysis pubis	▣	▣	▣	▣	☐	☐
40. Iliac crest	▣	▣	▣	▣	☐	☐

(continued)

	Procedure		Repeat		Competency	
	Yes	No	Yes	No	Yes	No
41. Hips	☐	☐	☐	☐	☐	☐
42. Stomach	☐	☐	☐	☐	☐	☐
43. Liver	☐	☐	☐	☐	☐	☐
44. Bowel gas	☐	☐	☐	☐	☐	☐
45. Obvious pathology	☐	☐	☐	☐	☐	☐

Comments:

_____

_____

_____   _____   _____
Procedure Evaluator Signature   Repeat Evaluator Signature   Competency Evaluator Signature

_____   _____   _____
Date   Date   Date

END DECUBITUS ABDOMEN EVALUATION

Dorsal Decubitus Abdomen

The objective of this evaluation is to determine the student's competency level when performing specific radiographic examinations.

Student Name: _____

Procedure Grade	Repeat Grade	Competency Grade

PATIENT INFORMATION OR SIMULATED PROCEDURE *(circle if simulated)*

	Procedure	Repeat	Competency
Age			
Medical Record No.			
Ability to Cooperate			
Condition/Pathology			
Technical Factors Used			
Exposure Index			

FACILITY PREPARATION
The student:

	Procedure Yes	No	Repeat Yes	No	Competency Yes	No
1. Examines the radiographic room and cleans/straightens it before escorting the patient in.	☐	☐	☐	☐	☐	☐
2. Has all equipment and supplies (patient gown, pillow, markers, etc.) readily available before escorting the patient in.	☐	☐	☐	☐	☐	☐
3. Is able to manipulate all radiographic equipment with ease, and centers the central ray to the cassette/receptor.	☐	☐	☐	☐	☐	☐
4. Adjusts the tube to the proper SID.	☐	☐	☐	☐	☐	☐
5. Selects a cassette/receptor of the appropriate size.	☐	☐	☐	☐	☐	☐

Comments:

_____

_____

PATIENT PREPARATION
The student:

	Procedure Yes	No	Repeat Yes	No	Competency Yes	No
6. Identifies the correct patient and examination according to the requisition while establishing a good rapport with him or her.	☐	☐	☐	☐	☐	☐
7. Obtains and documents the patient's history before the examination.	☑	☑	☑	☑	☐	☐
8. Explains the examination in terms the patient fully understands, and properly communicates with the patient throughout the examination.	☐	☐	☐	☐	☐	☐
9. Asks female patients of childbearing age the date of their last menstrual period and documents this; inquires about the possibility of pregnancy and has them sign pregnancy consent forms.	☐	☐	☐	☐	☐	☐
10. Removes all obscuring objects (snaps, zippers, belt, etc.) so as *not* to produce radiographic artifacts.	☐	☐	☐	☐	☐	☐
11. Respects the patient's modesty and provides ample comfort for him or her.	☐	☐	☐	☐	☐	☐

(continued)

Comments:

_____

_____

PATIENT POSITIONING OF A DORSAL DECUBITUS ABDOMEN
The student:

	Procedure		Repeat		Competency	
	Yes	No	Yes	No	Yes	No
12. Places the patient in supine/recumbent position, with the patient "built up" to adequately demonstrate the posterior surface.	☐	☐	☐	☐	☐	☐
13. Selects the appropriate receptor or places the grid/cassette lengthwise, as close to the patient as possible. For conventional cassettes, the flash must be at the bottom and away from any anatomy.	☐	☐	☐	☐	☐	☐
14. Instructs the patient to raise his or her arms above the area of the abdomen.	☐	☐	☐	☐	☐	☐
15. Centers the central ray 1–2 inches anteriorly to the midaxillary plane.	☐	☐	☐	☐	☐	☐
16. Directs the central ray perpendicularly at the level of the iliac crest.	☐	☐	☐	☐	☐	☐

Comments:

_____

_____

IMPORTANT DETAILS
The student:

	Procedure		Repeat		Competency	
	Yes	No	Yes	No	Yes	No
17. Instills confidence in the patient by exhibiting self-confidence throughout the examination.	☐	☐	☐	☐	☐	☐
18. Places a lead marker in the appropriate area of the cassette/receptor (top/bottom/anteriorly/laterally), where it will be visualized on the finished radiograph, on the proper anatomical side (R/L), and in the appropriate position (face up/face down), depending on the patient's position.	☐	☐	☐	☐	☐	☐
19. Provides radiation protection (shield) for the patient (when appropriate), self, and others (closes doors).	☐	☐	☐	☐	☐	☐
20. Applies proper collimation and makes adjustments as necessary.	☐	☐	☐	☐	☐	☐
21. Properly measures the patient along the course of the central ray.	☐	☐	☐	☐	☐	☐
22. Sets the proper exposure technique:	☐	☐	☐	☐	☐	☐

Conventional systems
- Sets the proper kVp, mA, and time and makes adjustments as necessary.

or

CR or DR systems
- Identifies the patient on the work-list (or manually types the patient information into the system).
- Selects appropriate body region, specific body part, and accurate view/projection.
- Double-checks preset parameters:
  — Adult vs. pediatric patients
    ○ Small, medium, or large
  — Bucky/receptor (upright vs. table) *or* non-Bucky
  — AEC vs. fixed
    ○ If AEC, checks ion chambers
    ○ Density setting
  — kVp and mA; adjusts if necessary
  — Focal spot/filament size

23. Exposes the cassette/receptor after telling the patient to hold still and after giving the patient proper breathing instructions (expiration) *for each projection.*	☐	☐	☐	☐	☐	☐

	Procedure		Repeat		Competency	
	Yes	No	Yes	No	Yes	No
24. Provides each radiograph with the proper patient identification (flash) and/or processes each cassette (image) without difficulty (regardless of technology—film, CR, or DR).	☑	☑	☑	☑	☐	☐
25. Properly completes the examination by filling out all necessary paperwork, entering the examination in the computer, having the images checked by the appropriate staff members, and informing the patient that he or she is finished.	☑	☑	☑	☑	☐	
26. Exhibits the ability to adapt to new and difficult situations if and when necessary.	☑	☑	☑	☑	☐	☐
27. Accepts constructive criticism and uses it to his or her advantage.	☐	☐	☐	☐	☐	☐
28. Leaves the radiographic room neat and clean for the next examination.	☑	☑	☑	☑	☐	☐
29. Completes the examination within a reasonable time frame.	☐	☐	☐	☐	☐	☐

Comments:

RADIOGRAPHIC IMAGE QUALITY

The student is able to critique his or her radiographs as to whether they demonstrate:

	Procedure		Repeat		Competency	
	Yes	No	Yes	No	Yes	No
30. Proper technique/optimal density	☑	☑	☑	☑	☐	☐
31. Enhanced detail, without evidence of motion and without any visible artifacts	☑	☑	☑	☑	☐	☐
32. Proper positioning (all anatomy included, evidence of proper centering/alignment, etc.)	☑	☑	☑	☑	☐	☐
33. Proper marker placement	☑	☑	☑	☑	☐	☐
34. Evidence of proper collimation and radiation protection	☑	☑	☑	☑	☐	☐
35. Long vs. short scale of contrast	☑	☑	☑	☑	☐	☐

Comments:

ABDOMEN ANATOMY

The student is able to identify:

	Procedure		Repeat		Competency	
	Yes	No	Yes	No	Yes	No
36. Diaphragm	☑	☑	☑	☑	☐	☐
37. Lumbar vertebrae	☑	☑	☑	☑	☐	☐
38. Sacrum	☑	☑	☑	☑	☐	☐
39. Iliac crest	☑	☑	☑	☑	☐	☐
40. Bowel gas	☑	☑	☑	☑	☐	☐
41. Obvious pathology	☑	☑	☑	☑	☐	☐

Comments:

Procedure Evaluator Signature   Repeat Evaluator Signature   Competency Evaluator Signature

Date   Date   Date

END DORSAL DECUITUS ABDOMEN EVALUATION

Student Name:_____

Procedure Grade	Repeat Grade	Competency Grade

PATIENT INFORMATION OR SIMULATED PROCEDURE *(circle if simulated)*

	Procedure	Repeat	Competency
Age			
Medical Record No.			
Ability to Cooperate			
Condition/Pathology			
Technical Factors Used			
Exposure Index			

FACILITY PREPARATION
The student:

	Procedure Yes	Procedure No	Repeat Yes	Repeat No	Competency Yes	Competency No
1. Examines the radiographic room and cleans/straightens it before escorting the patient in.	☐	☐	☐	☐	☐	☐
2. Has all equipment and supplies (patient gown, pillow, markers, etc.) readily available before escorting the patient in.	☐	☐	☐	☐	☐	☐
3. Is able to manipulate all radiographic equipment with ease, and centers the central ray to the cassette/receptor *for all projections.*	☐	☐	☐	☐	☐	☐
4. Adjusts the tube to the proper SID *for each projection.*	☐	☐	☐	☐	☐	☐
5. Selects cassette/receptor of the appropriate sizes for all projections.	☐	☐	☐	☐	☐	☐

Comments:

_____

_____

PATIENT PREPARATION
The student:

	Procedure Yes	Procedure No	Repeat Yes	Repeat No	Competency Yes	Competency No
6. Identifies the correct patient and examination according to the requisition while establishing a good rapport with him or her.	☐	☐	☐	☐	☐	☐
7. Obtains and documents the patient's history before the examination.	▨	▨	▨	▨	☐	☐
8. Explains the examination in terms the patient fully understands, and properly communicates with the patient throughout the examination.	☐	☐	☐	☐	☐	☐
9. Asks female patients of childbearing age the date of their last menstrual period and documents this; inquires about the possibility of pregnancy and has them sign pregnancy consent forms.	☐	☐	☐	☐	☐	☐
10. Removes all obscuring objects (snaps, zippers, belt, etc.) so as *not* to produce radiographic artifacts.	☐	☐	☐	☐	☐	☐
11. Respects the patient's modesty and provides ample comfort for him or her.	☐	☐	☐	☐	☐	☐

(continued)

Comments:

_____

_____

PATIENT POSITIONING FOR AN OBSTRUCTION SERIES
Chest
The student:

	Procedure		Repeat		Competency	
	Yes	No	Yes	No	Yes	No
12. Places the patient's chest in contact with the upright Bucky/receptor if erect (or supine on the radiographic table).	☐	☐	☐	☐	☐	☐
13. Selects the appropriate receptor or places the cassette lenghtwise or crosswise, depending on the patient's body type, and ensures that the upper border of the cassette/receptor is 1–2 inches above the patient's shoulders. For conventional cassettes, the flash must be at the top and away from any anatomy.	☐	☐	☐	☐	☐	☐
14. Instructs the patient to roll his or her shoulders forward.	☐	☐	☐	☐	☐	☐
15. Centers the central ray to the midsagittal plane of the body.	☐	☐	☐	☐	☐	☐
16. Directs the central ray perpendicularly at the level of the seventh thoracic vertebra.	☐	☐	☐	☐	☐	☐

Supine Abdomen (To Include Symphysis)
The student:

	Procedure		Repeat		Competency	
	Yes	No	Yes	No	Yes	No
17. Places the patient in the supine position, without rotation on the radiographic table, and with his or her arms at his or her sides.	☐	☐	☐	☐	☐	☐
18. Selects the appropriate receptor or places the cassette lengthwise. For conventional cassettes, the flash must be at the bottom and away from any anatomy.	☐	☐	☐	☐	☐	☐
19. Centers the central ray to the midsagittal plane of the body.	☐	☐	☐	☐	☐	☐
20. Directs the central ray perpendicularly at the level of the iliac crest.	☐	☐	☐	☐	☐	☐

Erect Abdomen (To Include Diaphragms)
The student:

	Procedure		Repeat		Competency	
	Yes	No	Yes	No	Yes	No
21. Places the patient in the erect position, with his or her back in contact with the upright Bucky/receptor, without rotation, and with his or her arms at his or her sides.	☐	☐	☐	☐	☐	☐
22. Selects the appropriate receptor or places the cassette lengthwise. For conventional cassettes, the flash must be at the bottom and away from any anatomy.	☐	☐	☐	☐	☐	☐
23. Centers the central ray to the midsagittal plane of the body.	☐	☐	☐	☐	☐	☐
24. Directs the central ray perpendicularly at a level 1–3 in. above the iliac crest.	☐	☐	☐	☐	☐	☐

Comments:

_____

_____

IMPORTANT DETAILS
The student:

	Procedure		Repeat		Competency	
	Yes	No	Yes	No	Yes	No
25. Instills confidence in the patient by exhibiting self-confidence throughout the examination.	☐	☐	☐	☐	☐	☐

	Procedure		Repeat		Competency	
	Yes	No	Yes	No	Yes	No
26. Places a lead marker in the appropriate area of the cassette/receptor (top/bottom/anteriorly/laterally), where it will be visualized on the finished radiograph, on the proper anatomical side (R/L), and in the appropriate position (face up/face down), depending on the patient's position.	☐	☐	☐	☐	☐	☐
27. Provides radiation protection (shield) for the patient (when appropriate), self, and others (closes doors).	☐	☐	☐	☐	☐	☐
28. Applies proper collimation and makes adjustments as necessary.	☐	☐	☐	☐	☐	☐
29. Properly measures the patient along the course of the central ray *for each projection*	☐	☐	☐	☐	☐	☐
30. Sets the proper exposure technique:	☐	☐	☐	☐	☐	☐

30. Sets the proper exposure technique:

Conventional systems
- Sets the proper kVp, mA, and time, and makes adjustments as necessary.

or

CR or DR systems
- Identifies the patient on the work-list (or manually types the patient information into the system).
- Selects appropriate body region, specific body part, and accurate view/projection.
- Double-checks preset parameters:
  — Adult vs. pediatric patients
    ○ Small, medium, or large
  — Bucky/receptor (upright vs. table) *or* non-Bucky
  — AEC vs. fixed
    ○ If AEC, checks ion chambers
    ○ Density setting
  — kVp and mA; adjusts if necessary
  — Focal spot/filament size

	Procedure		Repeat		Competency	
31. Exposes the cassette/receptor after telling the patient to hold still and after giving the patient proper breathing instructions (expiration) *for each projection.*	☐	☐	☐	☐	☐	☐
32. Provides each radiograph with the proper patient identification (flash) and/or processes each cassette (image) without difficulty (regardless of technology—film, CR, or DR).	▨	▨	▨	▨	☐	☐
33. Properly completes the examination by filling out all necessary paper-work, entering the examination in the computer, having the images checked by the appropriate staff members, and informing the patient that he or she is finished.	▨	▨	▨	▨	☐	
34. Exhibits the ability to adapt to new and difficult situations if and when necessary.	▨	▨	▨	▨	☐	☐
35. Accepts constructive criticism and uses it to his or her advantage.	☐	☐	☐	☐	☐	☐
36. Leaves the radiographic room neat and clean for the next examination.	▨	▨	▨	▨	☐	☐
37. Completes the examination within a reasonable time frame.	☐	☐	☐	☐	☐	☐

Comments:

_____

_____

RADIOGRAPHIC IMAGE QUALITY
The student is able to critique his or her radiographs as to whether they demonstrate:

	Procedure		Repeat		Competency	
	Yes	No	Yes	No	Yes	No
38. Proper technique/optimal density	▨	▨	▨	▨	☐	☐

(continued)

	Procedure		Repeat		Competency	
	Yes	No	Yes	No	Yes	No
39. Enhanced detail, without evidence of motion and without any visible artifacts	☐	☐	☐	☐	☐	☐
40. Proper positioning (all anatomy included, evidence of proper centering/ alignment, etc.)	☐	☐	☐	☐	☐	☐
41. Proper marker placement	☐	☐	☐	☐	☐	☐
42. Evidence of proper collimation and radiation protection	☐	☐	☐	☐	☐	☐
43. Long vs. short scale of contrast	☐	☐	☐	☐	☐	☐

Comments:

_____

_____

ABDOMEN ANATOMY
The student is able to identify:

	Procedure		Repeat		Competency	
	Yes	No	Yes	No	Yes	No
44. Kidneys	☐	☐	☐	☐	☐	☐
45. Psoas muscles	☐	☐	☐	☐	☐	☐
46. Bladder	☐	☐	☐	☐	☐	☐
47. Diaphragm	☐	☐	☐	☐	☐	☐
48. Symphysis pubis	☐	☐	☐	☐	☐	☐
49. Iliac crest	☐	☐	☐	☐	☐	☐
50. Hips	☐	☐	☐	☐	☐	☐
51. Stomach	☐	☐	☐	☐	☐	☐
52. Liver	☐	☐	☐	☐	☐	☐
53. Bowel gas	☐	☐	☐	☐	☐	☐
54. Apices	☐	☐	☐	☐	☐	☐
55. Costophrenic angles	☐	☐	☐	☐	☐	☐
56. Mediastinum	☐	☐	☐	☐	☐	☐
57. Aortic knob	☐	☐	☐	☐	☐	☐
58. Obvious pathology	☐	☐	☐	☐	☐	☐

Comments:

_____

_____

Procedure Evaluator Signature	Repeat Evaluator Signature	Competency Evaluator Signature
Date	Date	Date

END OBSTRUCTION SERIES EVALUATION

Student Name:_____

	Procedure Grade	Repeat Grade	Competency Grade

PATIENT INFORMATION OR SIMULATED PROCEDURE *(circle if simulated)*

	Procedure	Repeat	Competency
Age			
Medical Record No.			
Ability to Cooperate			
Condition/Pathology			
Technical Factors Used			
Exposure Index			

FACILITY PREPARATION
The student:

	Procedure Yes	Procedure No	Repeat Yes	Repeat No	Competency Yes	Competency No
1. Examines the radiographic room and cleans/straightens it before escorting the patient in.	☐	☐	☐	☐	☐	☐
2. Has all equipment and supplies (patient gown, pillow, markers, etc.) readily available before escorting the patient in.	☐	☐	☐	☐	☐	☐
3. Is able to manipulate all radiographic equipment with ease, and centers the central ray to the cassette/receptor.	☐	☐	☐	☐	☐	☐
4. Adjusts the tube to the proper SID.	☐	☐	☐	☐	☐	☐
5. Selects a cassette/receptor of the appropriate size.	☐	☐	☐	☐	☐	☐

Comments:

_____

_____

PATIENT PREPARATION
The student:

	Procedure Yes	Procedure No	Repeat Yes	Repeat No	Competency Yes	Competency No
6. Identifies the correct patient and examination according to the requisition while establishing a good rapport with the patient.	☐	☐	☐	☐	☐	☐
7. Obtains and documents the patient's history before the examination.	☒	☒	☒	☒	☐	☐
8. Explains the examination in terms the patient fully understands, and properly communicates with the patient throughout the examination.	☐	☐	☐	☐	☐	☐
9. Asks female patients of childbearing age the date of their last menstrual period and documents this; inquires about the possibility of pregnancy and has them sign pregnancy consent forms.	☐	☐	☐	☐	☐	☐
10. Removes all obscuring objects (snaps, zippers, belt, etc.) so as *not* to produce radiographic artifacts.	☐	☐	☐	☐	☐	☐
11. Respects the patient's modesty and provides ample comfort for him or her.	☐	☐	☐	☐	☐	☐

(continued)

Comments:

_____

_____

PATIENT POSITIONING OF LATERAL ABDOMEN
The student:

	Procedure		Repeat		Competency	
	Yes	No	Yes	No	Yes	No
12. Places the patient in the left lateral position on the radiographic table, without rotation.	☐	☐	☐	☐	☐	☐
13. Selects the appropriate receptor or places the cassette lengthwise. For conventional cassettes, the flash must be at the bottom and away from any anatomy.	☐	☐	☐	☐	☐	☐
14. Raises the patient's arms up above the area of the abdomen.	☐	☐	☐	☐	☐	☐
15. Adjusts the position of the patient so that the central ray is centered 1–2 inches anterior to the midaxillary plane.	☐	☐	☐	☐	☐	☐
16. Directs the central ray perpendicularly at the level of the iliac crest.	☐	☐	☐	☐	☐	☐

Comments:

_____

_____

IMPORTANT DETAILS
The student:

	Procedure		Repeat		Competency	
	Yes	No	Yes	No	Yes	No
17. Instills confidence in the patient by exhibiting self-confidence throughout the examination.	☐	☐	☐	☐	☐	☐
18. Places a lead marker in the appropriate area of the cassette/receptor (top/bottom/anteriorly/laterally), where it will be visualized on the finished radiograph, on the proper anatomical side (R/L), and in the appropriate position (face up/face down), depending on the patient's position.	☐	☐	☐	☐	☐	☐
19. Provides radiation protection (shield) for the patient (when appropriate), self, and others (closes doors).	☐	☐	☐	☐	☐	☐
20. Applies proper collimation and makes adjustments as necessary.	☐	☐	☐	☐	☐	☐
21. Properly measures the patient along the course of the central ray.	☐	☐	☐	☐	☐	☐
22. Sets the proper exposure technique:	☐	☐	☐	☐	☐	☐

22. Sets the proper exposure technique:

Conventional systems
- Sets the proper kVp, mA, and time, and makes adjustments as necessary.

or

CR or DR systems
- Identifies the patient on the work-list (or manually types the patient information into the system).
- Selects appropriate body region, specific body part, and accurate view/projection.
- Double-checks preset parameters:
  — Adult vs. pediatric patients
   ○ Small, medium, or large
  — Bucky/receptor (upright vs. table) *or* non-Bucky
  — AEC vs. fixed
   ○ If AEC, checks ion chambers
   ○ Density setting
  — kVp and mA; adjusts if necessary
  — Focal spot/filament size

| 23. Exposes the cassette/receptor after telling the patient to hold still and after giving the patient proper breathing instructions (expiration) *for each projection.* | ☐ | ☐ | ☐ | ☐ | ☐ | ☐ |

	Procedure Yes	Procedure No	Repeat Yes	Repeat No	Competency Yes	Competency No
24. Provides each radiograph with the proper patient identification (flash) and/or processes each cassette (image) without difficulty (regardless of technology—film, CR, or DR).	■	■	■	■	□	□
25. Properly completes the examination by filling out all necessary paperwork, entering the examination in the computer, having the images checked by the appropriate staff members, and informing the patient that he or she is finished.	■	■	■	■	□	
26. Exhibits the ability to adapt to new and difficult situations if and when necessary.	■	■	■	■	□	□
27. Accepts constructive criticism and uses it to his or her advantage.	□	□	□	□	□	□
28. Leaves the radiographic room neat and clean for the next examination.	■	■	■	■	□	□
29. Completes the examination within a reasonable time frame.	□	□	□	□	□	□

Comments:

_____

_____

RADIOGRAPHIC IMAGE QUALITY

The student is able to critique his or her radiographs as to whether they demonstrate:

	Procedure Yes	Procedure No	Repeat Yes	Repeat No	Competency Yes	Competency No
30. Proper technique/optimal density	■	■	■	■	□	□
31. Enhanced detail, without evidence of motion and without any visible artifacts	■	■	■	■	□	□
32. Proper positioning (all anatomy included, evidence of proper centering/alignment, etc.)	■	■	■	■	□	□
33. Proper marker placement	■	■	■	■	□	□
34. Evidence of proper collimation and radiation protection	■	■	■	■	□	□
35. Long vs. short scale of contrast	■	■	■	■	□	□

Comments:

_____

_____

ABDOMEN ANATOMY

The student is able to identify:

	Procedure Yes	Procedure No	Repeat Yes	Repeat No	Competency Yes	Competency No
36. Diaphragm	■	■	■	■	□	□
37. Lumbar vertebrae	■	■	■	■	□	□
38. Sacrum	■	■	■	■	□	□
39. Iliac crest	■	■	■	■	□	□
40. Bowel gas	■	■	■	■	□	□
41. Obvious pathology	■	■	■	■	□	□

Comments:

_____

_____

Procedure Evaluator Signature	Repeat Evaluator Signature	Competency Evaluator Signature
Date	Date	Date

END LATERAL ABDOMEN EVALUATION

Student Name:_____

Procedure Grade	Repeat Grade	Competency Grade

PATIENT INFORMATION OR SIMULATED PROCEDURE *(circle if simulated)*

	Procedure	Repeat	Competency
Age			
Medical Record No.			
Ability to Cooperate			
Condition/Pathology			
Technical Factors Used			
Exposure Index			

FACILITY PREPARATION
The student:

	Procedure Yes	No	Repeat Yes	No	Competency Yes	No
1. Examines the radiographic room and cleans/straightens it before escorting the patient in.	☐	☐	☐	☐	☐	☐
2. Has all equipment and supplies (patient gown, pillow, markers, etc.) readily available before escorting the patient in.	☐	☐	☐	☐	☐	☐
3. Is able to manipulate all radiographic equipment with ease, and centers the central ray to the cassette/receptor.	☐	☐	☐	☐	☐	☐
4. Adjusts the tube to the proper SID.	☐	☐	☐	☐	☐	☐
5. Selects a cassette/receptor of the appropriate size.	☐	☐	☐	☐	☐	☐

Comments:

_____

_____

PATIENT PREPARATION
The student:

	Procedure Yes	No	Repeat Yes	No	Competency Yes	No
6. Identifies the correct patient and examination according to the requisition while establishing a good rapport with him or her.	☐	☐	☐	☐	☐	☐
7. Obtains and documents the patient's history before the examination.	▧	▧	▧	▧	☐	☐
8. Explains the examination in terms the parent/guardian fully understands, and properly communicates with the patient and parent/guardian throughout the examination.	☐	☐	☐	☐	☐	☐
9. Asks the patient's mother/female guardian of childbearing age the date of her last menstrual period and documents this; inquires about the possibility of pregnancy if she intends to stay in the room during the exposure, and has her sign a pregnancy consent form.	☐	☐	☐	☐	☐	☐
10. Removes all obscuring objects (snaps, zippers, belt, etc.) so as *not* to produce radiographic artifacts.	☐	☐	☐	☐	☐	☐

(continued)

	Procedure		Repeat		Competency	
	Yes	No	Yes	No	Yes	No
11. Respects the patient's modesty and provides ample comfort for him or her.	☐	☐	☐	☐	☐	☐

Comments:

_____

_____

PATIENT POSITIONING OF A PEDIATRIC ABDOMEN (AGE 6 OR YOUNGER)
The student:

	Procedure		Repeat		Competency	
	Yes	No	Yes	No	Yes	No
12. Places the patient in the supine position, without rotation on the radiographic table, and with his or her arms at his or her sides.	☐	☐	☐	☐	☐	☐
13. Selects the appropriate receptor or places the cassette lengthwise. For conventional cassettes, the flash must be at the bottom and away from any anatomy.	☐	☐	☐	☐	☐	☐
14. Centers the central ray to the midsagittal plane of the body.	☐	☐	☐	☐	☐	☐
15. Directs the central ray perpendicularly at the level of the iliac crest.	☐	☐	☐	☐	☐	☐

Comments:

_____

_____

IMPORTANT DETAILS
The student:

	Procedure		Repeat		Competency	
	Yes	No	Yes	No	Yes	No
16. Instills confidence in the patient by exhibiting self-confidence throughout the examination.	☐	☐	☐	☐	☐	☐
18. Places a lead marker in the appropriate area of the cassette/receptor (top/bottom/anteriorly/laterally), where it will be visualized on the finished radiograph, on the proper anatomical side (right/left), and in the appropriate position (face up/face down), depending on the patient's position.	☐	☐	☐	☐	☐	☐
18. Provides radiation protection (shield) for the patient (when appropriate), self, and others (closes doors).	☐	☐	☐	☐	☐	☐
19. Applies proper collimation and makes adjustments as necessary.	☐	☐	☐	☐	☐	☐
20. Properly measures the patient along the course of the central ray.	☐	☐	☐	☐	☐	☐
21. Sets the proper exposure technique:	☐	☐	☐	☐	☐	☐

Conventional systems
- Sets the proper kVp, mA, and time, and makes adjustments as necessary.

or

CR or DR systems
- Identifies the patient on the work-list (or manually types the patient information into the system).
- Selects appropriate body region, specific body part, and accurate view/projection.
- Double-checks preset parameters:
  — Adult vs. pediatric patients
    ○ Small, medium, or large
  — Bucky/receptor (upright vs. table) *or* non-Bucky
  — AEC vs. fixed
    ○ If AEC, checks ion chambers
    ○ Density setting
  — kVp and mA; adjusts if necessary
  — Focal spot/filament size

	Procedure		Repeat		Competency	
	Yes	No	Yes	No	Yes	No
22. Exposes the cassette/receptor while watching for proper expiration, especially if the child is crying or there is other motion of the abdominal cavity, *for each projection.*	☐	☐	☐	☐	☐	☐
23. Provides each radiograph with the proper patient identification (flash) and/or processes each cassette (image) without difficulty (regardless of technology—film, CR, or DR).	☐	☐	☐	☐	☐	☐
24. Properly completes the examination by filling out all necessary paperwork, entering the examination in the computer, having the images checked by the appropriate staff members, and informing the patient and parent/guardian that they are finished.	☐	☐	☐	☐	☐	
25. Exhibits the ability to adapt to new and difficult situations if and when necessary.	☐	☐	☐	☐	☐	☐
26. Accepts constructive criticism and uses it to his or her advantage.	☐	☐	☐	☐	☐	☐
27. Leaves the radiographic room neat and clean for the next examination.	☐	☐	☐	☐	☐	☐
28. Completes the examination within a reasonable time frame.	☐	☐	☐	☐	☐	☐

Comments:

_____

_____

RADIOGRAPHIC IMAGE QUALITY
The student is able to critique his or her radiographs as to whether they demonstrate:

	Procedure		Repeat		Competency	
	Yes	No	Yes	No	Yes	No
29. Proper technique/optimal density	☐	☐	☐	☐	☐	☐
30. Enhanced detail, without evidence of motion and without any visible artifacts	☐	☐	☐	☐	☐	☐
31. Proper positioning (all anatomy included, evidence of proper centering/alignment, etc.)	☐	☐	☐	☐	☐	☐
32. Proper marker placement	☐	☐	☐	☐	☐	☐
33. Evidence of proper collimation and radiation protection	☐	☐	☐	☐	☐	☐
34. Long vs. short scale of contrast	☐	☐	☐	☐	☐	☐

Comments:

_____

_____

ABDOMEN ANATOMY
The student is able to identify:

	Procedure		Repeat		Competency	
	Yes	No	Yes	No	Yes	No
35. Kidneys	☐	☐	☐	☐	☐	☐
36. Psoas muscles	☐	☐	☐	☐	☐	☐
37. Bladder	☐	☐	☐	☐	☐	☐
38. Diaphragm	☐	☐	☐	☐	☐	☐
39. Symphysis pubis	☐	☐	☐	☐	☐	☐
40. Iliac crest	☐	☐	☐	☐	☐	☐
41. Hips	☐	☐	☐	☐	☐	☐
42. Stomach	☐	☐	☐	☐	☐	☐
43. Liver	☐	☐	☐	☐	☐	☐

(continued)

	Procedure		Repeat		Competency	
	Yes	No	Yes	No	Yes	No
44. Bowel gas	☐	☐	☐	☐	☐	☐
45. Obvious pathology	☐	☐	☐	☐	☐	☐

Comments:

_____

_____

_____

_____   _____   _____
Procedure Evaluator Signature   Repeat Evaluator Signature   Competency Evaluator Signature

_____   _____   _____
Date   Date   Date

END PEDIATRIC ABDOMEN (AGE 6 OR YOUNGER) EVALUATION

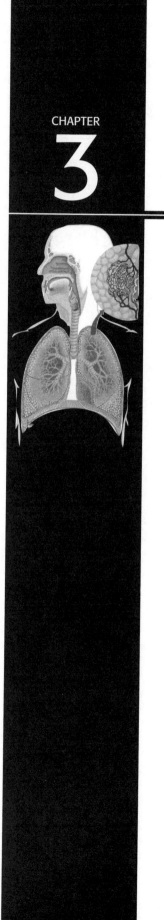

Chest

Student Name:_____

Procedure Grade	Repeat Grade	Competency Grade

PATIENT INFORMATION OR SIMULATED PROCEDURE *(circle if simulated)*

	Procedure	Repeat	Competency
Age			
Medical Record No.			
Ability to Cooperate			
Condition/Pathology			
Technical Factors Used			
Exposure Index			

FACILITY PREPARATION
The student:

	Procedure Yes	Procedure No	Repeat Yes	Repeat No	Competency Yes	Competency No
1. Examines the radiographic room and cleans/straightens it before escorting the patient in.	☐	☐	☐	☐	☐	☐
2. Has all equipment and supplies (patient gown, shield, markers, etc.) readily available before escorting the patient in.	☐	☐	☐	☐	☐	☐
3. Is able to manipulate all radiographic equipment with ease, and centers the central ray to the cassette/receptor *for both projections.*	☐	☐	☐	☐	☐	☐
4. Adjusts the tube to the proper source-to-image receptor distance (SID) *for each projection.*	☐	☐	☐	☐	☐	☐
5. Selects cassettes/receptor of the appropriate sizes *for both projections,* according to the patient's size and examination.	☐	☐	☐	☐	☐	☐

Comments:

_____

_____

PATIENT PREPARATION
The student:

	Procedure Yes	Procedure No	Repeat Yes	Repeat No	Competency Yes	Competency No
6. Identifies the correct patient and examination according to the requisition while establishing a good rapport with him or her.	☐	☐	☐	☐	☐	☐
7. Obtains and documents the patient's history before the examination.	☐	☐	☐	☐	☐	☐
8. Explains the examination in terms the patient fully understands, and properly communicates with the patient throughout the examination.	☐	☐	☐	☐	☐	☐
9. Asks female patients of childbearing age the date of their last menstrual period and documents this; inquires about the possibility of pregnancy and has them sign pregnancy consent forms.	☐	☐	☐	☐	☐	☐

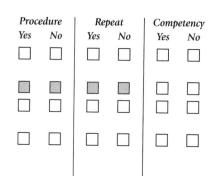

(continued)

	Procedure		Repeat		Competency	
	Yes	No	Yes	No	Yes	No
10. Removes all obscuring objects (snaps, zippers, necklaces, etc.) so as *not* to produce radiographic artifacts.	☐	☐	☐	☐	☐	☐
11. Respects the patient's modesty and provides ample comfort for him or her.	☐	☐	☐	☐	☐	☐

Comments:

_____

_____

PATIENT POSITIONING FOR A ROUTINE CHEST
PA Chest
The student:

	Procedure		Repeat		Competency	
	Yes	No	Yes	No	Yes	No
12. Places the patient's chest against the upright Bucky/receptor, without rotation.	☐	☐	☐	☐	☐	☐
13. Selects the appropriate receptor or places the cassette lengthwise or crosswise, depending on the patient's body type, the upper border of the cassette/receptor 1–2 inches above the patient's shoulders. For conventional cassettes, the flash must be at the top and away from any anatomy.	☐	☐	☐	☐	☐	☐
14. Instructs the patient to roll his or her shoulders forward.	☐	☐	☐	☐	☐	☐
15. Centers the central ray to the midsagittal plane of the body.	☐	☐	☐	☐	☐	☐
16. Directs the central ray perpendicularly at the level of the seventh thoracic vertebra.	☐	☐	☐	☐	☐	☐

Lateral Chest
The student:

	Procedure		Repeat		Competency	
	Yes	No	Yes	No	Yes	No
17. Places the patient in the left lateral position against the upright Bucky/receptor.	☐	☐	☐	☐	☐	☐
18. Places the cassette/receptor lengthwise 1–2 inches above the patient's shoulders. For conventional cassettes, the flash must be at the top and away from any anatomy.	☐	☐	☐	☐	☐	☐
19. Raises the patient's arms above the head as high as possible, and instructs the patient to grasp the bar.	☐	☐	☐	☐	☐	☐
20. Adjusts the position of the patient so that the central ray is centered to the midcoronal plane.	☐	☐	☐	☐	☐	☐
21. Directs the central ray perpendicularly to the upright Bucky/receptor at the level of the seventh thoracic vertebra.	☐	☐	☐	☐	☐	☐

Comments:

_____

_____

IMPORTANT DETAILS
The student:

	Procedure		Repeat		Competency	
	Yes	No	Yes	No	Yes	No
22. Instills confidence in the patient by exhibiting self-confidence throughout the examination.	☐	☐	☐	☐	☐	☐
23. Places a lead marker in the appropriate area of the cassette/receptor (top/bottom/anteriorly/laterally), where it will be visualized on the finished radiograph, on the proper anatomical side (right/left), and in the appropriate position (face up/face down), depending on the patient's position.	☐	☐	☐	☐	☐	☐

	Procedure		Repeat		Competency	
	Yes	No	Yes	No	Yes	No
24. Provides radiation protection (shield) for the patient, self, and others (closes doors).	☐	☐	☐	☐	☐	☐
25. Applies proper collimation and makes adjustments as necessary.	☐	☐	☐	☐	☐	☐
26. Properly measures the patient along the course of the central ray *for each projection.*	☐	☐	☐	☐	☐	☐
27. Sets the proper exposure technique:	☐	☐	☐	☐	☐	☐

Conventional systems
- Sets the proper kilovolts peak (kVp), milliamperage (mA), and time and makes adjustments as necessary.

or

CR or DR systems
- Identifies the patient on the work-list (or manually types the patient information into the system).
- Selects appropriate body region, specific body part, and accurate view/projection.
- Double-checks preset parameters:
  — Adult vs. pediatric patients
    ○ Small, medium, or large
  — Bucky/receptor (upright vs. table) or non-Bucky
  — Automatic exposure control (AEC) vs. fixed
    ○ If AEC, checks ion chambers
    ○ Density setting
  — kVp and mA; adjusts if necessary
  — Focal spot/filament size

	Procedure		Repeat		Competency	
28. Exposes the cassette/receptor after telling the patient to hold still and after giving him or her proper breathing instructions (inspiration) *for each projection.*	☐	☐	☐	☐	☐	☐
29. Provides each radiograph with the proper identification (flash) and/or processes each cassette (image) without difficulty (regardless of technology—film, CR, or DR).	▣	▣	▣	▣	☐	☐
30. Properly completes the examination by filling out all necessary paperwork, entering the examination in the computer, having the images checked by the appropriate staff members, and informing the patient that he or she is finished.	▣	▣	▣	▣	☐	☐
31. Exhibits the ability to adapt to new and difficult situations if and when necessary.	▣	▣	▣	▣	☐	☐
32. Accepts constructive criticism and uses it to his or her advantage.	☐	☐	☐	☐	☐	☐
33. Leaves the radiographic room neat and clean for the next examination.	▣	▣	▣	▣	☐	☐
34. Completes the examination within a reasonable time frame.	☐	☐	☐	☐	☐	☐

Comments:

_____

_____

RADIOGRAPHIC IMAGE QUALITY
The student is able to critique his or her radiographs as to whether they demonstrate:

	Procedure		Repeat		Competency	
	Yes	No	Yes	No	Yes	No
35. Proper technique/optimal density	▣	▣	▣	▣	☐	☐
36. Enhanced detail, without evidence of motion and without any visible artifacts	▣	▣	▣	▣	☐	☐
37. Proper positioning (all anatomy included, evidence of proper centering/ alignment, etc.)	▣	▣	▣	▣	☐	☐

(continued)

	Procedure		Repeat		Competency	
	Yes	No	Yes	No	Yes	No
38. Proper marker placement	☐	☐	☐	☐	☐	☐
39. Evidence of proper collimation and radiation protection	☐	☐	☐	☐	☐	☐
40. Long vs. short scale of contrast	☐	☐	☐	☐	☐	☐

Comments:

_____

_____

CHEST ANATOMY
The student is able to identify:

	Procedure		Repeat		Competency	
	Yes	No	Yes	No	Yes	No
41. Apices	☐	☐	☐	☐	☐	☐
42. Trachea	☐	☐	☐	☐	☐	☐
43. Heart	☐	☐	☐	☐	☐	☐
44. Mediastinum	☐	☐	☐	☐	☐	☐
45. Aortic knob/arch	☐	☐	☐	☐	☐	☐
46. Hilum	☐	☐	☐	☐	☐	☐
47. Costophrenic angles	☐	☐	☐	☐	☐	☐
48. Bases	☐	☐	☐	☐	☐	☐
49. Diaphragm	☐	☐	☐	☐	☐	☐
50. Clavicles	☐	☐	☐	☐	☐	☐
51. Sternoclavicular joints	☐	☐	☐	☐	☐	☐
52. Acromioclavicular joints	☐	☐	☐	☐	☐	☐
53. Ribs	☐	☐	☐	☐	☐	☐
54. Thoracic spine	☐	☐	☐	☐	☐	☐
55. Distal cervical spine	☐	☐	☐	☐	☐	☐
56. Scapula	☐	☐	☐	☐	☐	☐
57. Humeral head	☐	☐	☐	☐	☐	☐
58. Obvious pathology	☐	☐	☐	☐	☐	☐

Comments:

_____

_____

_____   _____   _____
Procedure Evaluator Signature   Repeat Evaluator Signature   Competency Evaluator Signature

_____   _____   _____
Date   Date   Date

END ROUTINE CHEST EVALUATION

Student Name:_____

Procedure Grade	Repeat Grade	Competency Grade

PATIENT INFORMATION OR SIMULATED PROCEDURE *(circle if simulated)*

	Procedure	Repeat	Competency
Age			
Medical Record No.			
Ability to Cooperate			
Condition/Pathology			
Technical Factors Used			
Exposure Index			

FACILITY PREPARATION
The student:

	Procedure Yes No	Repeat Yes No	Competency Yes No
1. Examines the radiographic room and cleans/straightens it before escorting the patient in.	☐ ☐	☐ ☐	☐ ☐
2. Has all equipment and supplies (patient gown, shield, markers, etc.) readily available before escorting the patient in.	☐ ☐	☐ ☐	☐ ☐
3. Is able to manipulate all radiographic equipment with ease, and centers the central ray to the cassette/receptor.	☐ ☐	☐ ☐	☐ ☐
4. Adjusts the tube to the proper SID.	☐ ☐	☐ ☐	☐ ☐
5. Selects a cassette/receptor of the appropriate size.	☐ ☐	☐ ☐	☐ ☐

Comments:

_____

_____

PATIENT PREPARATION
The student:

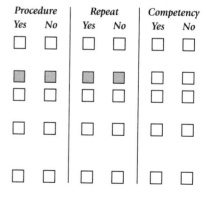

	Procedure Yes No	Repeat Yes No	Competency Yes No
6. Identifies the correct patient and examination according to the requisition while establishing a good rapport with him or her.	☐ ☐	☐ ☐	☐ ☐
7. Obtains and documents the patient's history before the examination.	■ ■	■ ■	☐ ☐
8. Explains the examination in terms the patient fully understands, and properly communicates with him or her throughout the examination.	☐ ☐	☐ ☐	☐ ☐
9. Asks female patients of childbearing age the date of their last menstrual period and documents this; inquires about the possibility of pregnancy and has them sign pregnancy consent forms.	☐ ☐	☐ ☐	☐ ☐
10. Removes all obscuring objects (snaps, zippers, necklaces, etc.) so as *not* to produce radiographic artifacts.	☐ ☐	☐ ☐	☐ ☐

(continued)

	Procedure		Repeat		Competency	
	Yes	No	Yes	No	Yes	No
11. Respects the patient's modesty and provides ample comfort and support for him or her.	☐	☐	☐	☐	☐	☐

Comments:

_____

_____

PATIENT POSITIONING FOR AN APICAL LORDOTIC CHEST
The student:

	Procedure		Repeat		Competency	
	Yes	No	Yes	No	Yes	No
12. Places the patient with his or her back against the upright Bucky/receptor, and instructs him or her to step forward approximately 1 foot.	☐	☐	☐	☐	☐	☐
13. Places one hand on the patient's lumbar region and assists him or her to arch back until he or she is in the lordotic position and the shoulders rest against the upright Bucky/receptor, or directs the central ray cephalad when necessary.	☐	☐	☐	☐	☐	☐
14. Selects the appropriate receptor or places the cassette lengthwise or crosswise, depending on the patient's body type, so that the upper border of the cassette/receptor is 1–2 inches above the patient's shoulders (or higher, if angling the central ray). For conventional cassettes, the flash must be at the top and away from any anatomy.	☐	☐	☐	☐	☐	☐
15. Centers the central ray to the midsagittal plane.	☐	☐	☐	☐	☐	☐
16. Directs the central ray perpendicularly (unless it is necessary to angle the central ray) to the level of midsternum.	☐	☐	☐	☐	☐	☐

Comments:

_____

_____

IMPORTANT DETAILS
The student:

	Procedure		Repeat		Competency	
	Yes	No	Yes	No	Yes	No
17. Instills confidence in the patient by exhibiting self-confidence throughout the examination.	☐	☐	☐	☐	☐	☐
18. Places a lead marker in the appropriate area of the cassette/receptor (top/bottom/anteriorly/laterally), where it will be visualized on the finished radiograph, on the proper anatomical side (right/left), and in the appropriate position (face up/face down), depending on the patient's position.	☐	☐	☐	☐	☐	☐
19. Provides radiation protection (shield) for the patient, self, and others (closes doors).	☐	☐	☐	☐	☐	☐
20. Applies proper collimation and makes adjustments as necessary.	☐	☐	☐	☐	☐	☐
21. Properly measures the patient along the course of the central ray.	☐	☐	☐	☐	☐	☐
22. Sets the proper exposure technique:	☐	☐	☐	☐	☐	☐

Conventional systems
- Sets the proper kVp, mA, and time and makes adjustments as necessary.

or

CR or DR systems
- Identifies the patient on the work-list (or manually types the patient information into the system).
- Selects appropriate body region, specific body part, and accurate view/projection.

	Procedure		Repeat		Competency	
	Yes	No	Yes	No	Yes	No

- Double-checks preset parameters:
  —Adult vs. pediatric patients
    ○ Small, medium, or large
  —Bucky/receptor (upright vs. table) or non-Bucky
  —AEC vs. fixed
    ○ If AEC, checks ion chambers
    ○ Density setting
  —kVp and mA; adjusts if necessary
  —Focal spot/filament size

	Procedure		Repeat		Competency	
	Yes	No	Yes	No	Yes	No
23. Exposes the cassette/receptor after telling the patient to hold still and after giving him or her proper breathing instructions (inspiration).	☐	☐	☐	☐	☐	☐
24. Provides each radiograph with the proper identification (flash) and/or processes each cassette (image) without difficulty (regardless of technology—film, CR, or DR).	☐	☐	☐	☐	☐	☐
25. Properly completes the examination by filling out all necessary paperwork, entering the examination in the computer, having the images checked by the appropriate staff members, and informing the patient that he or she is finished.	☐	☐	☐	☐	☐	☐
26. Exhibits the ability to adapt to new and difficult situations if and when necessary.	☐	☐	☐	☐	☐	☐
27. Accepts constructive criticism and uses it to his or her advantage.	☐	☐	☐	☐	☐	☐
28. Leaves the radiographic room neat and clean for the next examination.	☐	☐	☐	☐	☐	☐
29. Completes the examination within a reasonable time frame.	☐	☐	☐	☐	☐	☐

Comments:

RADIOGRAPHIC IMAGE QUALITY
The student is able to critique his or her radiographs as to whether they demonstrate:

	Procedure		Repeat		Competency	
	Yes	No	Yes	No	Yes	No
30. Proper technique/optimal density	☐	☐	☐	☐	☐	☐
31. Enhanced detail, without evidence of motion and without any visible artifacts	☐	☐	☐	☐	☐	☐
32. Proper positioning (all anatomy included, evidence of proper centering/alignment, etc.)	☐	☐	☐	☐	☐	☐
33. Proper marker placement	☐	☐	☐	☐	☐	☐
34. Evidence of proper collimation and radiation protection	☐	☐	☐	☐	☐	☐
35. Long vs. short scale of contrast	☐	☐	☐	☐	☐	☐

Comments:

CHEST ANATOMY
The student is able to identify:

	Procedure		Repeat		Competency	
	Yes	No	Yes	No	Yes	No
36. Apices	☐	☐	☐	☐	☐	☐
37. Trachea	☐	☐	☐	☐	☐	☐
38. Heart	☐	☐	☐	☐	☐	☐

(continued)

	Procedure		Repeat		Competency	
	Yes	No	Yes	No	Yes	No
39. Mediastinum	☐	☐	☐	☐	☐	☐
40. Aortic knob/arch	☐	☐	☐	☐	☐	☐
41. Hilum	☐	☐	☐	☐	☐	☐
42. Costophrenic angles	☐	☐	☐	☐	☐	☐
43. Bases	☐	☐	☐	☐	☐	☐
44. Diaphragm	☐	☐	☐	☐	☐	☐
45. Clavicles	☐	☐	☐	☐	☐	☐
46. Sternoclavicular joints	☐	☐	☐	☐	☐	☐
47. Acromioclavicular joints	☐	☐	☐	☐	☐	☐
48. Ribs	☐	☐	☐	☐	☐	☐
49. Thoracic spine	☐	☐	☐	☐	☐	☐
50. Distal cervical spine	☐	☐	☐	☐	☐	☐
51. Scapula	☐	☐	☐	☐	☐	☐
52. Humeral head	☐	☐	☐	☐	☐	☐
53. Obvious pathology	☐	☐	☐	☐	☐	☐

Comments:

_____

_____

_____

Procedure Evaluator Signature	Repeat Evaluator Signature	Competency Evaluator Signature

Date	Date	Date

END LORDOTIC CHEST EVALUATION

The objective c
specific radiog   forming

Student Name:_____

Procedure Grade	Repeat Grade	Competency Grade

PATIENT INFORMATION OR SIMULATED PROCEDURE *(circle if simulated)*

	Procedure	Repeat	Competency
Age			
Medical Record No.			
Ability to Cooperate			
Condition/Pathology			
Technical Factors Used			
Exposure Index			

FACILITY PREPARATION
The student:

	Procedure Yes No	Repeat Yes No	Competency Yes No
1. Examines the radiographic room and cleans/straightens it before escorting the patient in.	☐ ☐	☐ ☐	☐ ☐
2. Has all equipment and supplies (patient gown, shield, markers, etc.) readily available before escorting the patient in.	☐ ☐	☐ ☐	☐ ☐
3. Is able to manipulate all radiographic equipment with ease, and centers the central ray to the cassette/receptor *for both projections.*	☐ ☐	☐ ☐	☐ ☐
4. Adjusts the tube to the proper SID *for each projection.*	☐ ☐	☐ ☐	☐ ☐
5. Selects cassettes/receptor of the appropriate sizes *for both projections,* according to the patient's size and examination.	☐ ☐	☐ ☐	☐ ☐

Comments:

_____

_____

PATIENT PREPARATION
The student:

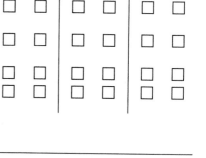

	Procedure Yes No	Repeat Yes No	Competency Yes No
6. Identifies the correct patient and examination according to the requisition while establishing a good rapport with him or her.	☐ ☐	☐ ☐	☐ ☐
7. Obtains and documents the patient's history before the examination.	▦ ▦	▦ ▦	☐ ☐
8. Explains the examination in terms the patient fully understands, and properly communicates with the patient throughout the examination.	☐ ☐	☐ ☐	☐ ☐
9. Asks female patients of childbearing age the date of their last menstrual period and documents this; inquires about the possibility of pregnancy and has them sign pregnancy consent forms.	☐ ☐	☐ ☐	☐ ☐
10. Removes all obscuring objects (snaps, zippers, necklaces, etc.) so as *not* to produce radiographic artifacts.	☐ ☐	☐ ☐	☐ ☐

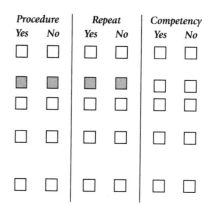

(continued)

45

	Procedure		Repeat		Competency	
	Yes	No	Yes	No	Yes	No
11. Respects the patient's modesty and provides ample comfort for him or her.	☐	☐	☐	☐	☐	☐

Comments:

_____

_____

PATIENT POSITIONING FOR A BILATERAL DECUBITUS CHEST
Left Lateral Decubitus
The student:

	Procedure		Repeat		Competency	
	Yes	No	Yes	No	Yes	No
12. Places the patient in the left lateral recumbent position, without rotation and with the patient "built up" to adequately demonstrate the left side.	☐	☐	☐	☐	☐	☐
13. Selects the appropriate receptor or places the cassette lengthwise or crosswise, depending on the patient's body type, so that the upper border of the cassette/receptor is 1–2 inches above the patient's shoulders. For conventional cassettes, the flash must be at the top and away from any anatomy.	☐	☐	☐	☐	☐	☐
14. Instructs the patient to raise his or her arms above his or her head, and adjusts the thorax to a true lateral position, making sure there is no rotation.	☐	☐	☐	☐	☐	☐
15 Adjusts the patient as close as possible to the cassette/receptor.	☐	☐	☐	☐	☐	☐
16. Using a horizontal beam, centers the central ray to the midsagittal plane.	☐	☐	☐	☐	☐	☐
17. Directs the central ray perpendicularly to the level of the seventh thoracic vertebra (if the patient is PA, centers 3 inches below the jugular notch).	☐	☐	☐	☐	☐	☐

Right Lateral Decubitus
The student:

	Procedure		Repeat		Competency	
	Yes	No	Yes	No	Yes	No
18. Selects the appropriate receptor or places the patient in the right lateral recumbent position, without rotation and with the patient "built up" to adequately demonstrate the right side.	☐	☐	☐	☐	☐	☐
19. Selects the appropriate receptor or places the cassette lengthwise or crosswise, depending on the patient's body type, so that the upper border of the cassette/receptor is 1–2 inches above the patient's shoulders. For conventional cassettes, the flash must be at the top and away from any anatomy.	☐	☐	☐	☐	☐	☐
20. Instructs the patient to raise his or her arms above his or her head, and adjusts the thorax to a true lateral position, making sure there is no rotation.	☐	☐	☐	☐	☐	☐
21. Adjusts the patient as close as possible to the cassette/receptor.	☐	☐	☐	☐	☐	☐
22. Using a horizontal beam, centers the central ray to the midsagittal plane.	☐	☐	☐	☐	☐	☐
23. Directs the central ray perpendicularly to the level of the seventh thoracic vertebra (if the patient is PA, centers the ray 3 inches below the jugular notch).	☐	☐	☐	☐	☐	☐

Comments:

_____

_____

IMPORTANT DETAILS
The student:

	Procedure Yes	Procedure No	Repeat Yes	Repeat No	Competency Yes	Competency No
24. Instills confidence in the patient by exhibiting self-confidence throughout the examination.	☐	☐	☐	☐	☐	☐
25. Places a lead marker in the appropriate area of the cassette/receptor (top/bottom/anteriorly/laterally), where it will be visualized on the finished radiograph, on the proper anatomical side (right/left), and in the appropriate position (face up/face down), depending on the patient's position.	☐	☐	☐	☐	☐	☐
26. Provides radiation protection (shield) for the patient, self, and others (closes doors).	☐	☐	☐	☐	☐	☐
27. Applies proper collimation and makes adjustments as necessary.	☐	☐	☐	☐	☐	☐
28. Properly measures the patient along the course of the central ray *for each projection.*	☐	☐	☐	☐	☐	☐
29. Sets the proper exposure technique:	☐	☐	☐	☐	☐	☐

29. (continued)

Conventional systems
- Sets the proper kVp, mA, and time and makes adjustments as necessary.

or

CR or DR systems
- Identifies the patient on the work-list (or manually types the patient information into the system).
- Selects appropriate body region, specific body part, and accurate view/projection.
- Double-checks preset parameters:
  —Adult vs. pediatric patients
    ○ Small, medium, or large
  —Bucky/receptor (upright vs. table) *or* non-Bucky
  —AEC vs. fixed
    ○ If AEC, checks ion chambers
    ○ Density setting
  —kVp and mA; adjusts if necessary
  —Focal spot/filament size

	Procedure Yes	Procedure No	Repeat Yes	Repeat No	Competency Yes	Competency No
30. Exposes the cassette/receptor after telling the patient to hold still and after giving him or her proper breathing instructions (inspiration) for each projection.	☐	☐	☐	☐	☐	☐
31. Provides each radiograph with the proper identification (flash) and/or processes each cassette (image) without difficulty (regardless of technology—film, CR, or DR).	▨	▨	▨	▨	☐	☐
32. Properly completes the examination by filling out all necessary paperwork, entering the examination in the computer, having the images checked by the appropriate staff members, and informing the patient that he or she is finished.	▨	▨	▨	▨	☐	☐
33. Exhibits the ability to adapt to new and difficult situations if and when necessary.	▨	▨	▨	▨	☐	☐
34. Accepts constructive criticism and uses it to his or her advantage.	☐	☐	☐	☐	☐	☐
35. Leaves the radiographic room neat and clean for the next examination.	▨	▨	▨	▨	☐	☐
36. Completes the examination within a reasonable time frame.	☐	☐	☐	☐	☐	☐

Comments:

_____

_____

(continued)

RADIOGRAPHIC IMAGE QUALITY
The student is able to critique his or her radiographs as to whether they demonstrate:

	Procedure		Repeat		Competency	
	Yes	No	Yes	No	Yes	No
37. Proper technique/optimal density	☐	☐	☐	☐	☐	☐
38. Enhanced detail, without evidence of motion and without any visible artifacts	☐	☐	☐	☐	☐	☐
39. Proper positioning (all anatomy included, evidence of proper centering/ alignment, etc.)	☐	☐	☐	☐	☐	☐
40. Proper marker placement	☐	☐	☐	☐	☐	☐
41. Evidence of proper collimation and radiation protection	☐	☐	☐	☐	☐	☐
42. Long vs. short scale of contrast	☐	☐	☐	☐	☐	☐

Comments:

_____

_____

CHEST ANATOMY
The student is able to identify:

	Procedure		Repeat		Competency	
	Yes	No	Yes	No	Yes	No
43. Apices	☐	☐	☐	☐	☐	☐
44. Trachea	☐	☐	☐	☐	☐	☐
45. Heart	☐	☐	☐	☐	☐	☐
46. Mediastinum	☐	☐	☐	☐	☐	☐
47. Aortic knob/arch	☐	☐	☐	☐	☐	☐
48. Hilum	☐	☐	☐	☐	☐	☐
49. Costophrenic angles	☐	☐	☐	☐	☐	☐
50. Bases	☐	☐	☐	☐	☐	☐
51. Diaphragm	☐	☐	☐	☐	☐	☐
52. Clavicles	☐	☐	☐	☐	☐	☐
53. Sternoclavicular joints	☐	☐	☐	☐	☐	☐
54. Acromioclavicular joints	☐	☐	☐	☐	☐	☐
55. Ribs	☐	☐	☐	☐	☐	☐
56. Thoracic spine	☐	☐	☐	☐	☐	☐
57. Distal cervical spine	☐	☐	☐	☐	☐	☐
58. Scapula	☐	☐	☐	☐	☐	☐
59. Humeral head	☐	☐	☐	☐	☐	☐
60. Obvious pathology	☐	☐	☐	☐	☐	☐

Comments:

_____

_____

_____   _____   _____
Procedure Evaluator Signature   Repeat Evaluator Signature   Competency Evaluator Signature

_____   _____   _____
Date   Date   Date

END BILATERAL DECUBITUS CHEST EVALUATION

Student Name:_____

Procedure Grade	Repeat Grade	Competency Grade

PATIENT INFORMATION OR SIMULATED PROCEDURE *(circle if simulated)*

	Procedure	Repeat	Competency
Age			
Medical Record No.			
Ability to Cooperate			
Condition/Pathology			
Technical Factors Used			
Exposure Index			

FACILITY PREPARATION
The student:

	Procedure Yes No	Repeat Yes No	Competency Yes No
1. Examines the radiographic room and cleans/straightens it before escorting the patient in.	☐ ☐	☐ ☐	☐ ☐
2. Has all equipment and supplies (patient gown, shield, markers, etc.) readily available before escorting the patient in.	☐ ☐	☐ ☐	☐ ☐
3. Is able to manipulate all radiographic equipment with ease, and centers the central ray to the cassette/receptor *for both projections.*	☐ ☐	☐ ☐	☐ ☐
4. Adjusts the tube to the proper SID *for each projection.*	☐ ☐	☐ ☐	☐ ☐
5. Selects cassettes/receptor of the appropriate sizes *for both projections,* according to the patient's size and examination.	☐ ☐	☐ ☐	☐ ☐

Comments:

_____

_____

PATIENT PREPARATION
The student:

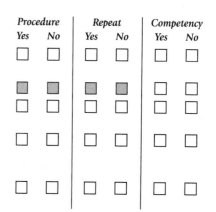

	Procedure Yes No	Repeat Yes No	Competency Yes No
6. Identifies the correct patient and examination according to the requisition while establishing a good rapport with him or her.	☐ ☐	☐ ☐	☐ ☐
7. Obtains and documents the patient's history before the examination.	▣ ▣	▣ ▣	☐ ☐
8. Explains the examination in terms the patient fully understands, and properly communicates with the patient throughout the examination.	☐ ☐	☐ ☐	☐ ☐
9. Asks female patients of childbearing age the date of their last menstrual period and documents this; inquires about the possibility of pregnancy and has them sign pregnancy consent forms.	☐ ☐	☐ ☐	☐ ☐
10. Removes all obscuring objects (snaps, zippers, necklaces, etc.) so as *not* to produce radiographic artifacts.	☐ ☐	☐ ☐	☐ ☐

(continued)

	Procedure		Repeat		Competency	
	Yes	No	Yes	No	Yes	No
11. Respects the patient's modesty and provides ample comfort for him or her.	☐	☐	☐	☐	☐	☐

Comments:

_____

_____

PATIENT POSITIONING FOR A BILATERAL OBLIQUE CHEST
Left Anterior Oblique
The student:

	Procedure		Repeat		Competency	
	Yes	No	Yes	No	Yes	No
12. Places the patient in the oblique position at a 45° angle (55–60° for cardiac series).	☐	☐	☐	☐	☐	☐
13. Selects the appropriate receptor or places the cassette lengthwise or crosswise, depending on the patient's body type, so that the upper border of the cassette/receptor is 1–2 inches above the patient's shoulders. For conventional cassettes, the flash must be at the top and away from any anatomy.	☐	☐	☐	☐	☐	☐
14. Places the left shoulder and breast in contact with the upright Bucky/receptor, with the right arm raised to shoulder level and the left hand on the hip.	☐	☐	☐	☐	☐	☐
15. Centers the central ray midway between the lateral surfaces of the chest, making sure both lungs will be fully demonstrated on the radiograph.	☐	☐	☐	☐	☐	☐
16. Centers the central ray perpendicularly at the level of the seventh thoracic vertebra.	☐	☐	☐	☐	☐	☐

Right Anterior Oblique
The student:

	Procedure		Repeat		Competency	
	Yes	No	Yes	No	Yes	No
17. Places the patient in the oblique position at a 45° angle.	☐	☐	☐	☐	☐	☐
18. Selects the appropriate receptor or places the cassette lengthwise or crosswise, depending on the patient's body type, so that the upper border of the cassette/receptor is 1–2 inches above the patient's shoulders. For conventional cassettes, the flash must be at the top and away from any anatomy.	☐	☐	☐	☐	☐	☐
19. Places the right shoulder and breast in contact with the upright Bucky/receptor, with the left arm raised to shoulder level and the right hand on the hip.	☐	☐	☐	☐	☐	☐
20. Centers the central ray midway between the lateral surfaces of the chest, making sure both lungs will be fully demonstrated on the radiograph.	☐	☐	☐	☐	☐	☐
21. Centers the central ray perpendicularly at the level of the seventh thoracic vertebra.	☐	☐	☐	☐	☐	☐

Comments:

_____

_____

IMPORTANT DETAILS
The student:

	Procedure		Repeat		Competency	
	Yes	No	Yes	No	Yes	No
22. Instills confidence in the patient by exhibiting self-confidence throughout the examination.	☐	☐	☐	☐	☐	☐
23. Places a lead marker in the appropriate area of the cassette/receptor (top/bottom/anteriorly/laterally), where it will be visualized on the finished radiograph, on the proper anatomical side (right/left), and	☐	☐	☐	☐	☐	☐

	Procedure		Repeat		Competency	
	Yes	No	Yes	No	Yes	No
in the appropriate position (face up/face down), depending on the patient's position.						
24. Provides radiation protection (shield) for the patient, self, and others (closes doors).	☐	☐	☐	☐	☐	☐
25. Applies proper collimation and makes adjustments as necessary.	☐	☐	☐	☐	☐	☐
26. Properly measures the patient along the course of the central ray *for each projection.*	☐	☐	☐	☐	☐	☐
27. Sets the proper exposure technique:	☐	☐	☐	☐	☐	☐

Conventional systems
- Sets the proper kVp, mA, and time and makes adjustments as necessary.

or

CR or DR systems
- Identifies the patient on the work-list (or manually types the patient information into the system).
- Selects appropriate body region, specific body part, and accurate view/ projection.
- Double-checks preset parameters:
  —Adult vs. pediatric patients
    ○ Small, medium, or large
  —Bucky/receptor (upright vs. table) *or* non-Bucky
  —AEC vs. fixed
    ○ If AEC, checks ion chambers
    ○ Density setting
  —kVp and mA; adjusts if necessary
  —Focal spot/filament size

	Procedure		Repeat		Competency	
28. Exposes the cassette/receptor after telling the patient to hold still and after giving him or her proper breathing instructions (inspiration) *for each projection.*	☐	☐	☐	☐	☐	☐
29. Provides each radiograph with the proper identification (flash) and/or processes each cassette (image) without difficulty (regardless of technology—film, CR, or DR).	☐	☐	☐	☐	☐	☐
30. Properly completes the examination by filling out all necessary paperwork, entering the examination in the computer, having the images checked by the appropriate staff members, and informing the patient that he or she is finished.	☐	☐	☐	☐	☐	☐
31. Exhibits the ability to adapt to new and difficult situations if and when necessary.	☐	☐	☐	☐	☐	☐
32. Accepts constructive criticism and uses it to his or her advantage.	☐	☐	☐	☐	☐	☐
33. Leaves the radiographic room neat and clean for the next examination.	☐	☐	☐	☐	☐	☐
34. Completes the examination within a reasonable time frame.	☐	☐	☐	☐	☐	☐

Comments:

_____

_____

RADIOGRAPHIC IMAGE QUALITY

The student is able to critique his or her radiographs as to whether they demonstrate:

	Procedure		Repeat		Competency	
	Yes	No	Yes	No	Yes	No
35. Proper technique/optimal density	☐	☐	☐	☐	☐	☐
36. Enhanced detail, without evidence of motion and without any visible artifacts	☐	☐	☐	☐	☐	☐
37. Proper positioning (all anatomy included, evidence of proper centering/ alignment, etc.)	☐	☐	☐	☐	☐	☐

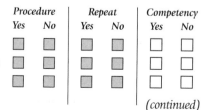

(continued)

	Procedure		Repeat		Competency	
	Yes	No	Yes	No	Yes	No
38. Proper marker placement	☐	☐	☐	☐	☐	☐
39. Evidence of proper collimation and radiation protection	☐	☐	☐	☐	☐	☐
40. Long vs. short scale of contrast	☐	☐	☐	☐	☐	☐

Comments:

_____

_____

CHEST ANATOMY
The student is able to identify:

	Procedure		Repeat		Competency	
	Yes	No	Yes	No	Yes	No
41. Apices	☐	☐	☐	☐	☐	☐
42. Trachea	☐	☐	☐	☐	☐	☐
43. Heart	☐	☐	☐	☐	☐	☐
44. Mediastinum	☐	☐	☐	☐	☐	☐
45. Aortic knob/arch	☐	☐	☐	☐	☐	☐
46. Hilum	☐	☐	☐	☐	☐	☐
47. Costophrenic angles	☐	☐	☐	☐	☐	☐
48. Bases	☐	☐	☐	☐	☐	☐
49. Diaphragm	☐	☐	☐	☐	☐	☐
50. Clavicles	☐	☐	☐	☐	☐	☐
51. Sternoclavicular joints	☐	☐	☐	☐	☐	☐
52. Acromioclavicular joints	☐	☐	☐	☐	☐	☐
53. Ribs	☐	☐	☐	☐	☐	☐
54. Thoracic spine	☐	☐	☐	☐	☐	☐
55. Distal cervical spine	☐	☐	☐	☐	☐	☐
56. Scapula	☐	☐	☐	☐	☐	☐
57. Humeral head	☐	☐	☐	☐	☐	☐
58. Obvious pathology	☐	☐	☐	☐	☐	☐

Comments:

_____

_____

_____   _____   _____
Procedure Evaluator Signature   Repeat Evaluator Signature   Competency Evaluator Signature

_____   _____   _____
Date   Date   Date

END BILATERAL OBLIQUE CHEST EVALUATION

Student Name:_____

Procedure Grade	Repeat Grade	Competency Grade

PATIENT INFORMATION OR SIMULATED PROCEDURE *(circle if simulated)*

	Procedure	Repeat	Competency
Age			
Medical Record No.			
Ability to Cooperate			
Condition/Pathology			
Technical Factors Used			
Exposure Index			

FACILITY PREPARATION
The student:

	Procedure Yes	Procedure No	Repeat Yes	Repeat No	Competency Yes	Competency No
1. Examines the radiographic room and cleans/straightens it before escorting the patient in.	☐	☐	☐	☐	☐	☐
2. Has all equipment and supplies (patient gown, shield, markers, etc.) readily available before escorting the patient in.	☐	☐	☐	☐	☐	☐
3. Is able to manipulate all radiographic equipment with ease, and centers the central ray to the cassette/receptor.	☐	☐	☐	☐	☐	☐
4. Adjusts the tube to the proper SID.	☐	☐	☐	☐	☐	☐
5. Selects a cassette/receptor of the appropriate size.	☐	☐	☐	☐	☐	☐

Comments:

_____

_____

PATIENT PREPARATION
The student:

	Procedure Yes	Procedure No	Repeat Yes	Repeat No	Competency Yes	Competency No
6. Identifies the correct patient and examination according to the requisition while establishing a good rapport with him or her.	☐	☐	☐	☐	☐	☐
7. Obtains and documents the patient's history before the examination.	▓	▓	▓	▓	☐	☐
8. Explains the examination in terms the patient fully understands, and properly communicates with the patient.	☐	☐	☐	☐	☐	☐
9. Asks female patients of childbearing age the date of their last menstrual period and documents this; inquires about the possibility of pregnancy and has them sign pregnancy consent forms	☐	☐	☐	☐	☐	☐
10. Removes all obscuring objects (snaps, zippers, necklaces, etc.) so as *not* to produce radiographic artifacts.	☐	☐	☐	☐	☐	☐
11. Respects the patient's modesty and provides ample comfort for him or her.	☐	☐	☐	☐	☐	☐

(continued)

Comments:

_____

_____

PATIENT POSITIONING FOR A WHEELCHAIR CHEST
Erect AP
The student:

	Procedure		Repeat		Competency	
	Yes	No	Yes	No	Yes	No
12. Adjusts the patient so that he or she is as erect as possible, without rotation.	☐	☐	☐	☐	☐	☐
13. Selects the appropriate receptor or places the cassette lengthwise or crosswise, depending on the patient's body type, so that the upper border of the cassette/receptor 1–2 inches above the patient's shoulders. For conventional cassettes, the flash must be at the top and away from any anatomy.	☐	☐	☐	☐	☐	☐
14. Centers the central ray to the midsagittal plane.	☐	☐	☐	☐	☐	☐
15. Directs the central ray perpendicularly (unless it is necessary to angle, according to the patient's position) to the level of the seventh thoracic vertebra.	☐	☐	☐	☐	☐	☐

Lateral Chest
The student:

	Procedure		Repeat		Competency	
	Yes	No	Yes	No	Yes	No
16. Places the patient in the left lateral position against the upright Bucky/receptor.	☐	☐	☐	☐	☐	☐
17. Selects the appropriate receptor or places the cassette lengthwise, the upper border of the cassette/receptor 1–2 inches above the patient's shoulders. For conventional cassettes, the flash must be at the top and away from any anatomy.	☐	☐	☐	☐	☐	☐
18. Instructs the patient to sit up in the erect position as much as possible, while assisting him or her to raise the arms above the head as high as possible.	☐	☐	☐	☐	☐	☐
19. Adjusts the position of the patient so that the central ray is centered to the midcoronal plane.	☐	☐	☐	☐	☐	☐
20. Directs the central ray perpendicularly to the upright Bucky/receptor at the seventh thoracic vertebra.	☐	☐	☐	☐	☐	☐

Comments:

_____

_____

IMPORTANT DETAILS
The student:

	Procedure		Repeat		Competency	
	Yes	No	Yes	No	Yes	No
21. Instills confidence in the patient by exhibiting self-confidence throughout the examination.	☐	☐	☐	☐	☐	☐
22. Places a lead marker in the appropriate area of the cassette/receptor (top/bottom/anteriorly/laterally), where it will be visualized on the finished radiograph, on the proper anatomical side (right/left), and in the appropriate position (face up/face down), depending on the patient's position.	☐	☐	☐	☐	☐	☐
23. Provides radiation protection (shield) for the patient, self, and others (closes doors).	☐	☐	☐	☐	☐	☐
24. Applies proper collimation and makes adjustments as necessary.	☐	☐	☐	☐	☐	☐

	Procedure		Repeat		Competency	
	Yes	No	Yes	No	Yes	No
25. Properly measures the patient along the course of the central ray.	☐	☐	☐	☐	☐	☐
26. Sets the proper exposure technique:	☐	☐	☐	☐	☐	☐

Conventional systems
- Sets the proper kVp, mA, and time and makes adjustments as necessary.

or

CR or DR systems
- Identifies the patient on the work-list (or manually types the patient information into the system).
- Selects appropriate body region, specific body part, and accurate view/projection.
- Double-checks preset parameters:
  —Adult vs. pediatric patients
  ○ Small, medium, or large
  —Bucky/receptor (upright vs. table) *or* non-Bucky
  —AEC vs. fixed
  ○ If AEC, checks ION chambers
  ○ Density setting
  —kVp and mA; adjusts if necessary
  —Focal spot/filament size

	Procedure		Repeat		Competency	
	Yes	No	Yes	No	Yes	No
27. Exposes the cassette/receptor after telling the patient to hold still and after giving him or her proper breathing instructions (inspiration).	☐	☐	☐	☐	☐	☐
28. Provides each radiograph with the proper identification (flash) and/or processes each cassette (image) without difficulty (regardless of technology—film, CR, or DR).	▣	▣	▣	▣	☐	☐
29. Properly completes the examination by filling out all necessary paperwork, entering the examination in the computer, having the images checked by the appropriate staff members, and informing the patient that he or she is finished.	▣	▣	▣	▣	☐	☐
30. Exhibits the ability to adapt to new and difficult situations if and when necessary.	▣	▣	▣	▣	☐	☐
31. Accepts constructive criticism and uses it to his or her advantage.	☐	☐	☐	☐	☐	☐
32. Leaves the radiographic room neat and clean for the next examination.	▣	▣	▣	▣	☐	☐
33. Completes the examination within a reasonable time frame.	☐	☐	☐	☐	☐	☐

Comments:

_____

RADIOGRAPHIC IMAGE QUALITY

The student is able to critique his or her radiographs as to whether they demonstrate:

	Procedure		Repeat		Competency	
	Yes	No	Yes	No	Yes	No
34. Proper technique/optimal density	▣	▣	▣	▣	☐	☐
35. Enhanced detail, without evidence of motion and without any visible artifacts	▣	▣	▣	▣	☐	☐
36. Proper positioning (all anatomy included, evidence of proper centering/alignment, etc.)	▣	▣	▣	▣	☐	☐
37. Proper marker placement	▣	▣	▣	▣	☐	☐
38. Evidence of proper collimation and radiation protection	▣	▣	▣	▣	☐	☐
39. Long vs. short scale of contrast	▣	▣	▣	▣	☐	☐

Comments:

_____

(continued)

CHEST ANATOMY
The student is able to identify:

	Procedure		Repeat		Competency	
	Yes	No	Yes	No	Yes	No
40. Apices	☐	☐	☐	☐	☐	☐
41. Trachea	☐	☐	☐	☐	☐	☐
42. Heart	☐	☐	☐	☐	☐	☐
43. Mediastinum	☐	☐	☐	☐	☐	☐
44. Aortic knob/arch	☐	☐	☐	☐	☐	☐
45. Hilum	☐	☐	☐	☐	☐	☐
46. Costophrenic angles	☐	☐	☐	☐	☐	☐
47. Bases	☐	☐	☐	☐	☐	☐
48. Diaphragm	☐	☐	☐	☐	☐	☐
49. Clavicles	☐	☐	☐	☐	☐	☐
50. Sternoclavicular joints	☐	☐	☐	☐	☐	☐
51. Acromioclavicular joints	☐	☐	☐	☐	☐	☐
52. Ribs	☐	☐	☐	☐	☐	☐
53. Thoracic spine	☐	☐	☐	☐	☐	☐
54. Distal cervical spine	☐	☐	☐	☐	☐	☐
55. Scapula	☐	☐	☐	☐	☐	☐
56. Humeral head	☐	☐	☐	☐	☐	☐
57. Obvious pathology	☐	☐	☐	☐	☐	☐

Comments:

_____

_____

_____ _____ _____
Procedure Evaluator Signature   Repeat Evaluator Signature   Competency Evaluator Signature

_____ _____ _____
Date   Date   Date

END WHEELCHAIR CHEST EVALUATION

Student Name:_____

Procedure Grade	Repeat Grade	Competency Grade

PATIENT INFORMATION OR SIMULATED PROCEDURE *(circle if simulated)*

	Procedure	Repeat	Competency
Age			
Medical Record No.			
Ability to Cooperate			
Condition/Pathology			
Technical Factors Used			
Exposure Index			

FACILITY PREPARATION
The student:

	Procedure Yes	No	Repeat Yes	No	Competency Yes	No
1. Examines the radiographic room and cleans/straightens it before escorting the patient in.	☐	☐	☐	☐	☐	☐
2. Has all equipment and supplies (patient gown, shield, markers, etc.) readily available before escorting the patient in.	☐	☐	☐	☐	☐	☐
3. Is able to manipulate all radiographic equipment with ease, and centers the central ray to the cassette/receptor.	☐	☐	☐	☐	☐	☐
4. Adjusts the tube to the proper SID.	☐	☐	☐	☐	☐	☐
5. Selects a cassette/receptor of the appropriate size.	☐	☐	☐	☐	☐	☐

Comments:

_____

_____

PATIENT PREPARATION
The student:

	Procedure Yes	No	Repeat Yes	No	Competency Yes	No
6. Identifies the correct patient and examination according to the requisition while establishing a good rapport with him or her.	☐	☐	☐	☐	☐	☐
7. Obtains and documents the patient's history before the examination.	☐	☐	☐	☐	☐	☐
8. Explains the examination in terms the patient fully understands, and properly communicates with the patient throughout the examination.	☐	☐	☐	☐	☐	☐
9. Asks female patients of childbearing age the date of their last menstrual period and documents this; inquires about the possibility of pregnancy and has them sign pregnancy consent forms	☐	☐	☐	☐	☐	☐
10. Removes all obscuring objects (snaps, zippers, necklaces, etc.) so as *not* to produce radiographic artifacts.	☐	☐	☐	☐	☐	☐
11. Respects the patient's modesty and provides ample comfort for him or her.	☐	☐	☐	☐	☐	☐

(continued)

Comments:

_____

_____

PATIENT POSITIONING FOR A STRETCHER CHEST
AP Supine
The student:

	Procedure		Repeat		Competency	
	Yes	No	Yes	No	Yes	No
12. Adjusts the patient so that he or she is supine without rotation and with the patient "built-up" to adequately demonstrate the posterior wall.	☐	☐	☐	☐	☐	☐
13. Selects the appropriate receptor or places the cassette lengthwise or crosswise, depending on the patient's body type, so that the upper border of the cassette/receptor is 1–2 inches above the patient's shoulders. For conventional cassettes, the flash must be at the top and away from any anatomy.	☐	☐	☐	☐	☐	☐
14. Centers the central ray to the midsagittal plane.	☐	☐	☐	☐	☐	☐
15. Directs the central ray perpendicularly (unless it is necessary to angle, according to the patient's position) to the level of the seventh thoracic vertebra.	☐	☐	☐	☐	☐	☐

Lateral/Dorsal/Ventral Decubitus
The student:

	Procedure		Repeat		Competency	
	Yes	No	Yes	No	Yes	No
16. Places the patient in the supine/recumbent position, without rotation and with the affected side against the cassette/receptor.	☐	☐	☐	☐	☐	☐
17. Selects the appropriate receptor or places the cassette lengthwise, the upper border of the cassette/receptor 1–2 inches above the patient's shoulders. For conventional cassettes, the flash must be at the top and away from any anatomy.	☐	☐	☐	☐	☐	☐
18. Instructs and assists the patient to raise his or her arms as high as possible.	☐	☐	☐	☐	☐	☐
19. Adjusts the patient as close as possible to the cassette/receptor.	☐	☐	☐	☐	☐	☐
20. Using a horizontal beam, centers the central ray to the midcoronal plane.	☐	☐	☐	☐	☐	☐
21. Directs the central ray perpendicularly 3–4 inches below the jugular notch.	☐	☐	☐	☐	☐	☐

Comments:

_____

_____

IMPORTANT DETAILS
The student:

	Procedure		Repeat		Competency	
	Yes	No	Yes	No	Yes	No
22. Instills confidence in the patient by exhibiting self-confidence throughout the examination.	☐	☐	☐	☐	☐	☐
23. Places a lead marker in the appropriate area of the cassette/receptor (top/bottom/anteriorly/laterally), where it will be visualized on the finished radiograph, on the proper anatomical side (right/left), and in the appropriate position (face up/face down), depending on the patient's position.	☐	☐	☐	☐	☐	☐
24. Provides radiation protection (shield) for the patient, self, and others (closes doors).	☐	☐	☐	☐	☐	☐
25. Applies proper collimation and makes adjustments as necessary.	☐	☐	☐	☐	☐	☐
26. Properly measures the patient along the course of the central ray.	☐	☐	☐	☐	☐	☐

	Procedure		Repeat		Competency	
	Yes	No	Yes	No	Yes	No
27. Sets the proper exposure technique:	☐	☐	☐	☐	☐	☐

27. Sets the proper exposure technique:

Conventional systems
- Sets the proper kVp, mA, and time and makes adjustments as necessary.

or

CR or DR systems
- Identifies the patient on the work-list (or manually types the patient information into the system).
- Selects appropriate body region, specific body part, and accurate view/ projection.
- Double-checks preset parameters:
  —Adult vs. pediatric patients
  - Small, medium, or large
  —Bucky/receptor (upright vs. table) *or* non-Bucky
  —AEC vs. fixed
  - If AEC, checks ion chambers
  - Density setting
  —kVp and mA; adjusts if necessary
  —Focal spot/filament size

	Procedure		Repeat		Competency	
	Yes	No	Yes	No	Yes	No
28. Exposes the cassette/receptor after telling the patient to hold still and after giving him or her proper breathing instructions (inspiration).	☐	☐	☐	☐	☐	☐
29. Provides each radiograph with the proper identification (flash) and/or processes each cassette (image) without difficulty (regardless of technology—film, CR, or DR).	▨	▨	▨	▨	☐	☐
30. Properly completes the examination by filling out all necessary paperwork, entering the examination in the computer, having the images checked by the appropriate staff members, and informing the patient that he or she is finished.	▨	▨	▨	▨	☐	☐
31. Exhibits the ability to adapt to new and difficult situations if and when necessary.	▨	▨	▨	▨	☐	☐
32. Accepts constructive criticism and uses it to his or her advantage.	☐	☐	☐	☐	☐	☐
33. Leaves the radiographic room neat and clean for the next examination.	▨	▨	▨	▨	☐	☐
34. Completes the examination within a reasonable time frame.	☐	☐	☐	☐	☐	☐

Comments:

_____

_____

RADIOGRAPHIC IMAGE QUALITY
The student is able to critique his or her radiographs as to whether they demonstrate:

	Procedure		Repeat		Competency	
	Yes	No	Yes	No	Yes	No
35. Proper technique/optimal density	▨	▨	▨	▨	☐	☐
36. Enhanced detail, without evidence of motion and without any visible artifacts	▨	▨	▨	▨	☐	☐
37. Proper positioning (all anatomy included, evidence of proper centering/ alignment, etc.)	▨	▨	▨	▨	☐	☐
38. Proper marker placement	▨	▨	▨	▨	☐	☐
39. Evidence of proper collimation and radiation protection	▨	▨	▨	▨	☐	☐
40. Long vs. short scale of contrast	▨	▨	▨	▨	☐	☐

Comments:

_____

_____

(continued)

CHEST ANATOMY
The student is able to identify:

	Procedure		Repeat		Competency	
	Yes	No	Yes	No	Yes	No
41. Apices	☐	☐	☐	☐	☐	☐
42. Trachea	☐	☐	☐	☐	☐	☐
43. Heart	☐	☐	☐	☐	☐	☐
44. Mediastinum	☐	☐	☐	☐	☐	☐
45. Aortic knob/arch	☐	☐	☐	☐	☐	☐
46. Hilum	☐	☐	☐	☐	☐	☐
47. Costophrenic angles	☐	☐	☐	☐	☐	☐
48. Bases	☐	☐	☐	☐	☐	☐
49. Diaphragm	☐	☐	☐	☐	☐	☐
50. Clavicles	☐	☐	☐	☐	☐	☐
51. Sternoclavicular joints	☐	☐	☐	☐	☐	☐
52. Acromioclavicular joints	☐	☐	☐	☐	☐	☐
53. Ribs	☐	☐	☐	☐	☐	☐
54. Thoracic spine	☐	☐	☐	☐	☐	☐
55. Distal cervical spine	☐	☐	☐	☐	☐	☐
56. Scapula	☐	☐	☐	☐	☐	☐
57. Humeral head	☐	☐	☐	☐	☐	☐
58. Obvious pathology	☐	☐	☐	☐	☐	☐

Comments:

_____

_____

_____   _____   _____
Procedure Evaluator Signature   Repeat Evaluator Signature   Competency Evaluator Signature

_____   _____   _____
Date   Date   Date

END STRETCHER CHEST EVALUATION

Student Name:_____

Procedure Grade	Repeat Grade	Competency Grade

PATIENT INFORMATION OR SIMULATED PROCEDURE *(circle if simulated)*

	Procedure	Repeat	Competency
Age			
Medical Record No.			
Ability to Cooperate			
Condition/Pathology			
Technical Factors Used			
Exposure Index			

FACILITY PREPARATION
The student:

	Procedure Yes No	Repeat Yes No	Competency Yes No
1. Examines the radiographic room and cleans/straightens it before escorting the patient in.	☐ ☐	☐ ☐	☐ ☐
2. Has all equipment and supplies (patient gown, shield, markers, immobilization devices, etc.) readily available before escorting the patient in.	☐ ☐	☐ ☐	☐ ☐
3. Is able to manipulate all radiographic equipment with ease, and centers the central ray to the cassette/receptor *for both projections.*	☐ ☐	☐ ☐	☐ ☐
4. Adjusts the tube to the proper SID *for each projection.*	☐ ☐	☐ ☐	☐ ☐
5. Selects cassettes/receptor of the appropriate sizes *for both projections,* according to the patient size and examination.	☐ ☐	☐ ☐	☐ ☐

Comments:

_____

_____

PATIENT PREPARATION
The student:

	Procedure Yes No	Repeat Yes No	Competency Yes No
6. Identifies the correct patient and examination according to the requisition while establishing a good rapport with him or her.	☐ ☐	☐ ☐	☐ ☐
7. Obtains and documents the patient's history before the examination.	▨ ▨	▨ ▨	☐ ☐
8. Explains the examination in terms the parent/guardian fully understands, and properly communicates with the patient and parent/guardian throughout the examination.	☐ ☐	☐ ☐	☐ ☐
9. If she intends to stay in the room during the exposure, asks the patient's mother/female guardian of childbearing age the date of her last menstrual period and documents this; inquires about the possibility of pregnancy and has her sign a pregnancy consent form.	☐ ☐	☐ ☐	☐ ☐

(continued)

	Procedure		Repeat		Competency	
	Yes	No	Yes	No	Yes	No
10. Removes all obscuring objects (snaps, zippers, necklaces, etc.) so as *not* to produce radiographic artifacts.	☐	☐	☐	☐	☐	☐
11. Respects the patient's modesty and provides ample comfort for him or her.	☐	☐	☐	☐	☐	☐

Comments:

_____

_____

PATIENT POSITIONING FOR A PEDIATRIC CHEST
AP or PA Chest
The student:

	Procedure		Repeat		Competency	
	Yes	No	Yes	No	Yes	No
12. Places the patient's chest or back in contact with the upright Bucky/receptor or supine on the radiographic table, without rotation.	☐	☐	☐	☐	☐	☐
13. Selects the appropriate receptor or places the cassette lengthwise, the upper border of the cassette/receptor 1–2 inches above the patient's shoulders, with the shoulders rolled forward if possible for PA. For conventional cassettes, the flash must be at the top and away from any anatomy.	☐	☐	☐	☐	☐	☐
14. Centers the central ray to the midsagittal plane of the body.	☐	☐	☐	☐	☐	☐
15. Directs the central ray perpendicularly at the level of the sixth and seventh thoracic vertebrae.	☐	☐	☐	☐	☐	☐

Lateral Chest
The student:

	Procedure		Repeat		Competency	
	Yes	No	Yes	No	Yes	No
16. Places the patient in the left lateral position, without rotation, against the upright Bucky/receptor, or keeps the patient in the supine position, built up for a crosstable lateral (ventral/dorsal decubitus).	▨	▨	▨	▨	☐	☐
17. Selects the appropriate receptor or places the cassette lengthwise, depending on the patient's body type, so that the upper border of the cassette/receptor is 1–2 inches above the patient's shoulders. For conventional cassettes, the flash must be at the top and away from any anatomy.	☐	☐	☐	☐	☐	☐
18. Raises and immobilizes the patient's arms above the head as high as possible.	☐	☐	☐	☐	☐	☐
19. Adjusts the position of the patient so that the centrral ray is centered to the midcoronal plane.	☐	☐	☐	☐	☐	☐
20. Directs the central ray perpendicularly to the radiographic cassette/receptor at the level of the sixth and seventh thoracic vertebrae.	☐	☐	☐	☐	☐	☐

Comments:

_____

IMPORTANT DETAILS
The student:

	Procedure		Repeat		Competency	
	Yes	No	Yes	No	Yes	No
21. Instills confidence in the patient and parent/guardian by exhibiting self-confidence throughout the examination.	☐	☐	☐	☐	☐	☐
22. Places a lead marker in the appropriate area of the cassette/receptor (top/bottom/anteriorly/laterally), where it will be visualized on the	☐	☐	☐	☐	☐	☐

	Procedure		Repeat		Competency	
	Yes	No	Yes	No	Yes	No

finished radiograph, on the proper anatomical side (right/left), and in the appropriate position (face up/face down), depending on the patient's position.

23. Provides radiation protection (shield) for the patient, parent/guardian, self, and others (closes doors).	☐	☐	☐	☐	☐	☐
24. Applies proper collimation from the mastoid tips to the iliac crests, and makes adjustments as necessary.	☐	☐	☐	☐	☐	☐
25. Properly measures the patient along the course of the central ray *for each projection.*	☐	☐	☐	☐	☐	☐
26. Sets the proper exposure technique:	☐	☐	☐	☐	☐	☐

Conventional systems
- Sets the proper kVp, mA, and time and makes adjustments as necessary.

or

CR or DR systems
- Identifies the patient on the work-list (or manually types the patient information into the system).
- Selects appropriate body region, specific body part, and accurate view/projection.
- Double-checks preset parameters:
  —Adult vs. pediatric patients
    ○ Small, medium, or large
  —Bucky/receptor (upright vs. table) *or* non-Bucky
  —AEC vs. fixed
    ○ If AEC, checks ion chambers
    ○ Density setting
  —kVp and mA; adjusts if necessary
  —Focal spot/filament size

27. Exposes the cassette/receptor while watching for proper inspiration, especially if the child is crying or there is other motion of the abdominal cavity, *for each projection.*	☐	☐	☐	☐	☐	☐
28. Provides each radiograph with the proper identification (flash) and/or processes each cassette (image) without difficulty (regardless of technology—film, CR, or DR).	▨	▨	▨	▨	☐	☐
29. Properly completes the examination by filling out all necessary paperwork, entering the examination in the computer, having the images checked by the appropriate staff members, and informing the patient that he or she is finished.	▨	▨	▨	▨	☐	☐
30. Exhibits the ability to adapt to new and difficult situations if and when necessary.	▨	▨	▨	▨	☐	☐
31. Accepts constructive criticism and uses it to his or her advantage.	☐	☐	☐	☐	☐	☐
32. Leaves the radiographic room neat and clean for the next examination.	▨	▨	▨	▨	☐	☐
33. Completes the examination within a reasonable time frame.	☐	☐	☐	☐	☐	☐

Comments:

_____

_____

RADIOGRAPHIC IMAGE QUALITY
The student is able to critique his or her radiographs as to whether they demonstrate:

	Procedure		Repeat		Competency	
	Yes	No	Yes	No	Yes	No
34. Proper technique/optimal density	▨	▨	▨	▨	☐	☐
35. Enhanced detail, without evidence of motion and without any visible artifacts	▨	▨	▨	▨	☐	☐

(continued)

	Procedure		Repeat		Competency	
	Yes	No	Yes	No	Yes	No
36. Proper positioning (all anatomy included, evidence of proper centering/ alignment, etc.)	☐	☐	☐	☐	☐	☐
37. Proper marker placement	☐	☐	☐	☐	☐	☐
38. Evidence of proper collimation and radiation protection	☐	☐	☐	☐	☐	☐
39. Long vs. short scale of contrast	☐	☐	☐	☐	☐	☐

Comments:

_____

_____

CHEST ANATOMY
The student is able to identify:

	Procedure		Repeat		Competency	
	Yes	No	Yes	No	Yes	No
40. Apices	☐	☐	☐	☐	☐	☐
41. Trachea	☐	☐	☐	☐	☐	☐
42. Heart	☐	☐	☐	☐	☐	☐
43. Mediastinum	☐	☐	☐	☐	☐	☐
44. Aortic knob/arch	☐	☐	☐	☐	☐	☐
45. Hilum	☐	☐	☐	☐	☐	☐
46. Costophrenic angles	☐	☐	☐	☐	☐	☐
47. Bases	☐	☐	☐	☐	☐	☐
48. Diaphragm	☐	☐	☐	☐	☐	☐
49. Clavicles	☐	☐	☐	☐	☐	☐
50. Sternoclavicular joints	☐	☐	☐	☐	☐	☐
51. Acromioclavicular joints	☐	☐	☐	☐	☐	☐
52. Ribs	☐	☐	☐	☐	☐	☐
53. Thoracic spine	☐	☐	☐	☐	☐	☐
54. Distal cervical spine	☐	☐	☐	☐	☐	☐
55. Scapula	☐	☐	☐	☐	☐	☐
56. Humeral head	☐	☐	☐	☐	☐	☐
57. Obvious pathology	☐	☐	☐	☐	☐	☐

Comments:

_____

_____

_____   _____   _____
Procedure Evaluator Signature   Repeat Evaluator Signature   Competency Evaluator Signature

_____   _____   _____
Date   Date   Date

END PEDIATRIC CHEST (AGE 6 OR YOUNGER) EVALUATION

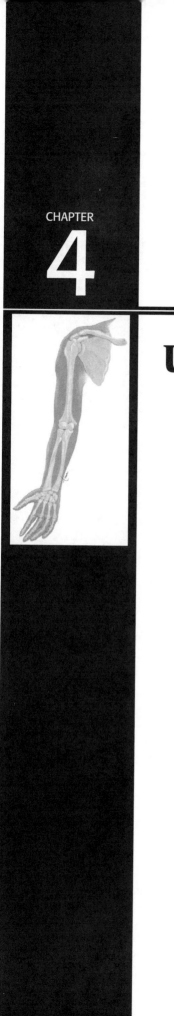

Upper Extremities

Finger/Thumb

The objective of this evaluation is to determine the student's competency level when performing specific radiographic examinations.

Student Name:_____

Procedure Grade	Repeat Grade	Competency Grade

PATIENT INFORMATION OR SIMULATED PROCEDURE *(circle if simulated)*

	Procedure	Repeat	Competency
Age			
Medical Record No.			
Ability to Cooperate			
Condition/Pathology			
Technical Factors Used			
Exposure Index			

FACILITY PREPARATION
The student:

	Procedure Yes No	Repeat Yes No	Competency Yes No
1. Examines the radiographic room and cleans/straightens it before escorting the patient in.	☐ ☐	☐ ☐	☐ ☐
2. Has all equipment and supplies (patient gown, pillow, markers, lead blockers, etc.) readily available before escorting the patient in.	☐ ☐	☐ ☐	☐ ☐
3. Is able to manipulate all radiographic equipment with ease, and centers the central ray to the cassette/receptor.	☐ ☐	☐ ☐	☐ ☐
4. Adjusts the tube to the proper SID.	☐ ☐	☐ ☐	☐ ☐
5. Selects a cassette/receptor of the appropriate size.	☐ ☐	☐ ☐	☐ ☐

Comments:

_____

_____

PATIENT PREPARATION
The student:

	Procedure Yes No	Repeat Yes No	Competency Yes No
6. Identifies the correct patient and examination according to the requisition while establishing a good rapport with him or her.	☐ ☐	☐ ☐	☐ ☐
7. Obtains and documents the patient's history before the examination.	☐ ☐	☐ ☐	☐ ☐
8. Explains the examination in terms the patient fully understands, and properly communicates with the patient throughout the examination.	☐ ☐	☐ ☐	☐ ☐
9. Asks female patients of childbearing age the date of their last menstrual period and documents this; inquires about the possibility of pregnancy and has them sign pregnancy consent forms.	☐ ☐	☐ ☐	☐ ☐
10. Removes all obscuring objects (snaps, zippers, belt, etc.) so as *not* to produce radiographic artifacts.	☐ ☐	☐ ☐	☐ ☐

(continued)

	Procedure		Repeat		Competency	
	Yes	No	Yes	No	Yes	No
11. Respects the patient's modesty and provides ample comfort for him or her.	☐	☐	☐	☐	☐	☐

Comments:

_____

_____

PATIENT POSITIONING FOR A FINGER/THUMB
Posteroanterior
The student:

	Procedure		Repeat		Competency	
	Yes	No	Yes	No	Yes	No
12. If using conventional film: divides the cassette into appropriate sections with lead blockers.	☐	☐	☐	☐	☐	☐
13. Instructs the patient to flatten his or her finger as much as possible.	☐	☐	☐	☐	☐	☐
14. Places the anterior surface of the finger on the appropriate area of the cassette/receptor (for a thumb, the student places the posterior surface of the thumb on the cassette/receptor by rotating the hand internally or externally).	☐	☐	☐	☐	☐	☐
15. Centers the anatomy of interest to the center of the cassette/receptor.	☐	☐	☐	☐	☐	☐
16. Centers the central ray perpendicularly to the proximal interphalangeal (PIP) joint for the finger or the metacarpophalangeal (MCP) joint for the thumb.	☐	☐	☐	☐	☐	☐

Oblique
The student:

	Procedure		Repeat		Competency	
	Yes	No	Yes	No	Yes	No
17. If using conventional film: adjusts the lead blockers to divide the cassette appropriately.	☐	☐	☐	☐	☐	☐
18. Instructs the patient to keep his or her finger as straight and flat as possible.	☐	☐	☐	☐	☐	☐
19. Using a wedge sponge if necessary, rotates the anterior surface of the finger 45° on the appropriate area of the cassette/receptor.	☐	☐	☐	☐	☐	☐
20. Centers the anatomy of interest to the center of the cassette/receptor.	☐	☐	☐	☐	☐	☐
21. Centers the central ray perpendicularly to the PIP joint for the finger or the MCP joint for the thumb.	☐	☐	☐	☐	☐	☐

Lateral
The student:

	Procedure		Repeat		Competency	
	Yes	No	Yes	No	Yes	No
22. If using conventional film: adjusts the lead blockers to divide the cassette appropriately.	☐	☐	☐	☐	☐	☐
23. Instructs the patient to keep his or her finger as straight as possible.	☐	☐	☐	☐	☐	☐
24. Rotates the finger 90° or until it is in the true lateral position on the appropriate area of the cassette/receptor, keeping it parallel with the cassette/receptor and using an immobilization device if necessary.	☐	☐	☐	☐	☐	☐
25. Centers the anatomy of interest to the center of the cassette/receptor.	☐	☐	☐	☐	☐	☐
26. Centers the central ray perpendicularly to the PIP joint for the finger or the MCP joint for the thumb.	☐	☐	☐	☐	☐	☐

Comments:

_____

_____

IMPORTANT DETAILS
The student:

	Procedure		Repeat		Competency	
	Yes	No	Yes	No	Yes	No
27. Instills confidence in the patient by exhibiting self-confidence throughout the examination.	☐	☐	☐	☐	☐	☐
28. Places a lead marker in the appropriate area of the cassette/receptor (top/bottom/anteriorly/laterally), where it will be visualized on the finished radiograph, on the proper anatomical side (right/left), and in the appropriate position (face up/face down), depending on the patient's position.	☐	☐	☐	☐	☐	☐
29. Provides radiation protection (shield) for the patient, self, and others (closes doors).	☐	☐	☐	☐	☐	☐
30. Applies proper collimation and makes adjustments as necessary.	☐	☐	☐	☐	☐	☐
31. Properly measures the patient along the course of the central ray *for each projection.*	☐	☐	☐	☐	☐	☐
32. Sets the proper exposure techniques:	☐	☐	☐	☐	☐	☐

32. Sets the proper exposure techniques:

Conventional systems
- Sets the proper kVp, mA, and time, and makes adjustments as necessary.

or

CR or DR systems
- Identifies the patient on the work-list (or manually types the patient information into the system).
- Selects appropriate body region, specific body part, and accurate view/projection.
- Double-checks preset parameters:
  — Adult vs. pediatric patients
    ○ Small, medium, or large
  — Bucky/receptor (upright vs. table) or non-Bucky
  — AEC vs. fixed
    ○ If AEC, checks ion chambers
    ○ Density setting
  — kVp and mA; adjusts if necessary
  — Focal spot/filament size

	Procedure		Repeat		Competency	
	Yes	No	Yes	No	Yes	No
33. Exposes the cassette/receptor after telling the patient to hold still and supporting and/or immobilizing the area of interest if necessary in order to keep the digit parallel to the cassette/receptor *for each projection.*	☐	☐	☐	☐	☐	☐
34. Provides each radiograph with the proper identification (flash) and/or processes each cassette (image) without difficulty (regardless of technology—film, CR, or DR).	▣	▣	▣	▣	☐	☐
35. Properly completes the examination by filling out all necessary paperwork, entering the examination in the computer, having the images checked by the appropriate staff members, and informing the patient that he or she is finished.	▣	▣	▣	▣	☐	☐
36. Exhibits the ability to adapt to new and difficult situations if and when necessary.	▣	▣	▣	▣	☐	☐
37. Accepts constructive criticism and uses it to his or her advantage.	☐	☐	☐	☐	☐	☐
38. Leaves the radiographic room neat and clean for the next examination.	▣	▣	▣	▣	☐	☐
39. Completes the examination within a reasonable time frame.	☐	☐	☐	☐	☐	☐

Comments:

_____

_____

(continued)

RADIOGRAPHIC IMAGE QUALITY
The student is able to critique his or her radiographs as to whether they demonstrate:

	Procedure Yes	No	Repeat Yes	No	Competency Yes	No
40. Proper technique/optimal density	☑	☑	☑	☑	☐	☐
41. Enhanced detail, without evidence of motion and without any visible artifacts	☑	☑	☑	☑	☐	☐
42. Proper positioning (all anatomy included, evidence of proper centering/alignment, etc.)	☑	☑	☑	☑	☐	☐
43. Proper marker placement	☑	☑	☑	☑	☐	☐
44. Evidence of proper collimation and radiation protection	☑	☑	☑	☑	☐	☐
45. Long vs. short scale of contrast	☑	☑	☑	☑	☐	☐

Comments:

_____

_____

FINGER ANATOMY
The student is able to identify:

	Procedure Yes	No	Repeat Yes	No	Competency Yes	No
46. Distal phalanx	☑	☑	☑	☑	☐	☐
47. Middle phalanx	☑	☑	☑	☑	☐	☐
48. Proximal phalanx	☑	☑	☑	☑	☐	☐
49. Distal interphalangeal joint	☑	☑	☑	☑	☐	☐
50. PIP joint	☑	☑	☑	☑	☐	☐
51. MCP joint	☑	☑	☑	☑	☐	☐
52. Metacarpal	☑	☑	☑	☑	☐	☐
53. Obvious pathology	☑	☑	☑	☑	☐	☐

Comments:

_____

_____

_____   _____   _____
Procedure Evaluator Signature   Repeat Evaluator Signature   Competency Evaluator Signature

_____   _____   _____
Date   Date   Date

END FINGER/THUMB EVALUATION

Student Name: _____

Procedure Grade	Repeat Grade	Competency Grade

PATIENT INFORMATION OR SIMULATED PROCEDURE *(circle if simulated)*

	Procedure	Repeat	Competency
Age			
Medical Record No.			
Ability to Cooperate			
Condition/Pathology			
Technical Factors Used			
Exposure Index			

FACILITY PREPARATION
The student:

	Procedure Yes	Procedure No	Repeat Yes	Repeat No	Competency Yes	Competency No
1. Examines the radiographic room and cleans/straightens it before escorting the patient in.	☐	☐	☐	☐	☐	☐
2. Has all equipment and supplies (patient gown, pillow, markers, lead blockers, etc.) readily available before escorting the patient in.	☐	☐	☐	☐	☐	☐
3. Is able to manipulate all radiographic equipment with ease, and centers the central ray to the cassette/receptor *for all projections.*	☐	☐	☐	☐	☐	☐
4. Adjusts the tube to the proper SID *for each projection.*	☐	☐	☐	☐	☐	☐
5. Selects cassettes/receptor of the appropriate sizes *for all projections,* according to the patient's size and examination.	☐	☐	☐	☐	☐	☐

Comments:

_____

_____

PATIENT PREPARATION
The student:

	Procedure Yes	Procedure No	Repeat Yes	Repeat No	Competency Yes	Competency No
6. Identifies the correct patient and examination according to the requisition while establishing a good rapport with him or her.	☐	☐	☐	☐	☐	☐
7. Obtains and documents the patient's history before the examination.	■	■	■	■	☐	☐
8. Explains the examination in terms the patient fully understands, and properly communicates with the patient throughout the examination.	☐	☐	☐	☐	☐	☐
9. Asks female patients of childbearing age the date of their last menstrual period and documents this; inquires about the possibility of pregnancy and has them sign pregnancy consent forms.	☐	☐	☐	☐	☐	☐
10. Removes all obscuring objects (snaps, zippers, belt, etc.) so as *not* to produce radiographic artifacts.	☐	☐	☐	☐	☐	☐

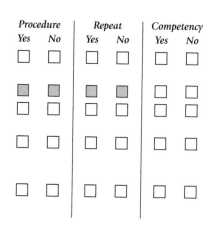

(continued)

	Procedure		Repeat		Competency	
	Yes	No	Yes	No	Yes	No
11. Respects the patient's modesty and provides ample comfort for him or her.	☐	☐	☐	☐	☐	☐

Comments:

_____

_____

PATIENT POSITIONING FOR A HAND
Posteroanterior
The student:

	Procedure		Repeat		Competency	
	Yes	No	Yes	No	Yes	No
12. If using conventional film: divides the cassette into appropriate sections with lead blockers.	☐	☐	☐	☐	☐	☐
13. Instructs the patient to flatten his or her hand as much as possible, resting it palm down.	☐	☐	☐	☐	☐	☐
14. Places the anterior surface of the hand on the appropriate area of the cassette/receptor.	☐	☐	☐	☐	☐	☐
15. Centers the anatomy of interest to the center of the cassette/receptor.	☐	☐	☐	☐	☐	☐
16. Centers the central ray perpendicularly to the third MCP joint.	☐	☐	☐	☐	☐	☐

Oblique
The student:

	Procedure		Repeat		Competency	
	Yes	No	Yes	No	Yes	No
17. If using conventional film: adjusts the lead blockers to divide the cassette appropriately.	☐	☐	☐	☐	☐	☐
18. Using a wedge sponge if necessary, rotates the hand 45° on the appropriate area of the cassette/receptor.	☐	☐	☐	☐	☐	☐
19. Centers the anatomy of interest to the center of the cassette/receptor.	☐	☐	☐	☐	☐	☐
20. Centers the central ray perpendicularly to the third MCP joint.	☐	☐	☐	☐	☐	☐

Lateral
The student:

	Procedure		Repeat		Competency	
	Yes	No	Yes	No	Yes	No
21. Selects a new cassette/receptor.	☐	☐	☐	☐	☐	☐
22. Instructs the patient to place the medical surface of the hand on the appropriate area of the cassette/receptor.	☐	☐	☐	☐	☐	☐
23. Adjusts the hand until it is in the true lateral position, keeping it as straight as possible and fanning the fingers when necessary.	☐	☐	☐	☐	☐	☐
24. Centers the anatomy of interest to the center of the cassette/receptor..	☐	☐	☐	☐	☐	☐
25. Centers the central ray perpendicularly to the second MCP joint	☐	☐	☐	☐	☐	☐

Comments:

_____

_____

IMPORTANT DETAILS
The student:

	Procedure		Repeat		Competency	
	Yes	No	Yes	No	Yes	No
26. Instills confidence in the patient by exhibiting self-confidence throughout the examination.	☐	☐	☐	☐	☐	☐

	Procedure		Repeat		Competency	
	Yes	No	Yes	No	Yes	No
27. Places a lead marker in the appropriate area of the cassette/receptor (top/bottom/anteriorly/laterally), where it will be visualized on the finished radiograph, on the proper anatomical side (right/left), and in the appropriate position (face up/face down), depending on the patient's position.	☐	☐	☐	☐	☐	☐
28. Provides radiation protection (shield) for the patient, self, and others (closes doors).	☐	☐	☐	☐	☐	☐
29. Applies proper collimation and makes adjustments as necessary.	☐	☐	☐	☐	☐	☐
30. Properly measures the patient along the course of the central ray *for each projection.*	☐	☐	☐	☐	☐	☐
31. Sets the proper exposure techniques:	☐	☐	☐	☐	☐	☐

31. Sets the proper exposure techniques:

Conventional systems
• Sets the proper kVp, mA, and time, and makes adjustments as necessary.

or

CR or DR systems
• Identifies the patient on the work-list (or manually types the patient information into the system).
• Selects appropriate body region, specific body part, and accurate view/ projection.
• Double-checks preset parameters:
—Adult vs. pediatric patients
  ○ Small, medium, or large
—Bucky/receptor (upright vs. table) or non-Bucky
—AEC vs. fixed
  ○ If AEC, checks ion chambers
  ○ Density setting
—kVp and mA; adjusts if necessary
—Focal spot/filament size

	Procedure		Repeat		Competency	
	Yes	No	Yes	No	Yes	No
32. Exposes the cassette/receptor after telling the patient to hold still and supporting and/or immobilizing the area of interest if necessary *for each projection.*	☐	☐	☐	☐	☐	☐
33. Provides each radiograph with the proper identification (flash) and/or processes each cassette (image) without difficulty (regardless of technology—film, CR, or DR).	▦	▦	▦	▦	☐	☐
34. Properly completes the examination by filling out all necessary paperwork, entering the examination in the computer, having the images checked by the appropriate staff members, and informing the patient that he or she is finished.	▦	▦	▦	▦	☐	☐
35. Exhibits the ability to adapt to new and difficult situations if and when necessary.	▦	▦	▦	▦	☐	☐
36. Accepts constructive criticism and uses it to his or her advantage.	☐	☐	☐	☐	☐	☐
37. Leaves the radiographic room neat and clean for the next examination.	▦	▦	▦	▦	☐	☐
38. Completes the examination within a reasonable time frame.	☐	☐	☐	☐	☐	☐

Comments:

_____

_____

(continued)

RADIOGRAPHIC IMAGE QUALITY
The student is able to critique his or her radiographs as to whether they demonstrate:

	Procedure		Repeat		Competency	
	Yes	No	Yes	No	Yes	No
39. Proper technique/optimal density	☐	☐	☐	☐	☐	☐
40. Enhanced detail, without evidence of motion and without any visible artifacts	☐	☐	☐	☐	☐	☐
41. Proper positioning (all anatomy included, evidence of proper centering/ alignment, etc.)	☐	☐	☐	☐	☐	☐
42. Proper marker placement	☐	☐	☐	☐	☐	☐
43. Evidence of proper collimation and radiation protection	☐	☐	☐	☐	☐	☐
44. Long vs. short scale of contrast	☐	☐	☐	☐	☐	☐

Comments:

_____

_____

HAND ANATOMY
The student is able to identify:

	Procedure		Repeat		Competency	
	Yes	No	Yes	No	Yes	No
45. Distal phalanx	☐	☐	☐	☐	☐	☐
46. Middle phalanx	☐	☐	☐	☐	☐	☐
47. Proximal phalanx	☐	☐	☐	☐	☐	☐
48. Distal interphalangeal joint	☐	☐	☐	☐	☐	☐
49. PIP joint	☐	☐	☐	☐	☐	☐
50. MCP joint	☐	☐	☐	☐	☐	☐
51. Metacarpal	☐	☐	☐	☐	☐	☐
52. Carpometacarpal joint	☐	☐	☐	☐	☐	☐
53. Carpal bone	☐	☐	☐	☐	☐	☐
54. Obvious pathology	☐	☐	☐	☐	☐	☐

Comments:

_____

_____

_____ _____ _____
Procedure Evaluator Signature   Repeat Evaluator Signature   Competency Evaluator Signature

_____ _____ _____
Date   Date   Date

END HAND EVALUATION

Anteroposterior Oblique Hand (Norgaard/Ball Catcher's Method)

The objective of this evaluation is to determine the student's competency level when performing specific radiographic examinations.

Student Name:_____

	Procedure Grade	Repeat Grade	Competency Grade

PATIENT INFORMATION OR SIMULATED PROCEDURE *(circle if simulated)*

	Procedure	Repeat	Competency
Age			
Medical Record No.			
Ability to Cooperate			
Condition/Pathology			
Technical Factors Used			
Exposure Index			

FACILITY PREPARATION
The student:

	Procedure Yes	No	Repeat Yes	No	Competency Yes	No
1. Examines the radiographic room and cleans/straightens it before escorting the patient in.	☐	☐	☐	☐	☐	☐
2. Has all equipment and supplies (patient gown, pillow, markers, lead blockers, etc.) readily available before escorting the patient in.	☐	☐	☐	☐	☐	☐
3. Is able to manipulate all radiographic equipment with ease, and centers the central ray to the cassette/receptor *for both projections.*	☐	☐	☐	☐	☐	☐
4. Adjusts the tube to the proper SID *for each projection.*	☐	☐	☐	☐	☐	☐
5. Selects cassettes/receptor of the appropriate sizes *for all projections,* according to the patient's size and examination.	☐	☐	☐	☐	☐	☐

Comments:

_____

_____

PATIENT PREPARATION
The student:

	Procedure Yes	No	Repeat Yes	No	Competency Yes	No
6. Identifies the correct patient and examination according to the requisition while establishing a good rapport with him or her.	☐	☐	☐	☐	☐	☐
7. Obtains and documents the patient's history before the examination.	▦	▦	▦	▦	☐	☐
8. Explains the examination in terms the patient fully understands, and properly communicates with the patient throughout the examination.	☐	☐	☐	☐	☐	☐
9. Asks female patients of childbearing age the date of their last menstrual period and documents this; inquires about the possibility of pregnancy and has them sign pregnancy consent forms.	☐	☐	☐	☐	☐	☐
10. Removes all obscuring objects (snaps, zippers, belt, etc.) so as *not* to produce radiographic artifacts.	☐	☐	☐	☐	☐	☐

(continued)

	Procedure		Repeat		Competency	
	Yes	No	Yes	No	Yes	No
11. Respects the patient's modesty and provides ample comfort for him or her.	☐	☐	☐	☐	☐	☐

Comments:

_____

PATIENT POSITIONING FOR AN AP OBLIQUE HAND, USING THE NORGAARD/BALL CATCHER'S METHOD
The student:

	Procedure		Repeat		Competency	
	Yes	No	Yes	No	Yes	No
12. With the patient seated at the end of the table, instructs him or her to rest both hands palm up.	☐	☐	☐	☐	☐	☐
13. Adjusts the position of the hands so that they are both half-supinated (at 45°).	☐	☐	☐	☐	☐	☐
14. Slightly extends the fingers and abducts the thumbs to avoid superimposition over the fingers.	☐	☐	☐	☐	☐	☐
15. Centers both hands so that they are evenly distributed over the center of the cassette/receptor.	☐	☐	☐	☐	☐	☐
16. Centers the center ray perpendicularly to the MCP joints at a point midway between the two hands.	☐	☐	☐	☐	☐	☐

Comments:

_____

IMPORTANT DETAILS
The student:

	Procedure		Repeat		Competency	
	Yes	No	Yes	No	Yes	No
17. Instills confidence in the patient by exhibiting self-confidence throughout the examination.	☐	☐	☐	☐	☐	☐
18. Places a lead marker in the appropriate area of the cassette/receptor (top/bottom/anteriorly/laterally), where it will be visualized on the finished radiograph, on the proper anatomical side (right/left), and in the appropriate position (face up/face down), depending on the patient's position.	☐	☐	☐	☐	☐	☐
19. Provides radiation protection (shield) for the patient, self, and others (closes doors).	☐	☐	☐	☐	☐	☐
20. Applies proper collimation and makes adjustments as necessary.	☐	☐	☐	☐	☐	☐
21. Properly measures the patient along the course of the central ray *for each projection.*	☐	☐	☐	☐	☐	☐
22. Sets the proper exposure techniques:	☐	☐	☐	☐	☐	☐

Conventional systems
- Sets the proper kVp, mA, and time and makes adjustments as necessary.

or

CR or DR systems
- Identifies the patient on the work-list (or manually types the patient information into the system).
- Selects appropriate body region, specific body part, and accurate view/projection.
- Double-checks preset parameters:
  —Adult vs. pediatric patients
    ○ Small, medium, or large
  —Bucky/receptor (upright vs. table) *or* non-Bucky

	Procedure		Repeat		Competency	
	Yes	No	Yes	No	Yes	No

   —AEC vs. fixed
      ○ If AEC, checks ion chambers
      ○ Density setting
   —kVp and mA; adjusts if necessary
   —Focal spot/filament size

	Procedure		Repeat		Competency	
	Yes	No	Yes	No	Yes	No
23. Exposes the cassette/receptor after telling the patient to hold still *for each projection.*	☐	☐	☐	☐	☐	☐
24. Provides each radiograph with the proper identification (flash) and/or processes each cassette (image) without difficulty (regardless of technology—film, CR, or DR).	☐	☐	☐	☐	☐	☐
25. Properly completes the examination by filling out all necessary paperwork, entering the examination in the computer, having the images checked by the appropriate staff members, and informing the patient that he or she is finished.	☐	☐	☐	☐	☐	☐
26. Exhibits the ability to adapt to new and difficult situations if and when necessary.	☐	☐	☐	☐	☐	☐
27. Accepts constructive criticism and uses it to his or her advantage.	☐	☐	☐	☐	☐	☐
28. Leaves the radiographic room neat and clean for the next examination.	☐	☐	☐	☐	☐	☐
29. Completes the examination within a reasonable time frame.	☐	☐	☐	☐	☐	☐

Comments:

_____

RADIOGRAPHIC IMAGE QUALITY

The student is able to critique his or her radiographs as to whether they demonstrate:

	Procedure		Repeat		Competency	
	Yes	No	Yes	No	Yes	No
30. Proper technique/optimal density	☐	☐	☐	☐	☐	☐
31. Enhanced detail, without evidence of motion and without any visible artifacts	☐	☐	☐	☐	☐	☐
32. Proper positioning (all anatomy included, evidence of proper centering/alignment, etc.)	☐	☐	☐	☐	☐	☐
33. Proper marker placement	☐	☐	☐	☐	☐	☐
34. Evidence of proper collimation and radiation protection	☐	☐	☐	☐	☐	☐
35. Long vs. short scale of contrast	☐	☐	☐	☐	☐	☐

Comments:

_____

HAND ANATOMY

The student is able to identify:

	Procedure		Repeat		Competency	
	Yes	No	Yes	No	Yes	No
36. Distal phalanges	☐	☐	☐	☐	☐	☐
37. Middle phalanges	☐	☐	☐	☐	☐	☐
38. Proximal phalanges	☐	☐	☐	☐	☐	☐
39. Distal interphalangeal joints	☐	☐	☐	☐	☐	☐
40. PIP joints	☐	☐	☐	☐	☐	☐
41. MCP joints	☐	☐	☐	☐	☐	☐

(continued)

	Procedure		Repeat		Competency	
	Yes	No	Yes	No	Yes	No
42. Metacarpals	☐	☐	☐	☐	☐	☐
43. Carpometacarpal joints	☐	☐	☐	☐	☐	☐
44. Carpal bones	☐	☐	☐	☐	☐	☐
45. Obvious pathology	☐	☐	☐	☐	☐	☐

Comments:

_____

_____

Procedure Evaluator Signature   Repeat Evaluator Signature   Competency Evaluator Signature

Date   Date   Date

END ANTEROPOSTERIOR OBLIQUE HAND (NORGAARD/BALL CATCHER'S METHOD) EVALUATION

Student Name:_____

	Procedure Grade	Repeat Grade	Competency Grade

PATIENT INFORMATION OR SIMULATED PROCEDURE *(circle if simulated)*

	Procedure	Repeat	Competency
Age			
Medical Record No.			
Ability to Cooperate			
Condition/Pathology			
Technical Factors Used			
Exposure Index			

FACILITY PREPARATION
The student:

	Procedure Yes	No	Repeat Yes	No	Competency Yes	No
1. Examines the radiographic room and cleans/straightens it before escorting the patient in.	☐	☐	☐	☐	☐	☐
2. Has all equipment and supplies (patient gown, pillow, markers, lead blockers, etc.) readily available before escorting the patient in.	☐	☐	☐	☐	☐	☐
3. Is able to manipulate all radiographic equipment with ease, and centers the central ray to the cassette/receptor *for all projections.*	☐	☐	☐	☐	☐	☐
4. Adjusts the tube to the proper SID *for each projection.*	☐	☐	☐	☐	☐	☐
5. Selects cassettes/receptor of the appropriate sizes *for all projections,* according to the patient's size and examination.	☐	☐	☐	☐	☐	☐

Comments:

_____

_____

PATIENT PREPARATION
The student:

	Procedure Yes	No	Repeat Yes	No	Competency Yes	No
6. Identifies the correct patient and examination according to the requisition while establishing a good rapport with him or her.	☐	☐	☐	☐	☐	☐
7. Obtains and documents the patient's history before the examination.	▓	▓	▓	▓	☐	☐
8. Explains the examination in terms the patient fully understands, and properly communicates with the patient throughout the examination.	☐	☐	☐	☐	☐	☐
9. Asks female patients of childbearing age the date of their last menstrual period and documents this; inquires about the possibility of pregnancy and has them sign pregnancy consent forms.	☐	☐	☐	☐	☐	☐
10. Removes all obscuring objects (snaps, zippers, belt, etc.) so as *not* to produce radiographic artifacts.	☐	☐	☐	☐	☐	☐

(continued)

	Procedure		Repeat		Competency	
	Yes	No	Yes	No	Yes	No
11. Respects the patient's modesty and provides ample comfort for him or her.	☐	☐	☐	☐	☐	☐

Comments:

_____

_____

PATIENT POSITIONING FOR A WRIST
Posteroanterior
The student:

	Procedure		Repeat		Competency	
	Yes	No	Yes	No	Yes	No
12. If using conventional film: divides the cassette into appropriate sections with lead blockers.	☐	☐	☐	☐	☐	☐
13. Instructs the patient to make a fist with his or her hand.	☐	☐	☐	☐	☐	☐
14. Places the anterior surface of the wrist on the appropriate area of the cassette/receptor.	☐	☐	☐	☐	☐	☐
15. Centers the anatomy of interest to the center of the cassette/receptor.	☐	☐	☐	☐	☐	☐
16. Centers the central ray perpendicularly to the midcarpal area.	☐	☐	☐	☐	☐	☐

Lateral
The student:

	Procedure		Repeat		Competency	
	Yes	No	Yes	No	Yes	No
17. If using conventional film: adjusts the lead blockers to divide the cassette appropriately.	☐	☐	☐	☐	☐	☐
18. Instructs the patient to bend his or her elbow 90° and place the medial surface of the wrist on the appropriate area of the cassette/receptor.	☐	☐	☐	☐	☐	☐
19. Adjusts the wrist until it is in the true lateral position, keeping it as straight as possible.	☐	☐	☐	☐	☐	☐
20. Has the patient's arm on the same level as the shoulder.	☐	☐	☐	☐	☐	☐
21. Centers the anatomy of interest to the center of the cassette/receptor.	☐	☐	☐	☐	☐	☐
22. Centers the central ray perpendicularly to the midcarpal area.	☐	☐	☐	☐	☐	☐

PA Oblique Lateral Rotation
The student:

	Procedure		Repeat		Competency	
	Yes	No	Yes	No	Yes	No
23. If using conventional film: selects a new cassette and adjusts the lead blockers to divide the cassette appropriately.	☐	☐	☐	☐	☐	☐
24. Using a wedge sponge if necessary, from the pronated position, rotates the wrist laterally (externally) 45° on the appropriate area of the cassette/receptor.	☐	☐	☐	☐	☐	☐
25. Centers the anatomy of interest to the center of the cassette/receptor.	☐	☐	☐	☐	☐	☐
26. Centers the central ray perpendicularly to the midcarpal area.	☐	☐	☐	☐	☐	☐

AP Oblique Medial Rotation
The student:

	Procedure		Repeat		Competency	
	Yes	No	Yes	No	Yes	No
27. If using conventional film: adjusts the lead blockers to divide the cassette appropriately.	☐	☐	☐	☐	☐	☐
28. Using a wedge sponge if necessary, from the AP position, rotates the wrist medially (internally) 45° on the appropriate area of the cassette/receptor.	☐	☐	☐	☐	☐	☐
29. Centers the anatomy of interest to the center of the cassette/receptor.	☐	☐	☐	☐	☐	☐
30. Centers the central ray perpendicularly to the midcarpal area.	☐	☐	☐	☐	☐	☐

Comments:

_____

_____

IMPORTANT DETAILS
The student:

	Procedure Yes	No	Repeat Yes	No	Competency Yes	No
31. Instills confidence in the patient by exhibiting self-confidence throughout the examination.	☐	☐	☐	☐	☐	☐
32. Places a lead marker in the appropriate area of the cassette/receptor (top/bottom/anteriorly/laterally), where it will be visualized on the finished radiograph, on the proper anatomical side (right/left), and in the appropriate position (face up/face down), depending on the patient's position.	☐	☐	☐	☐	☐	☐
33. Provides radiation protection (shield) for the patient, self, and others (closes doors).	☐	☐	☐	☐	☐	☐
34. Applies proper collimation and makes adjustments as necessary.	☐	☐	☐	☐	☐	☐
35. Properly measures the patient along the course of the central ray *for each projection.*	☐	☐	☐	☐	☐	☐
36. Sets the proper exposure techniques:	☐	☐	☐	☐	☐	☐

Conventional systems
• Sets the proper kVp, mA, and time, and makes adjustments as necessary.

or

CR or DR systems
• Identifies the patient on the work-list (or manually types the patient information into the system).
• Selects appropriate body region, specific body part, and accurate view/ projection.
• Double-checks preset parameters:
  —Adult vs. pediatric patients
    ○ Small, medium, or large
  —Bucky/receptor (upright vs. table) *or* non-Bucky
  —AEC vs. fixed
    ○ If AEC, checks ion chambers
    ○ Density setting
  —kVp and mA; adjusts if necessary
  —Focal spot/filament size

	Procedure Yes	No	Repeat Yes	No	Competency Yes	No
37. Exposes the cassette/receptor after telling the patient to hold still and supporting and/or immobilizing the area of interest if necessary *for each projection.*	☐	☐	☐	☐	☐	☐
38. Provides each radiograph with the proper identification (flash) and/or processes each cassette (image) without difficulty (regardless of technology—film, CR, or DR).	▣	▣	▣	▣	☐	☐
39. Properly completes the examination by filling out all necessary paperwork, entering the examination in the computer, having the images checked by the appropriate staff members, and informing the patient that he or she is finished.	▣	▣	▣	▣	☐	☐
40. Exhibits the ability to adapt to new and difficult situations if and when necessary.	▣	▣	▣	▣	☐	☐
41. Accepts constructive criticism and uses it to his or her advantage.	☐	☐	☐	☐	☐	☐
42. Leaves the radiographic room neat and clean for the next examination.	▣	▣	▣	▣	☐	☐
43. Completes the examination within a reasonable time frame.	☐	☐	☐	☐	☐	☐

(continued)

Comments:

_____

_____

_____

RADIOGRAPHIC IMAGE QUALITY
The student is able to critique his or her radiographs as to whether they demonstrate:

	Procedure		Repeat		Competency	
	Yes	No	Yes	No	Yes	No
44. Proper technique/optimal density	☐	☐	☐	☐	☐	☐
45. Enhanced detail, without evidence of motion and without any visible artifacts	☐	☐	☐	☐	☐	☐
46. Proper positioning (all anatomy included, evidence of proper centering/ alignment, etc.)	☐	☐	☐	☐	☐	☐
47. Proper marker placement	☐	☐	☐	☐	☐	☐
48. Evidence of proper collimation and radiation protection	☐	☐	☐	☐	☐	☐
49. Long vs. short scale of contrast	☐	☐	☐	☐	☐	☐

Comments:

_____

_____

WRIST ANATOMY
The student is able to identify:

	Procedure		Repeat		Competency	
	Yes	No	Yes	No	Yes	No
50. Carpometacarpal joints	☐	☐	☐	☐	☐	☐
51. Navicular/scaphoid	☐	☐	☐	☐	☐	☐
52. Lunate/semilunar	☐	☐	☐	☐	☐	☐
53. Triquetrum/cuneiform	☐	☐	☐	☐	☐	☐
54. Pisiform	☐	☐	☐	☐	☐	☐
55. Greater multangular/trapezium	☐	☐	☐	☐	☐	☐
56. Lesser multangular/trapezoid	☐	☐	☐	☐	☐	☐
57. Capitatum/os magnum	☐	☐	☐	☐	☐	☐
58. Hamate/unciform	☐	☐	☐	☐	☐	☐
59. Radius	☐	☐	☐	☐	☐	☐
60. Ulna	☐	☐	☐	☐	☐	☐
61. Distal radioulnar joint	☐	☐	☐	☐	☐	☐
62. Obvious pathology	☐	☐	☐	☐	☐	☐

Comments:

_____

_____

_____

Procedure Evaluator Signature	Repeat Evaluator Signature	Competency Evaluator Signature
Date	Date	Date

END WRIST EVALUATION

Student Name:_____

Procedure Grade	Repeat Grade	Competency Grade

PATIENT INFORMATION OR SIMULATED PROCEDURE *(circle if simulated)*

	Procedure	Repeat	Competency
Age			
Medical Record No.			
Ability to Cooperate			
Condition/Pathology			
Technical Factors Used			
Exposure Index			

FACILITY PREPARATION
The student:

	Procedure Yes No	Repeat Yes No	Competency Yes No
1. Examines the radiographic room and cleans/straightens it before escorting the patient in.	☐ ☐	☐ ☐	☐ ☐
2. Has all equipment and supplies (patient gown, pillow, markers, lead blockers, etc.) readily available before escorting the patient in.	☐ ☐	☐ ☐	☐ ☐
3. Is able to manipulate all radiographic equipment with ease, and centers the central ray to the cassette/receptor.	☐ ☐	☐ ☐	☐ ☐
4. Adjusts the tube to the proper SID.	☐ ☐	☐ ☐	☐ ☐
5. Selects a cassette/receptor of the appropriate size.	☐ ☐	☐ ☐	☐ ☐

Comments:

_____

_____

PATIENT PREPARATION
The student:

	Procedure Yes No	Repeat Yes No	Competency Yes No
6. Identifies the correct patient and examination according to the requisition while establishing a good rapport with him or her.	☐ ☐	☐ ☐	☐ ☐
7. Obtains and documents the patient's history before the examination.	▨ ▨	▨ ▨	☐ ☐
8. Explains the examination in terms the patient fully understands, and properly communicates with the patient throughout the examination.	☐ ☐	☐ ☐	☐ ☐
9. Asks female patients of childbearing age the date of their last menstrual period and documents this; inquires about the possibility of pregnancy and has them sign pregnancy consent forms	☐ ☐	☐ ☐	☐ ☐
10. Removes all obscuring objects (snaps, zippers, belt, etc.) so as *not* to produce radiographic artifacts.	☐ ☐	☐ ☐	☐ ☐
11. Respects the patient's modesty and provides ample comfort for him or her.	☐ ☐	☐ ☐	☐ ☐

(continued)

Comments:
_____

_____

PATIENT POSITIONING FOR A CARPAL CANAL OF THE WRIST
Inferosuperior Projection
The student:

	Procedure		Repeat		Competency	
	Yes	No	Yes	No	Yes	No
12. Instructs the patient to rest his or her forearm prone so that it lies parallel to the long axis of the radiographic table.	☐	☐	☐	☐	☐	☐
13. Instructs the patient to hyperextend his or her wrist so that the hand/palm is as near to vertical as possible, keeping the anterior surface of the forearm in contact with the cassette/receptor/table.	☐	☐	☐	☐	☐	☐
14. Rotates the hand slightly toward the radial side.	☐	☐	☐	☐	☐	☐
15. Centers the anatomy of interest to the center of the cassette/receptor.	☐	☐	☐	☐	☐	☐
16. Centers the central ray at an angle of 25–30° (toward the palm of the hand) to a point 1 inch distal to the base of the third metacarpal.	☐	☐	☐	☐	☐	☐

Superoinferior Projection
The student:

	Procedure		Repeat		Competency	
	Yes	No	Yes	No	Yes	No
17. Instructs the patient to stand with his or her back to the table, dorsiflex the wrist, and rest the hand on the table palm down, with the fingers pointing toward the body and the hand forming a right angle with the forearm.	☐	☐	☐	☐	☐	☐
18. Centers the anatomy of interest to the center of the cassette/receptor.	☐	☐	☐	☐	☐	☐
19. Centers the central ray at an angle of 0–30° to the wrist joint, entering the forearm and exiting the base of the palm of the hand.	☐	☐	☐	☐	☐	☐

Comments:
_____

_____

IMPORTANT DETAILS
The student:

	Procedure		Repeat		Competency	
	Yes	No	Yes	No	Yes	No
20. Instills confidence in the patient by exhibiting self-confidence throughout the examination.	☐	☐	☐	☐	☐	☐
21. Places a lead marker in the appropriate area of the cassette/receptor (top/bottom/anteriorly/laterally), where it will be visualized on the finished radiograph, on the proper anatomical side (right/left), and in the appropriate position (face up/face down), depending on the patient's position.	☐	☐	☐	☐	☐	☐
22. Provides radiation protection (shield) for the patient, self, and others (closes doors).	☐	☐	☐	☐	☐	☐
23. Applies proper collimation and makes adjustments as necessary.	☐	☐	☐	☐	☐	☐
24. Properly measures the patient along the course of the central ray *for each projection.*	☐	☐	☐	☐	☐	☐
25. Sets the proper exposure techniques:	☐	☐	☐	☐	☐	☐

Conventional systems
• Sets the proper kVp, mA, and time and makes adjustments as necessary.

or

	Procedure		Repeat		Competency	
	Yes	No	Yes	No	Yes	No

CR or DR systems
- Identifies the patient on the work-list (or manually types the patient information into the system).
- Selects appropriate body region, specific body part, and accurate view/ projection.
- Double-checks preset parameters:
  —Adult vs. pediatric patients
  　○ Small, medium, or large
  —Bucky/receptor (upright vs. table) *or* non-Bucky
  —AEC vs. fixed
  　○ If AEC, checks ion chambers
  　○ Density setting
  —kVp and mA; adjusts if necessary
  —Focal spot/filament size

	Procedure		Repeat		Competency	
26. Exposes the cassette/receptor after telling the patient to hold still and supporting and/or immobilizing the area of interest if necessary *for each projection.*	☐	☐	☐	☐	☐	☐
27. Provides each radiograph with the proper identification (flash) and/or processes each cassette (image) without difficulty (regardless of technology—film, CR, or DR).	▨	▨	▨	▨	☐	☐
28. Properly completes the examination by filling out all necessary paperwork, entering the examination in the computer, having the images checked by the appropriate staff members, and informing the patient that he or she is finished.	▨	▨	▨	▨	☐	☐
29. Exhibits the ability to adapt to new and difficult situations if and when necessary.	▨	▨	▨	▨	☐	☐
30. Accepts constructive criticism and uses it to his or her advantage.	☐	☐	☐	☐	☐	☐
31. Leaves the radiographic room neat and clean for the next examination.	▨	▨	▨	▨	☐	☐
32. Completes the examination within a reasonable time frame.	☐	☐	☐	☐	☐	☐

Comments:

RADIOGRAPHIC IMAGE QUALITY

The student is able to critique his or her radiographs as to whether they demonstrate:

	Procedure		Repeat		Competency	
	Yes	No	Yes	No	Yes	No
33. Proper technique/optimal density	▨	▨	▨	▨	☐	☐
34. Enhanced detail, without evidence of motion and without any visible artifacts	▨	▨	▨	▨	☐	☐
35. Proper positioning (all anatomy included, evidence of proper centering/ alignment, etc.)	▨	▨	▨	▨	☐	☐
36. Proper marker placement	▨	▨	▨	▨	☐	☐
37. Evidence of proper collimation and radiation protection	▨	▨	▨	▨	☐	☐
38. Long vs. short scale of contrast	▨	▨	▨	▨	☐	☐

Comments:

(continued)

WRIST ANATOMY
The student is able to identify:

	Procedure		Repeat		Competency	
	Yes	No	Yes	No	Yes	No
39. Navicular/scaphoid	☐	☐	☐	☐	☐	☐
40. Lunate/semilunar	☐	☐	☐	☐	☐	☐
41. Triquetrum/cuneiform	☐	☐	☐	☐	☐	☐
42. Pisiform	☐	☐	☐	☐	☐	☐
43. Lesser multangular/trapezoid	☐	☐	☐	☐	☐	☐
44. Greater multangular/trapezium	☐	☐	☐	☐	☐	☐
45. Capitatum/os magnum	☐	☐	☐	☐	☐	☐
46. Hamate/unciform	☐	☐	☐	☐	☐	☐
47. Obvious pathology	☐	☐	☐	☐	☐	☐

Comments:

_____

_____

_____   _____   _____
Procedure Evaluator Signature   Repeat Evaluator Signature   Competency Evaluator Signature

_____   _____   _____
Date   Date   Date

END CARPAL CANAL (TUNNEL) EVALUATION

86

Student Name:_____

	Procedure Grade	Repeat Grade	Competency Grade

PATIENT INFORMATION OR SIMULATED PROCEDURE *(circle if simulated)*

	Procedure	Repeat	Competency
Age			
Medical Record No.			
Ability to Cooperate			
Condition/Pathology			
Technical Factors Used			
Exposure Index			

FACILITY PREPARATION
The student:

	Procedure Yes	No	Repeat Yes	No	Competency Yes	No
1. Examines the radiographic room and cleans/straightens it before escorting the patient in.	☐	☐	☐	☐	☐	☐
2. Has all equipment and supplies (patient gown, pillow, markers, lead blockers, etc.) readily available before escorting the patient in.	☐	☐	☐	☐	☐	☐
3. Is able to manipulate all radiographic equipment with ease, and centers the central ray to the cassette/receptor.	☐	☐	☐	☐	☐	☐
4. Adjusts the tube to the proper SID.	☐	☐	☐	☐	☐	☐
5. Selects a cassette/receptor of the appropriate size.	☐	☐	☐	☐	☐	☐

Comments:

_____

_____

PATIENT PREPARATION
The student:

	Procedure Yes	No	Repeat Yes	No	Competency Yes	No
6. Identifies the correct patient and examination according to the requisition while establishing a good rapport with him or her.	☐	☐	☐	☐	☐	☐
7. Obtains and documents the patient's history before the examination.	■	■	■	■	☐	☐
8. Explains the examination in terms the patient fully understands, and properly communicates with the patient throughout the examination.	☐	☐	☐	☐	☐	☐
9. Asks female patients of childbearing age the date of their last menstrual period and documents this; inquires about the possibility of pregnancy and has them sign pregnancy consent forms.	☐	☐	☐	☐	☐	☐
10. Removes all obscuring objects (snaps, zippers, belt, etc.) so as *not* to produce radiographic artifacts.	☐	☐	☐	☐	☐	☐
11. Respects the patient's modesty and provides ample comfort for him or her.	☐	☐	☐	☐	☐	☐

(continued)

Comments:

_____

_____

PATIENT POSITIONING FOR A CARPAL BRIDGE OF THE WRIST
Posteroanterior
The student:

	Procedure		Repeat		Competency	
	Yes	No	Yes	No	Yes	No
12. Does *one* of the following:	☐	☐	☐	☐	☐	☐

    a. For a tangential projection, instructs the patient to stand and rest his or her hand on the table, palm up, with fingers pointing toward the body and the forearm forming a right angle with the hand.

    b. For a modified projection, instructs the patient to sit at the edge of the radiographic table with the arm elevated and supported, palm down, so that the wrist is flexed and the hand forms a right angle to the forearm.

	Procedure		Repeat		Competency	
13. Does *one* of the following:	☐	☐	☐	☐	☐	☐

    a. For a tangential projection, places the cassette/receptor under the posterior surface of the patient's hand.

    b. For a modified projection, places the cassette/receptor in a vertical position, adjacent to the back of the hand.

	Procedure		Repeat		Competency	
14. Centers the anatomy of interest to the center of the cassette/receptor.	☐	☐	☐	☐	☐	☐
15. Centers the central ray at a superoinferior angle of 45° (toward the hand) to a point 1.5 inches proximal to the wrist joint.	☐	☐	☐	☐	☐	☐

Comments:

_____

_____

IMPORTANT DETAILS
The student:

	Procedure		Repeat		Competency	
	Yes	No	Yes	No	Yes	No
16. Instills confidence in the patient by exhibiting self-confidence throughout the examination.	☐	☐	☐	☐	☐	☐
17. Places a lead marker in the appropriate area of the cassette/receptor (top/bottom/anteriorly/laterally), where it will be visualized on the finished radiograph, on the proper anatomical side (right/left), and in the appropriate position (face up/face down), depending on the patient's position.	☐	☐	☐	☐	☐	☐
18. Provides radiation protection (shield) for the patient, self, and others (closes doors).	☐	☐	☐	☐	☐	☐
19. Applies proper collimation and makes adjustments as necessary.	☐	☐	☐	☐	☐	☐
20. Properly measures the patient along the course of the central ray *for each projection.*	☐	☐	☐	☐	☐	☐
21. Sets the proper exposure techniques:	☐	☐	☐	☐	☐	☐

    Conventional systems
    • Sets the proper kVp, mA, and time and makes adjustments as necessary.

    or

    CR or DR systems
    • Identifies the patient on the work-list (or manually types the patient information into the system).

	Procedure		Repeat		Competency	
	Yes	No	Yes	No	Yes	No

- Selects appropriate body region, specific body part, and accurate view/projection.
- Double-checks preset parameters:
  —Adult vs. pediatric patients
  　○ Small, medium, or large
  —Bucky/receptor (upright vs. table) *or* non-Bucky
  —AEC vs. fixed
  　○ If AEC, checks ion chambers
  　○ Density setting
  —kVp and mA; adjusts if necessary
  —Focal spot/filament size

	Procedure		Repeat		Competency	
	Yes	No	Yes	No	Yes	No
22. Exposes the cassette/receptor after telling the patient to hold still and supporting and/or immobilizing the area of interest if necessary *for each projection.*	☐	☐	☐	☐	☐	☐
23. Provides each radiograph with the proper identification (flash) and/or processes each cassette (image) without difficulty (regardless of technology—film, CR, or DR).	☐	☐	☐	☐	☐	☐
24. Properly completes the examination by filling out all necessary paperwork, entering the examination in the computer, having the images checked by the appropriate staff members, and informing the patient that he or she is finished.	☐	☐	☐	☐	☐	☐
25. Exhibits the ability to adapt to new and difficult situations if and when necessary.	☐	☐	☐	☐	☐	☐
26. Accepts constructive criticism and uses it to his or her advantage.	☐	☐	☐	☐	☐	☐
27. Leaves the radiographic room neat and clean for the next examination.	☐	☐	☐	☐	☐	☐
28. Completes the examination within a reasonable time frame.	☐	☐	☐	☐	☐	☐

Comments:

_____

_____

RADIOGRAPHIC IMAGE QUALITY
The student is able to critique his or her radiographs as to whether they demonstrate:

	Procedure		Repeat		Competency	
	Yes	No	Yes	No	Yes	No
29. Proper technique/optimal density	☐	☐	☐	☐	☐	☐
30. Enhanced detail, without evidence of motion and without any visible artifacts	☐	☐	☐	☐	☐	☐
31. Proper positioning (all anatomy included, evidence of proper centering/alignment, etc.)	☐	☐	☐	☐	☐	☐
32. Proper marker placement	☐	☐	☐	☐	☐	☐
33. Evidence of proper collimation and radiation protection	☐	☐	☐	☐	☐	☐
34. Long vs. short scale of contrast	☐	☐	☐	☐	☐	☐

Comments:

_____

_____

WRIST ANATOMY
The student is able to identify:

	Procedure		Repeat		Competency	
	Yes	No	Yes	No	Yes	No
35. Navicular/scaphoid	☐	☐	☐	☐	☐	☐
36. Lunate/semilunar	☐	☐	☐	☐	☐	☐

(continued)

	Procedure		Repeat		Competency	
	Yes	No	Yes	No	Yes	No
37. Triquetrum/cuneiform	☐	☐	☐	☐	☐	☐
38. Greater multangular/trapezium	☐	☐	☐	☐	☐	☐
39. Capitatum/os magnum	☐	☐	☐	☐	☐	☐
40. Obvious pathology	☐	☐	☐	☐	☐	☐

Comments:

_____

_____

Procedure Evaluator Signature	Repeat Evaluator Signature	Competency Evaluator Signature

Date	Date	Date

Navicular/Scaphoid

The objective of this evaluation is to determine the student's competency level when performing specific radiographic examinations.

Student Name:_____

Procedure Grade	Repeat Grade	Competency Grade

PATIENT INFORMATION OR SIMULATED PROCEDURE *(circle if simulated)*

	Procedure	Repeat	Competency
Age			
Medical Record No.			
Ability to Cooperate			
Condition/Pathology			
Technical Factors Used			
Exposure Index			

FACILITY PREPARATION
The student:

	Procedure Yes	Procedure No	Repeat Yes	Repeat No	Competency Yes	Competency No
1. Examines the radiographic room and cleans/straightens it before escorting the patient in.	☐	☐	☐	☐	☐	☐
2. Has all equipment and supplies (patient gown, pillow, markers, lead blockers, etc.) readily available before escorting the patient in.	☐	☐	☐	☐	☐	☐
3. Is able to manipulate all radiographic equipment with ease, and centers the central ray to the cassette/receptor.	☐	☐	☐	☐	☐	☐
4. Adjusts the tube to the proper SID.	☐	☐	☐	☐	☐	☐
5. Selects a cassette/receptor of the appropriate size.	☐	☐	☐	☐	☐	☐

Comments:

_____

_____

PATIENT PREPARATION
The student:

	Procedure Yes	Procedure No	Repeat Yes	Repeat No	Competency Yes	Competency No
6. Identifies the correct patient and examination according to the requisition while establishing a good rapport with him or her.	☐	☐	☐	☐	☐	☐
7. Obtains and documents the patient's history before the examination.	☑	☑	☑	☑	☐	☐
8. Explains the examination in terms the patient fully understands, and properly communicates with the patient throughout the examination.	☐	☐	☐	☐	☐	☐
9. Asks female patients of childbearing age the date of their last menstrual period and documents this; inquires about the possibility of pregnancy and has them sign pregnancy consent forms.	☐	☐	☐	☐	☐	☐
10. Removes all obscuring objects (snaps, zippers, belt, etc.) so as *not* to produce radiographic artifacts.	☐	☐	☐	☐	☐	☐
11. Respects the patient's modesty and provides ample comfort for him or her.	☐	☐	☐	☐	☐	☐

(continued)

Comments:

_____

_____

PATIENT POSITIONING FOR FOR A NAVICULAR/SCAPHOID BONE OF A WRIST

The student:

	Procedure		Repeat		Competency	
	Yes	No	Yes	No	Yes	No
12. Instructs the patient to rest his or her forearm prone so that it lies parallel to the long axis of the radiographic table.	☐	☐	☐	☐	☐	☐
13. Does *one* of the following:	☐	☐	☐	☐	☐	☐
a. Places one end of the cassette/receptor on a support so that it forms a 20° angle toward the elbow.						
b. Keeps the cassette/receptor parallel to the table and angles the central ray toward the elbow.						
14. Adjusts the position of the wrist to extreme ulnar flexion.	☐	☐	☐	☐	☐	☐
15. Centers the anatomy of interest (the navicular) approximately 1/2 inch above the center of the cassette/receptor.	☐	☐	☐	☐	☐	☐
16. Centers the central ray to the navicular bone.	☐	☐	☐	☐	☐	☐

Comments:

_____

_____

IMPORTANT DETAILS

The student:

	Procedure		Repeat		Competency	
	Yes	No	Yes	No	Yes	No
17. Instills confidence in the patient by exhibiting self-confidence throughout the examination.	☐	☐	☐	☐	☐	☐
18. Places a lead marker in the appropriate area of the cassette/receptor (top/bottom/anteriorly/laterally), where it will be visualized on the finished radiograph, on the proper anatomical side (right/left), and in the appropriate position (face up/face down), depending on the patient's position.	☐	☐	☐	☐	☐	☐
19. Provides radiation protection (shield) for the patient, self, and others (closes doors).	☐	☐	☐	☐	☐	☐
20. Applies proper collimation and makes adjustments as necessary.	☐	☐	☐	☐	☐	☐
21. Properly measures the patient along the course of the central ray *for each projection.*	☐	☐	☐	☐	☐	☐
22. Sets the proper exposure techniques:	☐	☐	☐	☐	☐	☐

Conventional systems
- Sets the proper kVp, mA, and time and makes adjustments as necessary.

or

CR or DR systems
- Identifies the patient on the work-list (or manually types the patient information into the system).
- Selects appropriate body region, specific body part, and accurate view/projection.
- Double-checks preset parameters:
  —Adult vs. pediatric patients
     ○ Small, medium, or large
  —Bucky/receptor (upright vs. table) *or* non-Bucky

	Procedure		Repeat		Competency	
	Yes	No	Yes	No	Yes	No

—AEC vs. fixed
   ○ If AEC, checks ion chambers
   ○ Density setting
—kVp and mA; adjusts if necessary
—Focal spot/filament size

	Procedure		Repeat		Competency	
23. Exposes the cassette/receptor after telling the patient to hold still and supporting and/or immobilizing the area of interest if necessary *for each projection.*	☐	☐	☐	☐	☐	☐
24. Provides each radiograph with the proper identification (flash) and/or processes each cassette (image) without difficulty (regardless of technology—film, CR, or DR).	▣	▣	▣	▣	☐	☐
25. Properly completes the examination by filling out all necessary paperwork, entering the examination in the computer, having the images checked by the appropriate staff members, and informing the patient that he or she is finished.	▣	▣	▣	▣	☐	☐
26. Exhibits the ability to adapt to new and difficult situations if and when necessary.	▣	▣	▣	▣	☐	☐
27. Accepts constructive criticism and uses it to his or her advantage.	☐	☐	☐	☐	☐	☐
28. Leaves the radiographic room neat and clean for the next examination.	▣	▣	▣	▣	☐	☐
29. Completes the examination within a reasonable time frame.	☐	☐	☐	☐	☐	☐

Comments:

RADIOGRAPHIC IMAGE QUALITY
The student is able to critique his or her radiographs as to whether they demonstrate:

	Procedure		Repeat		Competency	
	Yes	No	Yes	No	Yes	No
30. Proper technique/optimal density	▣	▣	▣	▣	☐	☐
31. Enhanced detail, without evidence of motion and without any visible artifacts	▣	▣	▣	▣	☐	☐
32. Proper positioning (all anatomy included, evidence of proper centering/ alignment, etc.)	▣	▣	▣	▣	☐	☐
33. Proper marker placement	▣	▣	▣	▣	☐	☐
34. Evidence of proper collimation and radiation protection	▣	▣	▣	▣	☐	☐
35. Long vs. short scale of contrast	▣	▣	▣	▣	☐	☐

Comments:

WRIST ANATOMY
The student is able to identify:

	Procedure		Repeat		Competency	
	Yes	No	Yes	No	Yes	No
36. Navicular/scaphoid	▣	▣	▣	▣	☐	☐
37. Lunate/semilunar	▣	▣	▣	▣	☐	☐
38. Triquetrum/cuneiform	▣	▣	▣	▣	☐	☐
39. Pisiform	▣	▣	▣	▣	☐	☐
40. Greater multangular/trapezium	▣	▣	▣	▣	☐	☐
41. Lesser multangular/trapezoid	▣	▣	▣	▣	☐	☐

(continued)

	Procedure		Repeat		Competency	
	Yes	No	Yes	No	Yes	No
42. Capitatum/os magnum	☐	☐	☐	☐	☐	☐
43. Hamate/unciform	☐	☐	☐	☐	☐	☐
44. Distal radius and ulna	☐	☐	☐	☐	☐	☐
45. Proximal metacarpals	☐	☐	☐	☐	☐	☐
46. Obvious pathology	☐	☐	☐	☐	☐	☐

Comments:

_____

_____

_____   _____   _____
Procedure Evaluator Signature   Repeat Evaluator Signature   Competency Evaluator Signature

_____   _____   _____
Date   Date   Date

END NAVICULAR/SCAPHOID EVALUATION

The objective of this evaluation is to determine the student's competency level when performing specific radiographic examinations.

Student Name:_____

Procedure Grade	Repeat Grade	Competency Grade

PATIENT INFORMATION OR SIMULATED PROCEDURE *(circle if simulated)*

	Procedure	Repeat	Competency
Age			
Medical Record No.			
Ability to Cooperate			
Condition/Pathology			
Technical Factors Used			
Exposure Index			

FACILITY PREPARATION
The student:

	Procedure Yes	Procedure No	Repeat Yes	Repeat No	Competency Yes	Competency No
1. Examines the radiographic room and cleans/straightens it before escorting the patient in.	☐	☐	☐	☐	☐	☐
2. Has all equipment and supplies (patient gown, pillow, markers, lead blockers, etc.) readily available before escorting the patient in.	☐	☐	☐	☐	☐	☐
3. Is able to manipulate all radiographic equipment with ease, and centers the central ray to the cassette/receptor *for both projections.*	☐	☐	☐	☐	☐	☐
4. Adjusts the tube to the proper SID *for each projection.*	☐	☐	☐	☐	☐	☐
5. Selects cassettes/receptor of the appropriate sizes *for both projections,* according to the patient's size and examination.	☐	☐	☐	☐	☐	☐

Comments:

_____

_____

PATIENT PREPARATION
The student:

	Procedure Yes	Procedure No	Repeat Yes	Repeat No	Competency Yes	Competency No
6. Identifies the correct patient and examination according to the requisition while establishing a good rapport with him or her.	☐	☐	☐	☐	☐	☐
7. Obtains and documents the patient's history before the examination.	▨	▨	▨	▨	☐	☐
8. Explains the examination in terms the patient fully understands, and properly communicates with the patient throughout the examination.	☐	☐	☐	☐	☐	☐
9. Asks female patients of childbearing age the date of their last menstrual period and documents this; inquires about the possibility of pregnancy and has them sign pregnancy consent forms.	☐	☐	☐	☐	☐	☐
10. Removes all obscuring objects (snaps, zippers, belt, etc.) so as *not* to produce radiographic artifacts.	☐	☐	☐	☐	☐	☐

(continued)

	Procedure		Repeat		Competency	
	Yes	No	Yes	No	Yes	No
11. Respects the patient's modesty and provides ample comfort for him or her.	☐	☐	☐	☐	☐	☐

Comments:

_____

_____

PATIENT POSITIONING FOR A FOREARM
Anteroposterior
The student:

	Procedure		Repeat		Competency	
	Yes	No	Yes	No	Yes	No
12. If using conventional film: divides the cassette into appropriate sections with lead blockers, if appropriate.	☐	☐	☐	☐	☐	☐
13. Places the posterior surface of the forearm on the appropriate area of the cassette/receptor, with the elbow completely extended, and maintains supination of the hand, with a sandbag if necessary.	☐	☐	☐	☐	☐	☐
14. Places the entire arm at the same level as the shoulder.	☐	☐	☐	☐	☐	☐
15. Centers the anatomy of interest, including both joints, to the center of the cassette/receptor.	☐	☐	☐	☐	☐	☐
16. Centers the central ray perpendicularly to the midshaft of the forearm.	☐	☐	☐	☐	☐	☐

Lateral
The student:

	Procedure		Repeat		Competency	
	Yes	No	Yes	No	Yes	No
17. If using conventional film: adjusts the lead blockers to divide the cassette appropriately.	☐	☐	☐	☐	☐	☐
18. Rotates the wrist to the true lateral position while instructing the patient to bend his or her elbow 90° and placing the medial surface of the forearm on the appropriate area of the cassette/receptor.	☐	☐	☐	☐	☐	☐
19. Maintains the position of the patient's arm at the same level as the shoulder.	☐	☐	☐	☐	☐	☐
20. Centers the anatomy of interest, including both joints, to the center of the cassette/receptor.	☐	☐	☐	☐	☐	☐
21. Centers the central ray perpendicularly to the midshaft of the forearm.	☐	☐	☐	☐	☐	☐

Comments:

_____

_____

IMPORTANT DETAILS
The student:

	Procedure		Repeat		Competency	
	Yes	No	Yes	No	Yes	No
22. Instills confidence in the patient by exhibiting self-confidence throughout the examination.	☐	☐	☐	☐	☐	☐
23. Places a lead marker in the appropriate area of the cassette/receptor (top/bottom/anteriorly/laterally), where it will be visualized on the finished radiograph, on the proper anatomical side (right/left), and in the appropriate position (face up/face down), depending on the patient's position.	☐	☐	☐	☐	☐	☐
24. Provides radiation protection (shield) for the patient, self, and others (closes doors).	☐	☐	☐	☐	☐	☐
25. Applies proper collimation and makes adjustments as necessary.	☐	☐	☐	☐	☐	☐
26. Properly measures the patient along the course of the central ray *for each projection.*	☐	☐	☐	☐	☐	☐

	Procedure		Repeat		Competency	
	Yes	No	Yes	No	Yes	No
27. Sets the proper exposure techniques:	☐	☐	☐	☐	☐	☐

Conventional systems
- Sets the proper kVp, mA, and time and makes adjustments as necessary.

or

CR or DR systems
- Identifies the patient on the work-list (or manually types the patient information into the system).
- Selects appropriate body region, specific body part, and accurate view/projection.
- Double-checks preset parameters:
  —Adult vs. pediatric patients
    ○ Small, medium, or large
  —Bucky/receptor (upright vs. table) *or* non-Bucky
  —AEC vs. fixed
    ○ If AEC, checks ion chambers
    ○ Density setting
  —kVp and mA; adjusts if necessary
  —Focal spot/filament size

	Procedure		Repeat		Competency	
	Yes	No	Yes	No	Yes	No
28. Exposes the cassette/receptor after telling the patient to hold still and supporting and/or immobilizing the area of interest if necessary *for each projection.*	☐	☐	☐	☐	☐	☐
29. Provides each radiograph with the proper identification (flash) and/or processes each cassette (image) without difficulty (regardless of technology—film, CR, or DR).	▣	▣	▣	▣	☐	☐
30. Properly completes the examination by filling out all necessary paperwork, entering the examination in the computer, having the images checked by the appropriate staff members, and informing the patient that he or she is finished.	▣	▣	▣	▣	☐	☐
31. Exhibits the ability to adapt to new and difficult situations if and when necessary.	▣	▣	▣	▣	☐	☐
32. Accepts constructive criticism and uses it to his or her advantage.	☐	☐	☐	☐	☐	☐
33. Leaves the radiographic room neat and clean for the next examination.	▣	▣	▣	▣	☐	☐
34. Completes the examination within a reasonable time frame.	☐	☐	☐	☐	☐	☐

Comments:

RADIOGRAPHIC IMAGE QUALITY
The student is able to critique his or her radiographs as to whether they demonstrate:

	Procedure		Repeat		Competency	
	Yes	No	Yes	No	Yes	No
35. Proper technique/optimal density	▣	▣	▣	▣	☐	☐
36. Enhanced detail, without evidence of motion and without any visible artifacts	▣	▣	▣	▣	☐	☐
37. Proper positioning (all anatomy included, evidence of proper centering/alignment, etc.)	▣	▣	▣	▣	☐	☐
38. Proper marker placement	▣	▣	▣	▣	☐	☐
39. Evidence of proper collimation and radiation protection	▣	▣	▣	▣	☐	☐
40. Long vs. short scale of contrast	▣	▣	▣	▣	☐	☐

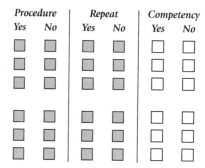

(continued)

Comments:

_____

_____

FOREARM ANATOMY
The student is able to identify:

	Procedure		Repeat		Competency	
	Yes	No	Yes	No	Yes	No
41. Radius	☐	☐	☐	☐	☐	☐
42. Ulna	☐	☐	☐	☐	☐	☐
43. Ulnar head	☐	☐	☐	☐	☐	☐
44. Styloid process of the radius	☐	☐	☐	☐	☐	☐
45. Radial tuberosity	☐	☐	☐	☐	☐	☐
46. Radial head and neck	☐	☐	☐	☐	☐	☐
47. Medial and lateral epicondyles	☐	☐	☐	☐	☐	☐
48. Olecranon process	☐	☐	☐	☐	☐	☐
49. Coronoid process	☐	☐	☐	☐	☐	☐
50. Carpal bones	☐	☐	☐	☐	☐	☐
51. Obvious pathology	☐	☐	☐	☐	☐	☐

Comments:

_____

_____

Procedure Evaluator Signature	Repeat Evaluator Signature	Competency Evaluator Signature

Date	Date	Date

END FOREARM EVALUATION

Student Name:_____

Procedure Grade	Repeat Grade	Competency Grade

PATIENT INFORMATION OR SIMULATED PROCEDURE *(circle if simulated)*

	Procedure	Repeat	Competency
Age			
Medical Record No.			
Ability to Cooperate			
Condition/Pathology			
Technical Factors Used			
Exposure Index			

FACILITY PREPARATION
The student:

	Procedure Yes No	Repeat Yes No	Competency Yes No
1. Examines the radiographic room and cleans/straightens it before escorting the patient in.	☐ ☐	☐ ☐	☐ ☐
2. Has all equipment and supplies (patient gown, pillow, markers, lead blockers, etc.) readily available before escorting the patient in.	☐ ☐	☐ ☐	☐ ☐
3. Is able to manipulate all radiographic equipment with ease, and centers the central ray to the cassette/receptor *for both projections.*	☐ ☐	☐ ☐	☐ ☐
4. Adjusts the tube to the proper SID *for each projection.*	☐ ☐	☐ ☐	☐ ☐
5. Selects cassettes/receptor of the appropriate sizes *for all projections,* according to the patient's size and examination.	☐ ☐	☐ ☐	☐ ☐

Comments:

_____

_____

PATIENT PREPARATION
The student:

	Procedure Yes No	Repeat Yes No	Competency Yes No
6. Identifies the correct patient and examination according to the requisition while establishing a good rapport with him or her.	☐ ☐	☐ ☐	☐ ☐
7. Obtains and documents the patient's history before the examination.	▣ ▣	▣ ▣	☐ ☐
8. Explains the examination in terms the patient fully understands, and properly communicates with the patient throughout the examination.	☐ ☐	☐ ☐	☐ ☐
9. Asks female patients of childbearing age the date of their last menstrual period and documents this; inquires about the possibility of pregnancy and has them sign pregnancy consent forms.	☐ ☐	☐ ☐	☐ ☐
10. Removes all obscuring objects (snaps, zippers, belt, etc.) so as *not* to produce radiographic artifacts.	☐ ☐	☐ ☐	☐ ☐
11. Respects the patient's modesty and provides ample comfort for him or her.	☐ ☐	☐ ☐	☐ ☐

(continued)

Comments:

_____

_____

PATIENT POSITIONING FOR AN ELBOW
Anteroposterior
The student:

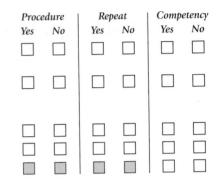

	Procedure		Repeat		Competency	
	Yes	No	Yes	No	Yes	No
12. If using conventional film: divides the cassette into appropriate sections with lead blockers.	☐	☐	☐	☐	☐	☐
13. Places the posterior surface of the elbow on the appropriate area of the cassette/receptor, with the elbow completely extended, and maintains supination of the hand, with a sandbag.	☐	☐	☐	☐	☐	☐
14. Places the entire arm at the same level as the shoulder.	☐	☐	☐	☐	☐	☐
15. Centers the elbow joint to the center of the casette/receptor.	☐	☐	☐	☐	☐	☐
16. Centers the central ray perpendicularly to the midelbow area.	☐	☐	☐	☐	☐	☐

Lateral
The student:

	Procedure		Repeat		Competency	
	Yes	No	Yes	No	Yes	No
17. If using conventional film: adjusts the lead blockers to divide the cassette appropriately.	☐	☐	☐	☐	☐	☐
18. Maintains the position of the patient's arm at the same level as the shoulder.	☐	☐	☐	☐	☐	☐
19. Rotates the elbow to the true lateral position, while instructing the patient to bend his or her elbow 90° and placing the medial surface of the elbow on the appropriate area of the cassette/receptor.	☐	☐	☐	☐	☐	☐
20. Places the wrist in the true lateral position.	☐	☐	☐	☐	☐	☐
21. Centers the elbow joint to the center of the cassette/receptor.	☐	☐	☐	☐	☐	☐
22. Centers the central ray perpendicularly to the midelbow area.	☐	☐	☐	☐	☐	☐

Internal/Medial Oblique
The student:

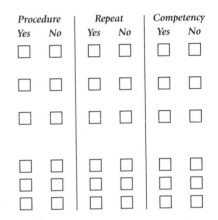

	Procedure		Repeat		Competency	
	Yes	No	Yes	No	Yes	No
23. If using conventional film: selects a new cassette and adjusts the lead blockers to divide the cassette appropriately.	☐	☐	☐	☐	☐	☐
24. Places the medial/posterior surface of the elbow on the appropriate area of the cassette/receptor, with the elbow completely extended.	☐	☐	☐	☐	☐	☐
25. Rotates the elbow internally until the epicondyles are at a 45° angle with the cassette/receptor, by pronating the hand.	☐	☐	☐	☐	☐	☐
26. Centers the elbow joint to the center of the cassette/receptor.	☐	☐	☐	☐	☐	☐
27. Centers the central ray perpendicularly to the midelbow area.	☐	☐	☐	☐	☐	☐

External/Lateral Oblique
The student:

	Procedure		Repeat		Competency	
	Yes	No	Yes	No	Yes	No
28. If using conventional film: adjusts the lead blockers to divide the cassette appropriately.	☐	☐	☐	☐	☐	☐
29. Places the lateral surface of the elbow on the appropriate area of the cassette/receptor, with the elbow completely extended.	☐	☐	☐	☐	☐	☐

	Procedure		Repeat		Competency	
	Yes	No	Yes	No	Yes	No
30. Rotates the elbow externally until the epicondyles are at a 45° angle with the cassette/receptor, representing extreme external rotation of the entire arm.	☐	☐	☐	☐	☐	☐
31. Centers the elbow joint to the center of the cassette/receptor.	☐	☐	☐	☐	☐	☐
32. Centers the central ray perpendicularly to the midelbow area.	☐	☐	☐	☐	☐	☐

Comments:

_____

_____

IMPORTANT DETAILS
The student:

	Procedure		Repeat		Competency	
	Yes	No	Yes	No	Yes	No
33. Instills confidence in the patient by exhibiting self-confidence throughout the examination.	☐	☐	☐	☐	☐	☐
34. Places a lead marker in the appropriate area of the cassette/receptor (top/bottom/anteriorly/laterally), where it will be visualized on the finished radiograph, on the proper anatomical side (right/left), and in the appropriate position (face up/face down), depending on the patient's position.	☐	☐	☐	☐	☐	☐
35. Provides radiation protection (shield) for the patient, self, and others (closes doors).	☐	☐	☐	☐	☐	☐
36. Applies proper collimation and makes adjustments as necessary.	☐	☐	☐	☐	☐	☐
37. Properly measures the patient along the course of the central ray *for each projection.*	☐	☐	☐	☐	☐	☐
38. Sets the proper exposure techniques:	☐	☐	☐	☐	☐	☐

Conventional systems
• Sets the proper kVp, mA, and time and makes adjustments as necessary.

or

CR or DR systems
• Identifies the patient on the work-list (or manually types the patient information into the system).
• Selects appropriate body region, specific body part, and accurate view/ projection.
• Double-checks preset parameters:
—Adult vs. pediatric patients
  ○ Small, medium, or large
—Bucky/receptor (upright vs. table) *or* non-Bucky
—AEC vs. fixed
  ○ If AEC, checks ion chambers
  ○ Density setting
—kVp and mA; adjusts if necessary
—Focal spot/filament size

	Procedure		Repeat		Competency	
39. Exposes the cassette/receptor after telling the patient to hold still and supporting and/or immobilizing the area of interest if necessary *for each projection.*	☐	☐	☐	☐	☐	☐
40. Provides each radiograph with the proper identification (flash) and/or processes each cassette (image) without difficulty (regardless of technology—film, CR, or DR).	▨	▨	▨	▨	☐	☐
41. Properly completes the examination by filling out all necessary paperwork, entering the examination in the computer, having the images checked by the appropriate staff members, and informing the patient that he or she is finished.	▨	▨	▨	▨	☐	☐

(continued)

	Procedure		Repeat		Competency	
	Yes	No	Yes	No	Yes	No
42. Exhibits the ability to adapt to new and difficult situations if and when necessary.	▢	▢	▢	▢	☐	☐
43. Accepts constructive criticism and uses it to his or her advantage.	☐	☐	☐	☐	☐	☐
44. Leaves the radiographic room neat and clean for the next examination.	▢	▢	▢	▢	☐	☐
45. Completes the examination within a reasonable time frame.	☐	☐	☐	☐	☐	☐

Comments:

_____

_____

RADIOGRAPHIC IMAGE QUALITY
The student is able to critique his or her radiographs as to whether they demonstrate:

	Procedure		Repeat		Competency	
	Yes	No	Yes	No	Yes	No
46. Proper technique/optimal density	▢	▢	▢	▢	☐	☐
47. Enhanced detail, without evidence of motion and without any visible artifacts	▢	▢	▢	▢	☐	☐
48. Proper positioning (all anatomy included, evidence of proper centering/ alignment, etc.)	▢	▢	▢	▢	☐	☐
49. Proper marker placement	▢	▢	▢	▢	☐	☐
50. Evidence of proper collimation and radiation protection	▢	▢	▢	▢	☐	☐
51. Long vs. short scale of contrast	▢	▢	▢	▢	☐	☐

Comments:

_____

_____

ELBOW ANATOMY
The student is able to identify:

	Procedure		Repeat		Competency	
	Yes	No	Yes	No	Yes	No
51. Humerus	▢	▢	▢	▢	☐	☐
52. Radius	▢	▢	▢	▢	☐	☐
53. Ulna	▢	▢	▢	▢	☐	☐
54. Trochlea	▢	▢	▢	▢	☐	☐
55. Capitulum	▢	▢	▢	▢	☐	☐
56. Radial tuberosity	▢	▢	▢	▢	☐	☐
57. Radial head and neck	▢	▢	▢	▢	☐	☐
58. Medial and lateral epicondyles	▢	▢	▢	▢	☐	☐
59. Olecranon process	▢	▢	▢	▢	☐	☐
60. Olecranon fossa	▢	▢	▢	▢	☐	☐
61. Coronoid process	▢	▢	▢	▢	☐	☐
62. Obvious pathology	▢	▢	▢	▢	☐	☐

Comments:

_____

_____

_____	_____	_____
Procedure Evaluator Signature	Repeat Evaluator Signature	Competency Evaluator Signature
_____	_____	_____
Date	Date	Date

END ELBOW EVALUATION

Student Name:_____

Procedure Grade	Repeat Grade	Competency Grade

PATIENT INFORMATION OR SIMULATED PROCEDURE *(circle if simulated)*

	Procedure	Repeat	Competency
Age			
Medical Record No.			
Ability to Cooperate			
Condition/Pathology			
Technical Factors Used			
Exposure Index			

FACILITY PREPARATION
The student:

	Procedure Yes / No	Repeat Yes / No	Competency Yes / No
1. Examines the radiographic room and cleans/straightens it before escorting the patient in.	☐ ☐	☐ ☐	☐ ☐
2. Has all equipment and supplies (patient gown, pillow, markers, lead blockers, etc.) readily available before escorting the patient in.	☐ ☐	☐ ☐	☐ ☐
3. Is able to manipulate all radiographic equipment with ease, and centers the central ray to the cassette/receptor *for both projections.*	☐ ☐	☐ ☐	☐ ☐
4. Adjusts the tube to the proper SID *for each projection.*	☐ ☐	☐ ☐	☐ ☐
5. Selects cassettes/receptor of the appropriate sizes *for both projections,* according to the patient's size and examination.	☐ ☐	☐ ☐	☐ ☐

Comments:

_____

_____

PATIENT PREPARATION
The student:

	Procedure Yes / No	Repeat Yes / No	Competency Yes / No
6. Identifies the correct patient and examination according to the requisition while establishing a good rapport with him or her.	☐ ☐	☐ ☐	☐ ☐
7. Obtains and documents the patient's history before the examination.	▨ ▨	▨ ▨	☐ ☐
8. Explains the examination in terms the patient fully understands, and properly communicates with the patient throughout the examination.	☐ ☐	☐ ☐	☐ ☐
9. Asks female patients of childbearing age the date of their last menstrual period and documents this; inquires about the possibility of pregnancy and has them sign pregnancy consent forms.	☐ ☐	☐ ☐	☐ ☐
10. Removes all obscuring objects (snaps, zippers, belt, etc.) so as *not* to produce radiographic artifacts.	☐ ☐	☐ ☐	☐ ☐
11. Respects the patient's modesty and provides ample comfort for him or her.	☐ ☐	☐ ☐	☐ ☐

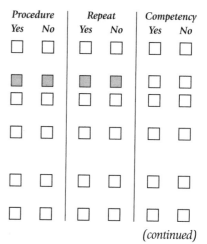

(continued)

Comments:

_____

_____

PATIENT POSITIONING FOR AN ELBOW IN THE ACUTE FLEXION POSITION (AXIAL PROJECTION)
Positioning to Visualize the Proximal Forearm
The student:

	Procedure		Repeat		Competency	
	Yes	No	Yes	No	Yes	No
12. If using conventional film: divides the cassette into appropriate sections with lead blockers.	☐	☐	☐	☐	☐	☐
13. Places the posterior surface of the humerus on the appropriate area of the cassette/receptor.	☐	☐	☐	☐	☐	☐
14. Centers the anatomy of interest to the center of the cassette/receptor.	☐	☐	☐	☐	☐	☐
15. Centers the central ray perpendicularly to the proximal forearm/ elbow joint.	☐	☐	☐	☐	☐	☐

Positioning to Visualize the Distal Humerus
The student:

	Procedure		Repeat		Competency	
	Yes	No	Yes	No	Yes	No
16. If using conventional film: adjusts the lead blockers to divide the cassette appropriately.	☐	☐	☐	☐	☐	☐
17. Places the posterior surface of the humerus on the appropriate area of the cassette/receptor.	☐	☐	☐	☐	☐	☐
18. Centers the anatomy of interest to the center of the cassette/receptor.	☐	☐	☐	☐	☐	☐
19. Centers the central ray perpendicularly to the humerus/elbow joint, approximately 2 inches superior to the olecranon process.	☐	☐	☐	☐	☐	☐

Comments:

_____

_____

IMPORTANT DETAILS
The student:

	Procedure		Repeat		Competency	
	Yes	No	Yes	No	Yes	No
20. Instills confidence in the patient by exhibiting self-confidence throughout the examination.	☐	☐	☐	☐	☐	☐
21. Places a lead marker in the appropriate area of the cassette/receptor (top/bottom/anteriorly/laterally), where it will be visualized on the finished radiograph, on the proper anatomical side (right/left), and in the appropriate position (face up/face down), depending on the patient's position.	☐	☐	☐	☐	☐	☐
22. Provides radiation protection (shield) for the patient, self, and others (closes doors).	☐	☐	☐	☐	☐	☐
23. Applies proper collimation and makes adjustments as necessary.	☐	☐	☐	☐	☐	☐
24. Properly measures the patient along the course of the central ray *for each projection.*	☐	☐	☐	☐	☐	☐
25. Sets the proper exposure techniques:	☐	☐	☐	☐	☐	☐

25. Sets the proper exposure techniques:

Conventional systems
- Sets the proper kVp, mA, and time and makes adjustments as necessary.

or

CR or DR systems
- Identifies the patient on the work-list (or manually types the patient information into the system).

	Procedure		Repeat		Competency	
	Yes	No	Yes	No	Yes	No

- Selects appropriate body region, specific body part, and accurate view/projection.
- Double-checks preset parameters:
  —Adult vs. pediatric patients
    ○ Small, medium, or large
  —Bucky/receptor (upright vs. table) *or* non-Bucky
  —AEC vs. fixed
    ○ If AEC, checks ion chambers
    ○ Density setting
  —kVp and mA; adjusts if necessary
  —Focal spot/filament size

Item	Procedure Yes	Procedure No	Repeat Yes	Repeat No	Competency Yes	Competency No
26. Exposes the cassette/receptor after telling the patient to hold still and supporting and/or immobilizing the area of interest if necessary *for each projection.*	☐	☐	☐	☐	☐	☐
27. Provides each radiograph with the proper identification (flash) and/or processes each cassette (image) without difficulty (regardless of technology—film, CR, or DR).	▣	▣	▣	▣	☐	☐
28. Properly completes the examination by filling out all necessary paperwork, entering the examination in the computer, having the images checked by the appropriate staff members, and informing the patient that he or she is finished.	▣	▣	▣	▣	☐	☐
29. Exhibits the ability to adapt to new and difficult situations if and when necessary.	▣	▣	▣	▣	☐	☐
30. Accepts constructive criticism and uses it to his or her advantage.	☐	☐	☐	☐	☐	☐
31. Leaves the radiographic room neat and clean for the next examination.	▣	▣	▣	▣	☐	☐
32. Completes the examination within a reasonable time frame.	☐	☐	☐	☐	☐	☐

Comments:

_____

_____

RADIOGRAPHIC IMAGE QUALITY
The student is able to critique his or her radiographs as to whether they demonstrate:

Item	Procedure Yes	Procedure No	Repeat Yes	Repeat No	Competency Yes	Competency No
33. Proper technique/optimal density	▣	▣	▣	▣	☐	☐
34. Enhanced detail, without evidence of motion and without any visible artifacts	▣	▣	▣	▣	☐	☐
35. Proper positioning (all anatomy included, evidence of proper centering/alignment, etc.)	▣	▣	▣	▣	☐	☐
36. Proper marker placement	▣	▣	▣	▣	☐	☐
37. Evidence of proper collimation and radiation protection	▣	▣	▣	▣	☐	☐
38. Long vs. short scale of contrast	▣	▣	▣	▣	☐	☐

Comments:

_____

_____

ELBOW ANATOMY
Proximal Forearm Projection
The student is able to identify:

Item	Procedure Yes	Procedure No	Repeat Yes	Repeat No	Competency Yes	Competency No
39. Humerus	▣	▣	▣	▣	☐	☐
40. Radius	▣	▣	▣	▣	☐	☐

(continued)

	Procedure		Repeat		Competency	
	Yes	No	Yes	No	Yes	No
41. Ulna	☐	☐	☐	☐	☐	☐
42. Radial tuberosity	☐	☐	☐	☐	☐	☐
43. Radial head and neck	☐	☐	☐	☐	☐	☐
44. Olecranon process	☐	☐	☐	☐	☐	☐

Distal Humerus Projection
The student is able to identify:

	Procedure		Repeat		Competency	
	Yes	No	Yes	No	Yes	No
45. Trochlea	☐	☐	☐	☐	☐	☐
46. Medial epicondyle	☐	☐	☐	☐	☐	☐
47. Olecranon process	☐	☐	☐	☐	☐	☐
48. Radial head	☐	☐	☐	☐	☐	☐
49. Capitulum	☐	☐	☐	☐	☐	☐
50. Obvious pathology	☐	☐	☐	☐	☐	☐

Comments:

_____

_____

_____

Procedure Evaluator Signature	Repeat Evaluator Signature	Competency Evaluator Signature

Date	Date	Date

END ACUTE FLEXION (AXIAL) ELBOW EVALUATION

The objective of this evaluation is to determine the student's competency level when performing specific radiographic examinations.

Student Name:_____

	Procedure Grade	Repeat Grade	Competency Grade

PATIENT INFORMATION OR SIMULATED PROCEDURE *(circle if simulated)*

	Procedure	Repeat	Competency
Age			
Medical Record No.			
Ability to Cooperate			
Condition/Pathology			
Technical Factors Used			
Exposure Index			

FACILITY PREPARATION
The student:

	Procedure Yes No	Repeat Yes No	Competency Yes No
1. Examines the radiographic room and cleans/straightens it before escorting the patient in.	☐ ☐	☐ ☐	☐ ☐
2. Has all equipment and supplies (patient gown, pillow, markers, lead blockers, etc.) readily available before escorting the patient in.	☐ ☐	☐ ☐	☐ ☐
3. Is able to manipulate all radiographic equipment with ease, and centers the central ray to the cassette/receptor *for both projections.*	☐ ☐	☐ ☐	☐ ☐
4. Adjusts the tube to the proper SID *for each projection.*	☐ ☐	☐ ☐	☐ ☐
5. Selects cassettes/receptor of the appropriate sizes *for both projections,* according to the patient's size and examination.	☐ ☐	☐ ☐	☐ ☐

Comments:

_____

_____

PATIENT PREPARATION
The student:

	Procedure Yes No	Repeat Yes No	Competency Yes No
6. Identifies the correct patient and examination according to the requisition while establishing a good rapport with him or her.	☐ ☐	☐ ☐	☐ ☐
7. Obtains and documents the patient's history before the examination.	☐ ☐	☐ ☐	☐ ☐
8. Explains the examination in terms the patient fully understands, and properly communicates with the patient throughout the examination.	☐ ☐	☐ ☐	☐ ☐
9. Asks female patients of childbearing age the date of their last menstrual period and documents this; inquires about the possibility of pregnancy and has them sign pregnancy consent forms.	☐ ☐	☐ ☐	☐ ☐
10. Removes all obscuring objects (snaps, zippers, belt, etc.) so as *not* to produce radiographic artifacts.	☐ ☐	☐ ☐	☐ ☐
11. Respects the patient's modesty and provides ample comfort for him or her.	☐ ☐	☐ ☐	☐ ☐

(continued)

Comments:

_____

_____

PATIENT POSITIONING FOR AN ELBOW THE PARTIAL FLEXION POSITION
Positioning to Visualize the Proximal Forearm
The student:

	Procedure Yes	No	Repeat Yes	No	Competency Yes	No
12. If using conventional film: divides the cassette into appropriate sections with lead blockers.	☐	☐	☐	☐	☐	☐
13. Has the patient either stand or sit, with the hand supinated	☐	☐	☐	☐	☐	☐
14. Places the elbow on the appropriate area of the cassette/receptor, with the forearm resting on its posterior surface	☐	☐	☐	☐	☐	☐
15. Centers the anatomy of interest to the center of the cassette/receptor	☐	☐	☐	☐	☐	☐
16. Centers the central ray perpendicularly to the elbow joint	☐	☐	☐	☐	☐	☐

Positioning to Visualize the Distal Humerus
The student:

	Procedure Yes	No	Repeat Yes	No	Competency Yes	No
17. If using conventional film: adjusts the lead blockers to divide the cassette/receptor appropriately	☐	☐	☐	☐	☐	☐
18. Has the patient sit with the elbow at the same level as the shoulder, while supporting the elevated forearm and supinated hand	☐	☐	☐	☐	☐	☐
19. Places the elbow on the appropriate area of the cassette/receptor, with the humerus resting on its posterior surface	☐	☐	☐	☐	☐	☐
20. Centers the anatomy of interest to the center of the cassette/receptor	☐	☐	☐	☐	☐	☐
21. Centers the central ray perpendicularly to the epicondyloid area of the humerus	☐	☐	☐	☐	☐	☐

Comments:

_____

_____

IMPORTANT DETAILS
The student:

	Procedure Yes	No	Repeat Yes	No	Competency Yes	No
22. Instills confidence in the patient by exhibiting self-confidence throughout the examination.	☐	☐	☐	☐	☐	☐
23. Places a lead marker in the appropriate area of the cassette/receptor (top/bottom/anteriorly/laterally), where it will be visualized on the finished radiograph, on the proper anatomical side (right/left), and in the appropriate position (face up/face down), depending on the patient's position.	☐	☐	☐	☐	☐	☐
24. Provides radiation protection (shield) for the patient, self, and others (closes doors).	☐	☐	☐	☐	☐	☐
25. Applies proper collimation and makes adjustments as necessary.	☐	☐	☐	☐	☐	☐
26. Properly measures the patient along the course of the central ray *for each projection.*	☐	☐	☐	☐	☐	☐
27. Sets the proper exposure techniques:	☐	☐	☐	☐	☐	☐

Conventional systems
• Sets the proper kVp, mA, and time and makes adjustments as necessary.

or

CR or DR systems
- Identifies the patient on the work-list (or manually types the patient information into the system).
- Selects appropriate body region, specific body part, and accurate view/ projection.
- Double-checks preset parameters:
  —Adult vs. pediatric patients
    ○ Small, medium, or large
  —Bucky/receptor (upright vs. table) *or* non-Bucky
  —AEC vs. fixed
    ○ If AEC, checks ion chambers
    ○ Density setting
  —kVp and mA; adjusts if necessary
  —Focal spot/filament size

	Procedure		Repeat		Competency	
	Yes	No	Yes	No	Yes	No
28. Exposes the cassette/receptor after telling the patient to hold still and supporting and/or immobilizing the area of interest if necessary *for each projection.*	☐	☐	☐	☐	☐	☐
29. Provides each radiograph with the proper identification (flash) and/or processes each cassette (image) without difficulty (regardless of technology—film, CR, or DR).	▨	▨	▨	▨	☐	☐
30. Properly completes the examination by filling out all necessary paperwork, entering the examination in the computer, having the images checked by the appropriate staff members, and informing the patient that he or she is finished.	▨	▨	▨	▨	☐	☐
31. Exhibits the ability to adapt to new and difficult situations if and when necessary.	▨	▨	▨	▨	☐	☐
32. Accepts constructive criticism and uses it to his or her advantage.	☐	☐	☐	☐	☐	☐
33. Leaves the radiographic room neat and clean for the next examination.	▨	▨	▨	▨	☐	☐
34. Completes the examination within a reasonable time frame.	☐	☐	☐	☐	☐	☐

Comments:

RADIOGRAPHIC IMAGE QUALITY
The student is able to critique his or her radiographs as to whether they demonstrate:

	Procedure		Repeat		Competency	
	Yes	No	Yes	No	Yes	No
35. Proper technique/optimal density	▨	▨	▨	▨	☐	☐
36. Enhanced detail, without evidence of motion and without any visible artifacts	▨	▨	▨	▨	☐	☐
37. Proper positioning (all anatomy included, evidence of proper centering/ alignment, etc.)	▨	▨	▨	▨	☐	☐
38. Proper marker placement	▨	▨	▨	▨	☐	☐
39. Evidence of proper collimation and radiation protection	▨	▨	▨	▨	☐	☐
40. Long vs. short scale of contrast	▨	▨	▨	▨	☐	☐

Comments:

(continued)

ELBOW ANATOMY
Proximal Forearm Projection
The student is able to identify:

	Procedure		Repeat		Competency	
	Yes	No	Yes	No	Yes	No
41. Humerus	☐	☐	☐	☐	☐	☐
42. Radius	☐	☐	☐	☐	☐	☐
43. Ulna	☐	☐	☐	☐	☐	☐
44. Radial tuberosity	☐	☐	☐	☐	☐	☐
45. Radial head and neck	☐	☐	☐	☐	☐	☐
46. Capitulum	☐	☐	☐	☐	☐	☐
47. Trochlea	☐	☐	☐	☐	☐	☐

Distal Humerus Projection
The student is able to identify:

	Procedure		Repeat		Competency	
	Yes	No	Yes	No	Yes	No
48. Trochlea	☐	☐	☐	☐	☐	☐
49. Lateral epicondyle	☐	☐	☐	☐	☐	☐
50. Olecranon process	☐	☐	☐	☐	☐	☐
51. Radial tuberosity	☐	☐	☐	☐	☐	☐
52. Capitulum	☐	☐	☐	☐	☐	☐
53. Obvious pathology	☐	☐	☐	☐	☐	☐

Comments:

_____

_____

Procedure Evaluator Signature	Repeat Evaluator Signature	Competency Evaluator Signature

Date	Date	Date

END PARTIAL FLEXION ELBOW EVALUATION

Radial Head

The objective of this evaluation is to determine the student's competency level when performing specific radiographic examinations.

Student Name:_____

Procedure Grade	Repeat Grade	Competency Grade

PATIENT INFORMATION OR SIMULATED PROCEDURE *(circle if simulated)*

	Procedure	Repeat	Competency
Age			
Medical Record No.			
Ability to Cooperate			
Condition/Pathology			
Technical Factors Used			
Exposure Index			

FACILITY PREPARATION
The student:

	Procedure Yes	No	Repeat Yes	No	Competency Yes	No
1. Examines the radiographic room and cleans/straightens it before escorting the patient in.	☐	☐	☐	☐	☐	☐
2. Has all equipment and supplies (patient gown, pillow, markers, lead blockers, etc.) readily available before escorting the patient in.	☐	☐	☐	☐	☐	☐
3. Is able to manipulate all radiographic equipment with ease, and centers the central ray to the cassette/receptor.	☐	☐	☐	☐	☐	☐
4. Adjusts the tube to the proper SID.	☐	☐	☐	☐	☐	☐
5. Selects cassettes/receptor of the appropriate size.	☐	☐	☐	☐	☐	☐

Comments:

_____

_____

PATIENT PREPARATION
The student:

	Procedure Yes	No	Repeat Yes	No	Competency Yes	No
6. Identifies the correct patient and examination according to the requisition while establishing a good rapport with him or her.	☐	☐	☐	☐	☐	☐
7. Obtains and documents the patient's history before the examination.	☒	☒	☒	☒	☐	☐
8. Explains the examination in terms the patient fully understands, and properly communicates with the patient throughout the examination.	☐	☐	☐	☐	☐	☐
9. Asks female patients of childbearing age the date of their last menstrual period and documents this; inquires about the possibility of pregnancy and has them sign pregnancy consent forms.	☐	☐	☐	☐	☐	☐
10. Removes all obscuring objects (snaps, zippers, belt, etc.) so as *not* to produce radiographic artifacts.	☐	☐	☐	☐	☐	☐
11. Respects the patient's modesty and provides ample comfort for him or her.	☐	☐	☐	☐	☐	☐

(continued)

Comments:

_____

_____

PATIENT POSITIONING FOR THE RADIAL HEAD OF THE ELBOW
The student:

	Procedure		Repeat		Competency	
	Yes	No	Yes	No	Yes	No
12. Places the elbow on the appropriate area of the cassette/receptor in the lateral position (flexed 90°), with the hand:	☐	☐	☐	☐	☐	☐

a. Pronated

b. Supinated as much as possible

c. Lateral, thumb up

d. Lateral, thumb down

(If the radial head is the primary area of interest, Greenspan and Norman suggest angling the central ray medially, from the elbow toward the shoulder, 45°.)

| 13. Centers the elbow joint to the center of the cassette/receptor. | ☐ | ☐ | ☐ | ☐ | ☐ | ☐ |
| 14. Directs the central ray perpendicularly to the elbow joint. | ☐ | ☐ | ☐ | ☐ | ☐ | ☐ |

Comments:

_____

_____

IMPORTANT DETAILS
The student:

	Procedure		Repeat		Competency	
	Yes	No	Yes	No	Yes	No
15. Instills confidence in the patient by exhibiting self-confidence throughout the examination.	☐	☐	☐	☐	☐	☐
16. Places a lead marker in the appropriate area of the cassette/receptor (top/bottom/anteriorly/laterally), where it will be visualized on the finished radiograph, on the proper anatomical side (right/left), and in the appropriate position (face up/face down), depending on the patient's position.	☐	☐	☐	☐	☐	☐
17. Provides radiation protection (shield) for the patient, self, and others (closes doors).	☐	☐	☐	☐	☐	☐
18. Applies proper collimation and makes adjustments as necessary.	☐	☐	☐	☐	☐	☐
19. Properly measures the patient along the course of the central ray *for each projection.*	☐	☐	☐	☐	☐	☐
20. Sets the proper exposure techniques:	☐	☐	☐	☐	☐	☐

Conventional systems
• Sets the proper kVp, mA, and time and makes adjustments as necessary.

or

CR or DR systems
• Identifies the patient on the work-list (or manually types the patient information into the system).
• Selects appropriate body region, specific body part, and accurate view/projection.
• Double-checks preset parameters:
 —Adult vs. pediatric patients
  ○ Small, medium, or large
 —Bucky/receptor (upright vs. table) *or* non-Bucky

	Procedure		Repeat		Competency	
	Yes	No	Yes	No	Yes	No

— AEC vs. fixed
  ○ If AEC, checks ion chambers
  ○ Density setting
— kVp and mA; adjusts if necessary
— Focal spot/filament size

	Procedure		Repeat		Competency	
	Yes	No	Yes	No	Yes	No
21. Exposes the cassette/receptor after telling the patient to hold still and supporting and/or immobilizing the area of interest if necessary *for each projection.*	☐	☐	☐	☐	☐	☐
22. Provides each radiograph with the proper identification (flash) and/or processes each cassette (image) without difficulty (regardless of technology—film, CR, or DR).	■	■	■	■	☐	☐
23. Properly completes the examination by filling out all necessary paperwork, entering the examination in the computer, having the images checked by the appropriate staff members, and informing the patient that he or she is finished.	■	■	■	■	☐	☐
24. Exhibits the ability to adapt to new and difficult situations if and when necessary.	■	■	■	■	☐	☐
25. Accepts constructive criticism and uses it to his or her advantage.	☐	☐	☐	☐	☐	☐
26. Leaves the radiographic room neat and clean for the next examination.	■	■	■	■	☐	☐
27. Completes the examination within a reasonable time frame.	☐	☐	☐	☐	☐	☐

Comments:

RADIOGRAPHIC IMAGE QUALITY

The student is able to critique his or her radiographs as to whether they demonstrate:

	Procedure		Repeat		Competency	
	Yes	No	Yes	No	Yes	No
28. Proper technique/optimal density	■	■	■	■	☐	☐
29. Enhanced detail, without evidence of motion and without any visible artifacts	■	■	■	■	☐	☐
30. Proper positioning (all anatomy included, evidence of proper centering/alignment, etc.)	■	■	■	■	☐	☐
31. Proper marker placement	■	■	■	■	☐	☐
32. Evidence of proper collimation and radiation protection	■	■	■	■	☐	☐
33. Long vs. short scale of contrast	■	■	■	■	☐	☐

Comments:

ELBOW ANATOMY

The student is able to identify:

	Procedure		Repeat		Competency	
	Yes	No	Yes	No	Yes	No
34. Humerus	■	■	■	■	☐	☐
35. Humeral epicondyles	■	■	■	■	☐	☐
36. Olecranon process	■	■	■	■	☐	☐
37. Radius	■	■	■	■	☐	☐
38. Radial head and neck	■	■	■	■	☐	☐

(continued)

	Procedure		Repeat		Competency	
	Yes	No	Yes	No	Yes	No
39. Ulna	☐	☐	☐	☐	☐	☐
40. Coronoid process	☐	☐	☐	☐	☐	☐
41. Obvious pathology	☐	☐	☐	☐	☐	☐

Comments:

_____

_____

_____   _____   _____
Procedure Evaluator Signature   Repeat Evaluator Signature   Competency Evaluator Signature

_____   _____   _____
Date   Date   Date

END RADIAL HEAD EVALUATION

The objective of this evaluation is to determine the student's competency level when performing specific radiographic examinations.

Student Name:_____

Procedure Grade	Repeat Grade	Competency Grade

PATIENT INFORMATION OR SIMULATED PROCEDURE *(circle if simulated)*

	Procedure	Repeat	Competency
Age			
Medical Record No.			
Ability to Cooperate			
Condition/Pathology			
Technical Factors Used			
Exposure Index			

FACILITY PREPARATION
The student:

	Procedure Yes No	Repeat Yes No	Competency Yes No
1. Examines the radiographic room and cleans/straightens it before escorting the patient in.	☐ ☐	☐ ☐	☐ ☐
2. Has all equipment and supplies (patient gown, pillow, markers, lead blockers, etc.) readily available before escorting the patient in.	☐ ☐	☐ ☐	☐ ☐
3. Is able to manipulate all radiographic equipment with ease, and centers the central ray to the cassette/receptor *for both projections.*	☐ ☐	☐ ☐	☐ ☐
4. Adjusts the tube to the proper SID *for each projection.*	☐ ☐	☐ ☐	☐ ☐
5. Selects cassettes/receptor of the appropriate sizes *for both projections,* according to the patient's size and examination.	☐ ☐	☐ ☐	☐ ☐

Comments:

_____

_____

PATIENT PREPARATION
The student:

	Procedure Yes No	Repeat Yes No	Competency Yes No
6. Identifies the correct patient and examination according to the requisition while establishing a good rapport with him or her.	☐ ☐	☐ ☐	☐ ☐
7. Obtains and documents the patient's history before the examination.	■ ■	■ ■	☐ ☐
8. Explains the examination in terms the patient fully understands, and properly communicates with the patient throughout the examination.	☐ ☐	☐ ☐	☐ ☐
9. Asks female patients of childbearing age the date of their last menstrual period and documents this; inquires about the possibility of pregnancy and has them sign pregnancy consent forms.	☐ ☐	☐ ☐	☐ ☐
10. Removes all obscuring objects (snaps, zippers, belt, etc.) so as *not* to produce radiographic artifacts.	☐ ☐	☐ ☐	☐ ☐

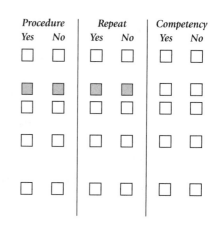

(continued)

	Procedure		Repeat		Competency	
	Yes	No	Yes	No	Yes	No
11. Respects the patient's modesty and provides ample comfort for him or her.	☐	☐	☐	☐	☐	☐

Comments:

_____

_____

PATIENT POSITIONING FOR A HUMERUS
Anteroposterior
The student:

	Procedure		Repeat		Competency	
	Yes	No	Yes	No	Yes	No
12. Places the patient in the supine position on the table, or in the erect position, with the patient's back against the upright Bucky/receptor.	☐	☐	☐	☐	☐	☐
13. Selects the appropriate receptor or places the cassette lengthwise to have a 1-inch margin from the top of the shoulder to the top of the cassette/receptor. For conventional cassettes, the flash must be away from any anatomy.	☐	☐	☐	☐	☐	☐
14. Supinates the hand to place the posterior surface of the humerus against the Bucky/receptor so that the epicondyles are parallel with the cassette/receptor.	☐	☐	☐	☐	☐	☐
15. Centers the anatomy of interest, including both joints, to the center of the cassette/receptor.	☐	☐	☐	☐	☐	☐
16. Centers the central ray perpendicularly to the midshaft of the humerus.	☐	☐	☐	☐	☐	☐

Lateral
The student:

	Procedure		Repeat		Competency	
	Yes	No	Yes	No	Yes	No
17. Rotates the arm internally to place the humerus in the lateral position so the epicondyles are perpendicular to the cassette/receptor.	☐	☐	☐	☐	☐	☐
18. Centers the anatomy of interest, including both joints, to the center of the cassette/receptor.	☐	☐	☐	☐	☐	☐
19. Centers the central ray perpendicularly to the midshaft of the humerus.	☐	☐	☐	☐	☐	☐

Comments:

_____

_____

IMPORTANT DETAILS
The student:

	Procedure		Repeat		Competency	
	Yes	No	Yes	No	Yes	No
20. Instills confidence in the patient by exhibiting self-confidence throughout the examination.	☐	☐	☐	☐	☐	☐
21. Places a lead marker in the appropriate area of the cassette/receptor (top/bottom/anteriorly/laterally), where it will be visualized on the finished radiograph, on the proper anatomical side (right/left), and in the appropriate position (face up/face down), depending on the patient's position.	☐	☐	☐	☐	☐	☐
22. Provides radiation protection (shield) for the patient, self, and others (closes doors).	☐	☐	☐	☐	☐	☐
23. Applies proper collimation and makes adjustments as necessary.	☐	☐	☐	☐	☐	☐
24. Properly measures the patient along the course of the central ray *for each projection.*	☐	☐	☐	☐	☐	☐
25. Sets the proper exposure techniques:	☐	☐	☐	☐	☐	☐

Conventional systems
- Sets the proper kVp, mA, and time and makes adjustments as necessary.

	Procedure		Repeat		Competency	
	Yes	No	Yes	No	Yes	No

or

CR or DR systems

- Identifies the patient on the work-list (or manually types the patient information into the system).
- Selects appropriate body region, specific body part, and accurate view/ projection.
- Double-checks preset parameters:
  —Adult vs. pediatric patients
    ○ Small, medium, or large
  —Bucky/receptor (upright vs. table) *or* non-Bucky
  —AEC vs. fixed
    ○ If AEC, checks ion chambers
    ○ Density setting
  —kVp and mA; adjusts if necessary
  —Focal spot/filament size

	Procedure		Repeat		Competency	
	Yes	No	Yes	No	Yes	No
26. Exposes the cassette/receptor after telling the patient to hold still and after giving the patient proper breathing instructions (expiration) and supporting or immobilizing the area of interest *for each projection.*	☐	☐	☐	☐	☐	☐
27. Provides each radiograph with the proper identification (flash) and/or processes each cassette (image) without difficulty (regardless of technology—film, CR, or DR).	☑	☑	☑	☑	☐	☐
28. Properly completes the examination by filling out all necessary paperwork, entering the examination in the computer, having the images checked by the appropriate staff members, and informing the patient that he or she is finished.	☑	☑	☑	☑	☐	☐
29. Exhibits the ability to adapt to new and difficult situations if and when necessary.	☑	☑	☑	☑	☐	☐
30. Accepts constructive criticism and uses it to his or her advantage.	☐	☐	☐	☐	☐	☐
31. Leaves the radiographic room neat and clean for the next examination.	☑	☑	☑	☑	☐	☐
32. Completes the examination within a reasonable time frame.	☐	☐	☐	☐	☐	☐

Comments:

RADIOGRAPHIC IMAGE QUALITY

The student is able to critique his or her radiographs as to whether they demonstrate:

	Procedure		Repeat		Competency	
	Yes	No	Yes	No	Yes	No
33. Proper technique/optimal density	☑	☑	☑	☑	☐	☐
34. Enhanced detail, without evidence of motion and without any visible artifacts	☑	☑	☑	☑	☐	☐
35. Proper positioning (all anatomy included, evidence of proper centering/ alignment, etc.)	☑	☑	☑	☑	☐	☐
36. Proper marker placement	☑	☑	☑	☑	☐	☐
37. Evidence of proper collimation and radiation protection	☑	☑	☑	☑	☐	☐
38. Long vs. short scale of contrast	☑	☑	☑	☑	☐	☐

Comments:

(continued)

HUMERUS ANATOMY
The student is able to identify:

	Procedure		Repeat		Competency	
	Yes	No	Yes	No	Yes	No
39. Proximal radius	☐	☐	☐	☐	☐	☐
40. Proximal ulna	☐	☐	☐	☐	☐	☐
41. Capitulum	☐	☐	☐	☐	☐	☐
42. Trochlea	☐	☐	☐	☐	☐	☐
43. Medial and lateral epicondyles	☐	☐	☐	☐	☐	☐
44. Humeral head	☐	☐	☐	☐	☐	☐
45. Anatomical and surgical necks	☐	☐	☐	☐	☐	☐
46. Greater and lesser tubercles	☐	☐	☐	☐	☐	☐
47. Glenoid fossa	☐	☐	☐	☐	☐	☐
48. Acromion process	☐	☐	☐	☐	☐	☐
49. Clavicle	☐	☐	☐	☐	☐	☐
50. Obvious pathology	☐	☐	☐	☐	☐	☐

Comments:

_____

_____

Procedure Evaluator Signature	Repeat Evaluator Signature	Competency Evaluator Signature
Date	Date	Date

END HUMERUS EVALUATION

Specific radiographic examinations.

Student Name:_____

Procedure Grade	Repeat Grade	Competency Grade

PATIENT INFORMATION OR SIMULATED PROCEDURE *(circle if simulated)*

	Procedure	Repeat	Competency
Age			
Medical Record No.			
Ability to Cooperate			
Condition/Pathology			
Technical Factors Used			
Exposure Index			

FACILITY PREPARATION
The student:

	Procedure Yes No	Repeat Yes No	Competency Yes No
1. Examines the radiographic room and cleans/straightens it before escorting the patient in.	☐ ☐	☐ ☐	☐ ☐
2. Has all equipment and supplies (patient gown, pillow, markers, lead blockers, etc.) readily available before escorting the patient in.	☐ ☐	☐ ☐	☐ ☐
3. Is able to manipulate all radiographic equipment with ease, and centers the central ray to the cassette/receptor *for all projections.*	☐ ☐	☐ ☐	☐ ☐
4. Adjusts the tube to the proper SID *for each projection.*	☐ ☐	☐ ☐	☐ ☐
5. Selects cassettes/receptor of the appropriate sizes *for all projections,* according to the patient's size and examination.	☐ ☐	☐ ☐	☐ ☐

Comments:

_____

_____

PATIENT PREPARATION
The student:

	Procedure Yes No	Repeat Yes No	Competency Yes No
6. Identifies the correct patient and examination according to the requisition while establishing a good rapport with him or her.	☐ ☐	☐ ☐	☐ ☐
7. Obtains and documents the patient's history before the examination.	▨ ▨	▨ ▨	☐ ☐
8. Explains the examination in terms the patient fully understands, and properly communicates with the patient throughout the examination.	☐ ☐	☐ ☐	☐ ☐
9. Asks female patients of childbearing age the date of their last menstrual period and documents this; inquires about the possibility of pregnancy and has them sign pregnancy consent forms.	☐ ☐	☐ ☐	☐ ☐
10. Removes all obscuring objects (snaps, zippers, belt, etc.) so as *not* to produce radiographic artifacts.	☐ ☐	☐ ☐	☐ ☐

(continued)

	Procedure		Repeat		Competency	
	Yes	No	Yes	No	Yes	No
11. Respects the patient's modesty and provides ample comfort for him or her.	☐	☐	☐	☐	☐	☐

Comments:

_____

_____

PATIENT POSITIONING FOR A SHOULDER
AP: Internal
The student:

	Procedure		Repeat		Competency	
	Yes	No	Yes	No	Yes	No
12. Places the patient in the supine position on the table, or in the erect position at the erect Bucky/receptor, with the arm slightly abducted.	☐	☐	☐	☐	☐	☐
13. Selects the appropriate receptor or places the cassette lengthwise so there is a 1-inch margin from the top of the shoulder to the top of the cassette/receptor. For conventional cassettes, the flash must be away from any anatomy.	☐	☐	☐	☐	☐	☐
14. Internally rotates the patient's hand to place the epicondyles of the humerus perpendicular with the cassette/receptor. (The patient might be most comfortable resting the back of his or her hand on the hip for support.)	☐	☐	☐	☐	☐	☐
15. Centers the anatomy of interest to the center of the cassette/receptor.	☐	☐	☐	☐	☐	☐
16. Centers the central ray perpendicularly, 1 inch inferior to the coracoid process.	☐	☐	☐	☐	☐	☐

AP: External
The student:

	Procedure		Repeat		Competency	
	Yes	No	Yes	No	Yes	No
17. Rotates the arm externally, and supinates the hand to the place the epicondyles parallel to the cassette/receptor.	☐	☐	☐	☐	☐	☐
18. Centers the anatomy of interest to the center of the cassette/receptor.	☐	☐	☐	☐	☐	☐
19. Centers the central ray perpendicularly, 1 inch inferior to the coracoid process.	☐	☐	☐	☐	☐	☐

Scapular Y (PA Oblique Shoulder) for the Glenohumeral Joint and Suspected Dislocation
The student:

	Procedure		Repeat		Competency	
	Yes	No	Yes	No	Yes	No
20. Places the patient in the PA oblique position, with the affected scapula against the Bucky/receptor.	☐	☐	☐	☐	☐	☐
21. Places the patient so that his or her arm hangs beside the body such that the humerus superimposes the wing of the scapula.	☐	☐	☐	☐	☐	☐
22. Grasps the axillary and vertebral borders of the scapula with one hand and adjusts the body to place the wing of the scapula perpendicular to the plane of the cassette/receptor.	☐	☐	☐	☐	☐	☐
23. Centers the anatomy of interest to the center of the cassette/receptor.	☐	☐	☐	☐	☐	☐
24. Centers the central ray perpendicularly to the vertebral border of the protruding scapula/glenohumeral joint.	☐	☐	☐	☐	☐	☐

Comments:

_____

_____

IMPORTANT DETAILS
The student:

	Procedure		Repeat		Competency	
	Yes	No	Yes	No	Yes	No
25. Instills confidence in the patient by exhibiting self-confidence throughout the examination.	☐	☐	☐	☐	☐	☐
26. Places a lead marker in the appropriate area of the cassette/receptor (top/bottom/anteriorly/laterally), where it will be visualized on the finished radiograph, on the proper anatomical side (right/left), and in the appropriate position (face up/face down), depending on the patient's position.	☐	☐	☐	☐	☐	☐
27. Provides radiation protection (shield) for the patient, self, and others (closes doors).	☐	☐	☐	☐	☐	☐
28. Applies proper collimation and makes adjustments as necessary.	☐	☐	☐	☐	☐	☐
29. Properly measures the patient along the course of the central ray *for each projection.*	☐	☐	☐	☐	☐	☐
30. Sets the proper exposure techniques:	☐	☐	☐	☐	☐	☐

30. (continued)

Conventional systems
- Sets the proper kVp, mA, and time, and makes adjustments as necessary.

or

CR or DR systems
- Identifies the patient on the work-list (or manually types the patient information into the system).
- Selects appropriate body region, specific body part, and accurate view/projection.
- Double-checks preset parameters:
  —Adult vs. pediatric patients
    ○ Small, medium, or large
  —Bucky/receptor (upright vs. table) *or* non-Bucky
  —AEC vs. fixed
    ○ If AEC, checks ion chambers
    ○ Density setting
  —kVp and mA; adjusts if necessary
  —Focal spot/filament size

	Procedure		Repeat		Competency	
31. Exposes the cassette/receptor after telling the patient to hold still and after giving the patient proper breathing instructions (expiration) *for each projection.*	☐	☐	☐	☐	☐	☐
32. Provides each radiograph with the proper identification (flash) and/or processes each cassette (image) without difficulty (regardless of technology—film, CR, or DR).	▣	▣	▣	▣	☐	☐
33. Properly completes the examination by filling out all necessary paperwork, entering the examination in the computer, having the images checked by the appropriate staff members, and informing the patient that he or she is finished.	▣	▣	▣	▣	☐	☐
34. Exhibits the ability to adapt to new and difficult situations if and when necessary.	▣	▣	▣	▣	☐	☐
35. Accepts constructive criticism and uses it to his or her advantage.	☐	☐	☐	☐	☐	☐
36. Leaves the radiographic room neat and clean for the next examination.	▣	▣	▣	▣	☐	☐
37. Completes the examination within a reasonable time frame.	☐	☐	☐	☐	☐	☐

Comments:

_____

_____

(continued)

RADIOGRAPHIC IMAGE QUALITY
The student is able to critique his or her radiographs as to whether they demonstrate:

	Procedure		Repeat		Competency	
	Yes	No	Yes	No	Yes	No
38. Proper technique/optimal density	☐	☐	☐	☐	☐	☐
39. Enhanced detail, without evidence of motion and without any visible artifacts	☐	☐	☐	☐	☐	☐
40. Proper positioning (all anatomy included, evidence of proper centering/alignment, etc.)	☐	☐	☐	☐	☐	☐
41. Proper marker placement	☐	☐	☐	☐	☐	☐
42. Evidence of proper collimation and radiation protection	☐	☐	☐	☐	☐	☐
43. Long vs. short scale of contrast	☐	☐	☐	☐	☐	☐

Comments:

_____

_____

SHOULDER ANATOMY
The student is able to identify:

	Procedure		Repeat		Competency	
	Yes	No	Yes	No	Yes	No
44. Upper scapula	☐	☐	☐	☐	☐	☐
45. Clavicle	☐	☐	☐	☐	☐	☐
46. Acromioclavicular joint	☐	☐	☐	☐	☐	☐
47. Acromion process	☐	☐	☐	☐	☐	☐
48. Greater and lesser tubercles	☐	☐	☐	☐	☐	☐
49. Humeral head	☐	☐	☐	☐	☐	☐
50. Anatomical and surgical necks	☐	☐	☐	☐	☐	☐
51. Glenoid fossa	☐	☐	☐	☐	☐	☐
52. Coracoid process	☐	☐	☐	☐	☐	☐
53. Obvious pathology	☐	☐	☐	☐	☐	☐

Comments:

_____

_____

Procedure Evaluator Signature	Repeat Evaluator Signature	Competency Evaluator Signature
Date	Date	Date

END SHOULDER EVALUATION

The objective of this evaluation is to determine the student's competency level when performing specific radiographic examinations.

Student Name:_____

	Procedure Grade	Repeat Grade	Competency Grade

PATIENT INFORMATION OR SIMULATED PROCEDURE *(circle if simulated)*

	Procedure	Repeat	Competency
Age			
Medical Record No.			
Ability to Cooperate			
Condition/Pathology			
Technical Factors Used			
Exposure Index			

FACILITY PREPARATION
The student:

	Procedure Yes	Procedure No	Repeat Yes	Repeat No	Competency Yes	Competency No
1. Examines the radiographic room and cleans/straightens it before escorting the patient in.	☐	☐	☐	☐	☐	☐
2. Has all equipment and supplies (patient gown, pillow, markers, lead blockers, etc.) readily available before escorting the patient in.	☐	☐	☐	☐	☐	☐
3. Is able to manipulate all radiographic equipment with ease, and centers the central ray to the cassette/receptor *for both projections.*	☐	☐	☐	☐	☐	☐
4. Adjusts the tube to the proper SID *for each projection.*	☐	☐	☐	☐	☐	☐
5. Selects cassettes/receptor of the appropriate sizes *for both projections,* according to the patient's size and examination.	☐	☐	☐	☐	☐	☐

Comments:

_____

_____

PATIENT PREPARATION
The student:

	Procedure Yes	Procedure No	Repeat Yes	Repeat No	Competency Yes	Competency No
6. Identifies the correct patient and examination according to the requisition while establishing a good rapport with him or her.	☐	☐	☐	☐	☐	☐
7. Obtains and documents the patient's history before the examination.	▦	▦	▦	▦	☐	☐
8. Explains the examination in terms the patient fully understands, and properly communicates with the patient throughout the examination.	☐	☐	☐	☐	☐	☐
9. Asks female patients of childbearing age the date of their last menstrual period and documents this; inquires about the possibility of pregnancy and has them sign pregnancy consent forms.	☐	☐	☐	☐	☐	☐
10. Removes all obscuring objects (snaps, zippers, belt, etc.) so as *not* to produce radiographic artifacts.	☐	☐	☐	☐	☐	☐

(continued)

	Procedure		Repeat		Competency	
	Yes	No	Yes	No	Yes	No
11. Respects the patient's modesty and provides ample comfort for him or her.	☐	☐	☐	☐	☐	☐

Comments:

_____

_____

PATIENT POSITIONING FOR A TRANSTHORACIC HUMERUS, USING THE TRAUMA/LAWRENCE METHOD

Anteroposterior
The student:

	Procedure		Repeat		Competency	
	Yes	No	Yes	No	Yes	No
12. Places the patient in the supine position on the table, or in the erect position, at the erect Bucky/receptor.	☐	☐	☐	☐	☐	☐
13. Selects the appropriate receptor or places the cassette lengthwise to have a 1-inch margin from the top of the shoulder to the top of the cassette/receptor. For conventional cassettes, the flash must be away from any anatomy.	☐	☐	☐	☐	☐	☐
14. Places the patient in the neutral position, with the posterior surface of the humerus against the Bucky/receptor.	☐	☐	☐	☐	☐	☐
15. Centers the anatomy of interest, including both joints, to the center of the cassette/receptor.	☐	☐	☐	☐	☐	☐
16. Centers the central ray perpendicularly to the midshaft of the humerus.	☐	☐	☐	☐	☐	☐

Transthoracic Lateral
The student:

	Procedure		Repeat		Competency	
	Yes	No	Yes	No	Yes	No
17. Places the patient in the lateral position, with the affected arm against the Bucky/receptor.	☐	☐	☐	☐	☐	☐
18. Raises the patient's uninjured arm above his or her head and elevates the same shoulder as much as possible, which depresses the injured side, thereby separating the shoulders and preventing superimposition.	☐	☐	☐	☐	☐	☐
19. Checks to be sure the epicondyles are perpendicular to the cassette/receptor.	☐	☐	☐	☐	☐	☐
20. Adjusts the rotation of the patient's body to project the humerus between the vertebral column and the sternum.	☐	☐	☐	☐	☐	☐
21. Adjusts the cassette/receptor to 2 inch above the top of the shoulder.	☐	☐	☐	☐	☐	☐
22. Centers the surgical neck to the center of the cassette/receptor.	☐	☐	☐	☐	☐	☐
23. Centers the central ray perpendicularly to the surgical neck of the humerus or angles 10–20° cephalad if necessary.	☐	☐	☐	☐	☐	☐

Comments:

_____

_____

IMPORTANT DETAILS
The student:

	Procedure		Repeat		Competency	
	Yes	No	Yes	No	Yes	No
24. Instills confidence in the patient by exhibiting self-confidence throughout the examination.	☐	☐	☐	☐	☐	☐
25. Places a lead marker in the appropriate area of the cassette/receptor (top/bottom/anteriorly/laterally), where it will be visualized on the finished radiograph, on the proper anatomical side (right/left), and in the appropriate position (face up/face down), depending on the patient's position.	☐	☐	☐	☐	☐	☐

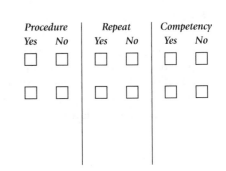

	Procedure		Repeat		Competency	
	Yes	No	Yes	No	Yes	No
26. Provides radiation protection (shield) for the patient, self, and others (closes doors).	☐	☐	☐	☐	☐	☐
27. Applies proper collimation and makes adjustments as necessary.	☐	☐	☐	☐	☐	☐
28. Properly measures the patient along the course of the central ray *for each projection.*	☐	☐	☐	☐	☐	☐
29. Sets the proper exposure techniques:	☐	☐	☐	☐	☐	☐

Conventional systems
- Sets the proper kVp, mA, and time, and makes adjustments as necessary.

or

CR or DR systems
- Identifies the patient on the work-list (or manually types the patient information into the system).
- Selects appropriate body region, specific body part, and accurate view/ projection.
- Double-checks preset parameters:
  —Adult vs. pediatric patients
   ○ Small, medium, or large
  —Bucky/receptor (upright vs. table) *or* non-Bucky
  —AEC vs. fixed
   ○ If AEC, checks ion chambers
   ○ Density setting
  —kVp and mA; adjusts if necessary
  —Focal spot/filament size

	Procedure		Repeat		Competency	
30. Exposes the cassette/receptor after telling the patient to hold still and after giving the patient proper breathing instructions (AP—expiration; lateral—full inspiration or breathing technique) *for each projection.*	☐	☐	☐	☐	☐	☐
31. Provides each radiograph with the proper identification (flash) and/or processes each cassette (image) without difficulty (regardless of technology—film, CR, or DR).	▨	▨	▨	▨	☐	☐
32. Properly completes the examination by filling out all necessary paperwork, entering the examination in the computer, having the images checked by the appropriate staff members, and informing the patient that he or she is finished.	▨	▨	▨	▨	☐	☐
33. Exhibits the ability to adapt to new and difficult situations if and when necessary.	▨	▨	▨	▨	☐	☐
34. Accepts constructive criticism and uses it to his or her advantage.	☐	☐	☐	☐	☐	☐
35. Leaves the radiographic room neat and clean for the next examination.	▨	▨	▨	▨	☐	☐
36. Completes the examination within a reasonable time frame.	☐	☐	☐	☐	☐	☐

Comments:

_____

_____

RADIOGRAPHIC IMAGE QUALITY
The student is able to critique his or her radiographs as to whether they demonstrate:

	Procedure		Repeat		Competency	
	Yes	No	Yes	No	Yes	No
37. Proper technique/optimal density	▨	▨	▨	▨	☐	☐
38. Enhanced detail, without evidence of motion and without any visible artifacts	▨	▨	▨	▨	☐	☐
39. Proper positioning (all anatomy included, evidence of proper centering/ alignment, etc.)	▨	▨	▨	▨	☐	☐

(continued)

	Procedure		Repeat		Competency	
	Yes	No	Yes	No	Yes	No
40. Proper marker placement	☐	☐	☐	☐	☐	☐
41. Evidence of proper collimation and radiation protection	☐	☐	☐	☐	☐	☐
42. Long vs. short scale of contrast	☐	☐	☐	☐	☐	☐

Comments:

HUMERUS ANATOMY
The student is able to identify:

	Procedure		Repeat		Competency	
	Yes	No	Yes	No	Yes	No
43. Greater and lesser tubercles	☐	☐	☐	☐	☐	☐
44. Thoracic vertebra	☐	☐	☐	☐	☐	☐
45. Acromion process	☐	☐	☐	☐	☐	☐
46. Clavicle	☐	☐	☐	☐	☐	☐
47. Humeral head	☐	☐	☐	☐	☐	☐
48. Anatomical and surgical necks	☐	☐	☐	☐	☐	☐
49. Obvious pathology	☐	☐	☐	☐	☐	☐

Comments:

Procedure Evaluator Signature   Repeat Evaluator Signature   Competency Evaluator Signature

Date   Date   Date

END TRAUMA SHOULDER – A EVALUATION

Student Name:_____

Procedure Grade	Repeat Grade	Competency Grade

PATIENT INFORMATION OR SIMULATED PROCEDURE *(circle if simulated)*

	Procedure	Repeat	Competency
Age			
Medical Record No.			
Ability to Cooperate			
Condition/Pathology			
Technical Factors Used			
Exposure Index			

FACILITY PREPARATION
The student:

	Procedure Yes	No	Repeat Yes	No	Competency Yes	No
1. Examines the radiographic room and cleans/straightens it before escorting the patient in.	☐	☐	☐	☐	☐	☐
2. Has all equipment and supplies (patient gown, pillow, markers, lead blockers, etc.) readily available before escorting the patient in.	☐	☐	☐	☐	☐	☐
3. Is able to manipulate all radiographic equipment with ease, and centers the central ray to the cassette/receptor *for all projections.*	☐	☐	☐	☐	☐	☐
4. Adjusts the tube to the proper SID *for each projection.*	☐	☐	☐	☐	☐	☐
5. Selects cassettes/receptor of the appropriate sizes *for all projections,* according to the patient's size and examination.	☐	☐	☐	☐	☐	☐

Comments:

_____

_____

PATIENT PREPARATION
The student:

	Procedure Yes	No	Repeat Yes	No	Competency Yes	No
6. Identifies the correct patient and examination according to the requisition while establishing a good rapport with him or her.	☐	☐	☐	☐	☐	☐
7. Obtains and documents the patient's history before the examination.	▦	▦	▦	▦	☐	☐
8. Explains the examination in terms the patient fully understands, and properly communicates with the patient throughout the examination.	☐	☐	☐	☐	☐	☐
9. Asks female patients of childbearing age the date of their last menstrual period and documents this; inquires about the possibility of pregnancy and has them sign pregnancy consent forms.	☐	☐	☐	☐	☐	☐
10. Removes all obscuring objects (snaps, zippers, belt, etc.) so as *not* to produce radiographic artifacts.	☐	☐	☐	☐	☐	☐

(continued)

	Procedure		Repeat		Competency	
	Yes	No	Yes	No	Yes	No
11. Respects the patient's modesty and provides ample comfort for him or her.	☐	☐	☐	☐	☐	☐

Comments:

_____

_____

PATIENT POSITIONING FOR A TRAUMA SHOULDER
AP: Neutral
The student:

	Procedure		Repeat		Competency	
	Yes	No	Yes	No	Yes	No
12. Places the patient in the supine position on the table, or in the erect position, at the erect Bucky/receptor.	☐	☐	☐	☐	☐	☐
13. Selects the appropriate receptor or places the cassettes so there is a 1-inch margin from the top of the shoulder to the top of the cassette/receptor. For conventional cassettes, the flash must be away from any anatomy.	☐	☐	☐	☐	☐	☐
14. Places the patient in the neutral position, with the posterior surface of the humerus against the Bucky/receptor.	☐	☐	☐	☐	☐	☐
15. Centers the anatomy of interest to the center of the cassette/receptor.	☐	☐	☐	☐	☐	☐
16. Centers the central ray perpendicularly, 1 inch inferior to the coracoid process.	☐	☐	☐	☐	☐	☐

PA Oblique/Y View
The student:

	Procedure		Repeat		Competency	
	Yes	No	Yes	No	Yes	No
17. Places the patient in the PA oblique position, with the affected scapula against the Bucky/receptor.	☐	☐	☐	☐	☐	☐
18. Places the patient so that his or her arm hangs beside the body so that the humerus superimposes the wing of the scapula.	☐	☐	☐	☐	☐	☐
19. Grasps the axillary and vertebral borders of the scapula with one hand, and adjusts the body to place the wing of the scapula perpendicular to the plane of the cassette/receptor.	☐	☐	☐	☐	☐	☐
20. Centers the anatomy of interest to the center of the cassette/receptor.	☐	☐	☐	☐	☐	☐
21. Centers the central ray perpendicularly to the vertebral border of the protruding scapula/glenohumeral joint.	☐	☐	☐	☐	☐	☐

Comments:

_____

_____

IMPORTANT DETAILS
The student:

	Procedure		Repeat		Competency	
	Yes	No	Yes	No	Yes	No
22. Instills confidence in the patient by exhibiting self-confidence throughout the examination.	☐	☐	☐	☐	☐	☐
23. Places a lead marker in the appropriate area of the cassette/receptor (top/bottom/anteriorly/laterally), where it will be visualized on the finished radiograph, on the proper anatomical side (right/left), and in the appropriate position (face up/face down), depending on the patient's position.	☐	☐	☐	☐	☐	☐
24. Provides radiation protection (shield) for the patient, self, and others (closes doors).	☐	☐	☐	☐	☐	☐
25. Applies proper collimation and makes adjustments as necessary.	☐	☐	☐	☐	☐	☐

	Procedure		Repeat		Competency	
	Yes	No	Yes	No	Yes	No
26. Properly measures the patient along the course of the central ray *for each projection.*	☐	☐	☐	☐	☐	☐
27. Sets the proper exposure techniques:	☐	☐	☐	☐	☐	☐

Conventional systems
- Sets the proper kVp, mA, and time, and makes adjustments as necessary.

or

CR or DR systems
- Identifies the patient on the work-list (or manually types the patient information into the system).
- Selects appropriate body region, specific body part, and accurate view/projection.
- Double-checks preset parameters:
  —Adult vs. pediatric patients
    ○ Small, medium, or large
  —Bucky/receptor (upright vs. table) *or* non-Bucky
  —AEC vs. fixed
    ○ If AEC, checks ion chambers
    ○ Density setting
  —kVp and mA; adjusts if necessary
  —Focal spot/filament size

	Procedure		Repeat		Competency	
28. Exposes the cassette/receptor after telling the patient to hold still and giving the patient proper breathing instructions (expiration) *for each projection.*	☐	☐	☐	☐	☐	☐
29. Provides each radiograph with the proper identification (flash) and/or processes each cassette (image) without difficulty (regardless of technology—film, CR, or DR).	▣	▣	▣	▣	☐	☐
30. Properly completes the examination by filling out all necessary paperwork, entering the examination in the computer, having the images checked by the appropriate staff members, and informing the patient that he or she is finished.	▣	▣	▣	▣	☐	☐
31. Exhibits the ability to adapt to new and difficult situations if and when necessary.	▣	▣	▣	▣	☐	☐
32. Accepts constructive criticism and uses it to his or her advantage.	☐	☐	☐	☐	☐	☐
33. Leaves the radiographic room neat and clean for the next examination.	▣	▣	▣	▣	☐	☐
34. Completes the examination within a reasonable time frame.	☐	☐	☐	☐	☐	☐

Comments:

RADIOGRAPHIC IMAGE QUALITY
The student is able to critique his or her radiographs as to whether they demonstrate:

	Procedure		Repeat		Competency	
	Yes	No	Yes	No	Yes	No
35. Proper technique/optimal density	▣	▣	▣	▣	☐	☐
36. Enhanced detail, without evidence of motion and without any visible artifacts	▣	▣	▣	▣	☐	☐
37. Proper positioning (all anatomy included, evidence of proper centering/alignment, etc.)	▣	▣	▣	▣	☐	☐
38. Proper marker placement	▣	▣	▣	▣	☐	☐
39. Evidence of proper collimation and radiation protection	▣	▣	▣	▣	☐	☐
40. Long vs. short scale of contrast	▣	▣	▣	▣	☐	☐

(continued)

Comments:

_____

_____

_____

SHOULDER ANATOMY
The student is able to identify:

	Procedure		Repeat		Competency	
	Yes	No	Yes	No	Yes	No
40. Scapula	☐	☐	☐	☐	☐	☐
41. Clavicle	☐	☐	☐	☐	☐	☐
42. Acromioclavicular joint	☐	☐	☐	☐	☐	☐
43. Acromion process	☐	☐	☐	☐	☐	☐
44. Humeral head	☐	☐	☐	☐	☐	☐
45. Glenoid fossa	☐	☐	☐	☐	☐	☐
46. Coracoid process	☐	☐	☐	☐	☐	☐
47. Obvious pathology	☐	☐	☐	☐	☐	☐

Comments:

_____

_____

_____

_____   _____   _____
Procedure Evaluator Signature   Repeat Evaluator Signature   Competency Evaluator Signature

_____   _____   _____
Date   Date   Date

END TRAUMA SHOULDER – B EVALUATION

Student Name:_____

Procedure Grade	Repeat Grade	Competency Grade

PATIENT INFORMATION OR SIMULATED PROCEDURE *(circle if simulated)*

	Procedure	Repeat	Competency
Age			
Medical Record No.			
Ability to Cooperate			
Condition/Pathology			
Technical Factors Used			
Exposure Index			

FACILITY PREPARATION
The student:

	Procedure Yes	Procedure No	Repeat Yes	Repeat No	Competency Yes	Competency No
1. Examines the radiographic room and cleans/straightens it before escorting the patient in.	☐	☐	☐	☐	☐	☐
2. Has all equipment and supplies (patient gown, pillow, markers, lead blockers, etc.) readily available before escorting the patient in.	☐	☐	☐	☐	☐	☐
3. Is able to manipulate all radiographic equipment with ease, and centers the central ray to the cassette/receptor *for all projections.*	☐	☐	☐	☐	☐	☐
4. Adjusts the tube to the proper SID *for each projection.*	☐	☐	☐	☐	☐	☐
5. Selects cassettes/receptor of the appropriate sizes *for all projections,* according to the patient's size and examination.	☐	☐	☐	☐	☐	☐

Comments:

_____

_____

PATIENT PREPARATION
The student:

	Procedure Yes	Procedure No	Repeat Yes	Repeat No	Competency Yes	Competency No
6. Identifies the correct patient and examination according to the requisition while establishing a good rapport with him or her.	☐	☐	☐	☐	☐	☐
7. Obtains and documents the patient's history before the examination.	☑	☑	☑	☑	☐	☐
8. Explains the examination in terms the patient fully understands, and properly communicates with the patient throughout the examination.	☐	☐	☐	☐	☐	☐
9. Asks female patients of childbearing age the date of their last menstrual period and documents this; inquires about the possibility of pregnancy and has them sign pregnancy consent forms.	☐	☐	☐	☐	☐	☐
10. Removes all obscuring objects (snaps, zippers, belt, etc.) so as *not* to produce radiographic artifacts.	☐	☐	☐	☐	☐	☐

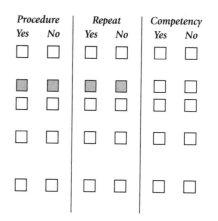

(continued)

	Procedure		Repeat		Competency	
	Yes	No	Yes	No	Yes	No
11. Respects the patient's modesty and provides ample comfort for him or her.	☐	☐	☐	☐	☐	☐

Comments:

_____

_____

PATIENT POSITIONING FOR A SHOULDER AXILLARY PROJECTION
Inferosuperior Axial Shoulder (Lawrence Method)
The student:

	Procedure		Repeat		Competency	
	Yes	No	Yes	No	Yes	No
12. Places the patient in the supine position on the table, elevating the head and shoulders about 3 inches.	☐	☐	☐	☐	☐	☐
13. Abducts the affected arm to form a right angle with the long axis of the body, while supporting the extended extremity.	☐	☐	☐	☐	☐	☐
14. Instructs the patient to turn his or her head away from the side being examined.	☐	☐	☐	☐	☐	☐
15. Selects the appropriate receptor or places the cassette/receptor in the vertical position next to the shoulder, as close to the neck as possible. For conventional cassettes, the flash must be away from any anatomy.	☐	☐	☐	☐	☐	☐
16. Directs the central ray perpendicularly to the cassette/receptor horizontally through the axilla, centered to the region of the AC articulation, and depending on the degree of abduction, angles the central ray medially if necessary.	☐	☐	☐	☐	☐	☐

Superoinferior Axial Shoulder
The student:

	Procedure		Repeat		Competency	
	Yes	No	Yes	No	Yes	No
17. Places the patient at the end of the table, seated in the erect position on a stool or chair high enough to enable him or her to extend the affected arm well over the cassette/receptor.	☐	☐	☐	☐	☐	☐
18. Abducts the affected arm to form a right angle with the long axis of the body.	☐	☐	☐	☐	☐	☐
19. Has the patient lean laterally over the cassette/receptor until the shoulder is over the midpoint of the cassette/receptor.	☐	☐	☐	☐	☐	☐
20. Rests the elbow on the table, with the hand in the neutral position and the elbow bent 90°.	☐	☐	☐	☐	☐	☐
21. Instructs the patient to turn his or her head away from the side being examined.	☐	☐	☐	☐	☐	☐
22. Adjusts any anterior or posterior leaning of the body to place the humeral epicondyles in the vertical position.	☐	☐	☐	☐	☐	☐
23. Selects the appropriate receptor or places the cassette/receptor under the shoulder, as much as possible. For conventional cassettes, the flash must be away from any anatomy.	☐	☐	☐	☐	☐	☐
24. Directs the central ray from the shoulder toward the elbow at an angle of 5–15°, centered to the shoulder joint.	☐	☐	☐	☐	☐	☐

Comments:

_____

_____

IMPORTANT DETAILS
The student:

	Procedure		Repeat		Competency	
	Yes	No	Yes	No	Yes	No
25. Instills confidence in the patient by exhibiting self-confidence throughout the examination.	☐	☐	☐	☐	☐	☐
26. Places a lead marker in the appropriate area of the cassette/receptor (top/bottom/anteriorly/laterally), where it will be visualized on the finished radiograph, on the proper anatomical side (right/left), and in the appropriate position (face up/face down), depending on the patient's position.	☐	☐	☐	☐	☐	☐
27. Provides radiation protection (shield) for the patient, self, and others (closes doors).	☐	☐	☐	☐	☐	☐
28. Applies proper collimation and makes adjustments as necessary.	☐	☐	☐	☐	☐	☐
29. Properly measures the patient along the course of the central ray *for each projection.*	☐	☐	☐	☐	☐	☐
30. Sets the proper exposure techniques:	☐	☐	☐	☐	☐	☐

Conventional systems
- Sets the proper kVp, mA, and time, and makes adjustments as necessary.

or

CR or DR systems
- Identifies the patient on the work-list (or manually types the patient information into the system).
- Selects appropriate body region, specific body part, and accurate view/projection.
- Double-checks preset parameters:
  —Adult vs. pediatric patients
    ○ Small, medium, or large
  —Bucky/receptor (upright vs. table) *or* non-Bucky
  —AEC vs. fixed
    ○ If AEC, checks ion chambers
    ○ Density setting
  —kVp and mA; adjusts if necessary
  —Focal spot/filament size

	Procedure		Repeat		Competency	
31. Exposes the cassette/receptor after telling the patient to hold still and after giving the patient proper breathing instructions (expiration) *for each projection.*	☐	☐	☐	☐	☐	☐
32. Provides each radiograph with the proper identification (flash) and/or processes each cassette (image) without difficulty (regardless of technology—film, CR, or DR).	▩	▩	▩	▩	☐	☐
33. Properly completes the examination by filling out all necessary paperwork, entering the examination in the computer, having the images checked by the appropriate staff members, and informing the patient that he or she is finished.	▩	▩	▩	▩	☐	☐
34. Exhibits the ability to adapt to new and difficult situations if and when necessary.	▩	▩	▩	▩	☐	☐
35. Accepts constructive criticism and uses it to his or her advantage.	☐	☐	☐	☐	☐	☐
36. Leaves the radiographic room neat and clean for the next examination.	▩	▩	▩	▩	☐	☐
37. Completes the examination within a reasonable time frame.	☐	☐	☐	☐	☐	☐

Comments:

_____

_____

(continued)

RADIOGRAPHIC IMAGE QUALITY
The student is able to critique his or her radiographs as to whether they demonstrate:

	Procedure Yes	Procedure No	Repeat Yes	Repeat No	Competency Yes	Competency No
38. Proper technique/optimal density	☐	☐	☐	☐	☐	☐
39. Enhanced detail, without evidence of motion and without any visible artifacts	☐	☐	☐	☐	☐	☐
40. Proper positioning (all anatomy included, evidence of proper centering/alignment, etc.)	☐	☐	☐	☐	☐	☐
41. Proper marker placement	☐	☐	☐	☐	☐	☐
42. Evidence of proper collimation and radiation protection	☐	☐	☐	☐	☐	☐
43. Long vs. short scale of contrast	☐	☐	☐	☐	☐	☐

Comments:

_____

_____

SHOULDER ANATOMY
The student is able to identify:

	Procedure Yes	Procedure No	Repeat Yes	Repeat No	Competency Yes	Competency No
44. Coracoid process	☐	☐	☐	☐	☐	☐
45. Clavicle	☐	☐	☐	☐	☐	☐
46. Acromion process	☐	☐	☐	☐	☐	☐
47. Lesser tubercles	☐	☐	☐	☐	☐	☐
48. Humeral head	☐	☐	☐	☐	☐	☐
49. Obvious pathology	☐	☐	☐	☐	☐	☐

Comments:

_____

_____

_____   _____   _____
Procedure Evaluator Signature   Repeat Evaluator Signature   Competency Evaluator Signature

_____   _____   _____
Date   Date   Date

END AXIAL SHOULDER EVALUATION

Student Name:_____

Procedure Grade	Repeat Grade	Competency Grade

PATIENT INFORMATION OR SIMULATED PROCEDURE *(circle if simulated)*

	Procedure	Repeat	Competency
Age			
Medical Record No.			
Ability to Cooperate			
Condition/Pathology			
Technical Factors Used			
Exposure Index			

FACILITY PREPARATION
The student:

	Procedure Yes No	Repeat Yes No	Competency Yes No
1. Examines the radiographic room and cleans/straightens it before escorting the patient in.	☐ ☐	☐ ☐	☐ ☐
2. Has all equipment and supplies (patient gown, pillow, markers, lead blockers, etc.) readily available before escorting the patient in.	☐ ☐	☐ ☐	☐ ☐
3. Is able to manipulate all radiographic equipment with ease, and centers the central ray to the cassette/receptor *for all projections*.	☐ ☐	☐ ☐	☐ ☐
4. Adjusts the tube to the proper SID *for each projection*.	☐ ☐	☐ ☐	☐ ☐
5. Selects cassettes/receptor of the appropriate sizes *for all projections*, according to the patient's size and examination.	☐ ☐	☐ ☐	☐ ☐

Comments:

_____

_____

PATIENT PREPARATION
The student:

	Procedure Yes No	Repeat Yes No	Competency Yes No
6. Identifies the correct patient and examination according to the requisition while establishing a good rapport with him or her.	☐ ☐	☐ ☐	☐ ☐
7. Obtains and documents the patient's history before the examination.	▨ ▨	▨ ▨	☐ ☐
8. Explains the examination in terms the patient fully understands, and properly communicates with the patient throughout the examination.	☐ ☐	☐ ☐	☐ ☐
9. Asks female patients of childbearing age the date of their last menstrual period and documents this; inquires about the possibility of pregnancy and has them sign pregnancy consent forms.	☐ ☐	☐ ☐	☐ ☐
10. Removes all obscuring objects (snaps, zippers, belt, etc.) so as *not* to produce radiographic artifacts.	☐ ☐	☐ ☐	☐ ☐

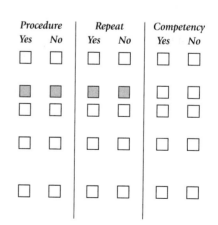

(continued)

	Procedure		Repeat		Competency	
	Yes	No	Yes	No	Yes	No
11. Respects the patient's modesty and provides ample comfort for him or her.	☐	☐	☐	☐	☐	☐

Comments:

_____

_____

PATIENT POSITIONING FOR THE GLENOID FOSSA (GRASHEY METHOD)
Anteroposterior
The student:

	Procedure		Repeat		Competency	
	Yes	No	Yes	No	Yes	No
12. Places the patient in the supine position on the table, or in the erect position, at the erect Bucky/receptor.	☐	☐	☐	☐	☐	☐
13. Selects the appropriate receptor or places the cassette lengthwise to have a 1-inch margin from the top of the shoulder to the top of the cassette/receptor. For conventional cassettes, the flash must be away from any anatomy.	☐	☐	☐	☐	☐	☐
14. Rotates the patient approximately 45° toward the affected side.	☐	☐	☐	☐	☐	☐
15. Adjust the degree of rotation so that the scapula is parallel with the receptor and the humeral head is in contact with it.	☐	☐	☐	☐	☐	☐
16. Abduct the arm and internally rotate the arm slightly.	☐	☐	☐	☐	☐	☐
17. Centers the anatomy of interest to the center of the cassette/receptor.	☐	☐	☐	☐	☐	☐
18. Centers the central ray perpendicularly to a point 2 inches medially and distally to the upper border of the shoulder.	☐	☐	☐	☐	☐	☐

Comments:

_____

_____

IMPORTANT DETAILS
The student:

	Procedure		Repeat		Competency	
	Yes	No	Yes	No	Yes	No
19. Instills confidence in the patient by exhibiting self-confidence throughout the examination.	☐	☐	☐	☐	☐	☐
20. Places a lead marker in the appropriate area of the cassette/receptor (top/bottom/anteriorly/laterally), where it will be visualized on the finished radiograph, on the proper anatomical side (right/left), and in the appropriate position (face up/face down), depending on the patient's position.	☐	☐	☐	☐	☐	☐
21. Provides radiation protection (shield) for the patient, self, and others (closes doors).	☐	☐	☐	☐	☐	☐
22. Applies proper collimation and makes adjustments as necessary.	☐	☐	☐	☐	☐	☐
23. Properly measures the patient along the course of the central ray *for each projection.*	☐	☐	☐	☐	☐	☐
24. Sets the proper exposure techniques:	☐	☐	☐	☐	☐	☐

24. Sets the proper exposure techniques:

Conventional systems
• Sets the proper kVp, mA, and time, and makes adjustments as necessary.

or

CR or DR systems
• Identifies the patient on the work-list (or manually types the patient information into the system).
• Selects appropriate body region, specific body part, and accurate view/projection.

- Double-checks preset parameters:
  - —Adult vs. pediatric patients
    - ○ Small, medium, or large
  - —Bucky/receptor (upright vs. table) *or* non-Bucky
  - —AEC vs. fixed
    - ○ If AEC, checks ion chambers
    - ○ Density setting
  - —kVp and mA; adjusts if necessary
  - —Focal spot/filament size

	Procedure		Repeat		Competency	
	Yes	No	Yes	No	Yes	No
25. Exposes the cassette/receptor after telling the patient to hold still and after giving patient proper breathing instructions (expiration) *for each projection.*	☐	☐	☐	☐	☐	☐
26. Provides each radiograph with the proper identification (flash) and/or processes each cassette (image) without difficulty (regardless of technology—film, CR, or DR).	▣	☐	▣	☐	☐	☐
27. Properly completes the examination by filling out all necessary paperwork, entering the examination in the computer, having the images checked by the appropriate staff members, and informing the patient that he or she is finished.	▣	☐	▣	☐	☐	☐
28. Exhibits the ability to adapt to new and difficult situations if and when necessary.	▣	▣	▣	▣	☐	☐
29. Accepts constructive criticism and uses it to his or her advantage.	☐	☐	☐	☐	☐	☐
30. Leaves the radiographic room neat and clean for the next examination.	▣	▣	▣	▣	☐	☐
31. Completes the examination within a reasonable time frame.	☐	☐	☐	☐	☐	☐

Comments:

_____

RADIOGRAPHIC IMAGE QUALITY
The student is able to critique his or her radiographs as to whether they demonstrate:

	Procedure		Repeat		Competency	
	Yes	No	Yes	No	Yes	No
32. Proper technique/optimal density	▣	▣	▣	▣	☐	☐
33. Enhanced detail, without evidence of motion and without any visible artifacts	▣	▣	▣	▣	☐	☐
34. Proper positioning (all anatomy included, evidence of proper centering/alignment, etc.)	▣	▣	▣	▣	☐	☐
35. Proper marker placement	▣	▣	▣	▣	☐	☐
36. Evidence of proper collimation and radiation protection	▣	▣	▣	▣	☐	☐
37. Long vs. short scale of contrast	▣	▣	▣	▣	☐	☐

Comments:

_____

SCAPULA ANATOMY
The student is able to identify:

	Procedure		Repeat		Competency	
	Yes	No	Yes	No	Yes	No
38. Glenoid fossa	▣	▣	▣	▣	☐	☐
39. Humerus	▣	▣	▣	▣	☐	☐
40. Clavicle	▣	▣	▣	▣	☐	☐

(continued)

	Procedure		Repeat		Competency	
	Yes	No	Yes	No	Yes	No
41. Scapula	☐	☐	☐	☐	☐	☐
42. Joint space between the humeral head and the fossa	☐	☐	☐	☐	☐	☐
43. Inferior angle of the scapula	☐	☐	☐	☐	☐	☐
44. Acromion	☐	☐	☐	☐	☐	☐
45. Obvious pathology	☐	☐	☐	☐	☐	☐

Comments:

_____

_____

_____

Procedure Evaluator Signature   Repeat Evaluator Signature   Competency Evaluator Signature

Date   Date   Date

END GLENOID FOSSA (GRASHEY METHOD) EVALUATION

The objective of this evaluation is to determine the student's competency level when performing specific radiographic examinations.

Student Name:_____

Procedure Grade	Repeat Grade	Competency Grade

PATIENT INFORMATION OR SIMULATED PROCEDURE *(circle if simulated)*

	Procedure	Repeat	Competency
Age			
Medical Record No.			
Ability to Cooperate			
Condition/Pathology			
Technical Factors Used			
Exposure Index			

FACILITY PREPARATION
The student:

	Procedure Yes No	Repeat Yes No	Competency Yes No
1. Examines the radiographic room and cleans/straightens it before escorting the patient in.	☐ ☐	☐ ☐	☐ ☐
2. Has all equipment and supplies (patient gown, pillow, markers, lead blockers, etc.) readily available before escorting the patient in.	☐ ☐	☐ ☐	☐ ☐
3. Is able to manipulate all radiographic equipment with ease, and centers the central ray to the cassette/receptor *for all projections*.	☐ ☐	☐ ☐	☐ ☐
4. Adjusts the tube to the proper SID *for each projection*.	☐ ☐	☐ ☐	☐ ☐
5. Selects cassettes/receptor of the appropriate sizes *for all projections*, according to the patient's size and examination.	☐ ☐	☐ ☐	☐ ☐

Comments:

_____

_____

PATIENT PREPARATION
The student:

	Procedure Yes No	Repeat Yes No	Competency Yes No
6. Identifies the correct patient and examination according to the requisition while establishing a good rapport with him or her.	☐ ☐	☐ ☐	☐ ☐
7. Obtains and documents the patient's history before the examination.	▨ ▨	▨ ▨	☐ ☐
8. Explains the examination in terms the patient fully understands, and properly communicates with the patient throughout the examination.	☐ ☐	☐ ☐	☐ ☐
9. Asks female patients of childbearing age the date of their last menstrual period and documents this; inquires about the possibility of pregnancy and has them sign pregnancy consent forms.	☐ ☐	☐ ☐	☐ ☐
10. Removes all obscuring objects (snaps, zippers, belt, etc.) so as *not* to produce radiographic artifacts.	☐ ☐	☐ ☐	☐ ☐

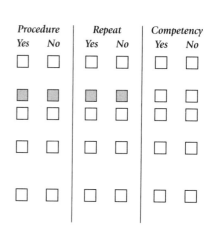

(continued)

	Procedure		Repeat		Competency	
	Yes	No	Yes	No	Yes	No
11. Respects the patient's modesty and provides ample comfort for him or her.	☐	☐	☐	☐	☐	☐

Comments:

_____

_____

PATIENT POSITIONING FOR A SCAPULA
Anteroposterior
The student:

	Procedure		Repeat		Competency	
	Yes	No	Yes	No	Yes	No
12. Places the patient in the supine position on the table, or in the erect position, at the erect Bucky/receptor.	☐	☐	☐	☐	☐	☐
13. Selects the appropriate receptor or places the cassette lengthwise to have a 1-inch margin from the top of the shoulder to the top of the cassette/receptor. For conventional cassettes, the flash must be away from any anatomy.	☐	☐	☐	☐	☐	☐
14. Abducts the affected arm to form a right angle to the body, to draw the scapula laterally.	☐	☐	☐	☐	☐	☐
15. Centers the anatomy of interest to the center of the cassette/receptor.	☐	☐	☐	☐	☐	☐
16. Centers the central ray perpendicularly to the midscapular area	☐	☐	☐	☐	☐	☐

Lateral: Scapular Y
The student:

	Procedure		Repeat		Competency	
	Yes	No	Yes	No	Yes	No
17. Places the patient in the erect PA oblique position, with the affected scapula against the Bucky/receptor.	☐	☐	☐	☐	☐	☐
18. Does one of the following:	☐	☐	☐	☐	☐	☐

   a. For delineation of the scapular body, extends the arm upward and rests the forearm on his or her head.

   b. For delineation of the acromion and coracoid processes, flexes the elbow of the affected side and places the hand on the anterior chest wall (with the affected side's hand, reaches up and grasps the opposite shoulder) or flexes the elbow of the affected side and rests the hand on his or her back at a level that prevents the shadow of the humerus from overlapping the scapula.

   c. For delineation of the glenohumeral joint for suspected dislocation scapular Y (PA oblique shoulder), places the patient so that his or her arm hangs beside the body such that the humerus superimposes the wing of the scapula.

	Procedure		Repeat		Competency	
19. Grasps the axillary and vertebral borders of the scapula with one hand, and adjusts the body to place the wing of the scapula perpendicular to the plane of the cassette/receptor.	☐	☐	☐	☐	☐	☐
20. Centers the anatomy of interest to the center of the cassette/receptor.	☐	☐	☐	☐	☐	☐
21. Centers the central ray perpendicularly to the vertebral border of the protruding scapula/glenohumeral joint.	☐	☐	☐	☐	☐	☐

Comments:

_____

_____

IMPORTANT DETAILS
The student:

	Procedure		Repeat		Competency	
	Yes	No	Yes	No	Yes	No
22. Instills confidence in the patient by exhibiting self-confidence throughout the examination.	☐	☐	☐	☐	☐	☐
23. Places a lead marker in the appropriate area of the cassette/receptor (top/bottom/anteriorly/laterally), where it will be visualized on the finished radiograph, on the proper anatomical side (right/left), and in the appropriate position (face up/face down), depending on the patient's position.	☐	☐	☐	☐	☐	☐
24. Provides radiation protection (shield) for the patient, self, and others (closes doors).	☐	☐	☐	☐	☐	☐
25. Applies proper collimation and makes adjustments as necessary.	☐	☐	☐	☐	☐	☐
26. Properly measures the patient along the course of the central ray *for each projection.*	☐	☐	☐	☐	☐	☐
27. Sets the proper exposure techniques:	☐	☐	☐	☐	☐	☐

Conventional systems
* Sets the proper kVp, mA, and time, and makes adjustments as necessary.

or

CR or DR systems
* Identifies the patient on the work-list (or manually types the patient information into the system).
* Selects appropriate body region, specific body part, and accurate view/ projection.
* Double-checks preset parameters:
  —Adult vs. pediatric patients
    ○ Small, medium, or large
  —Bucky/receptor (upright vs. table) *or* non-Bucky
  —AEC vs. fixed
    ○ If AEC, checks ion chambers
    ○ Density setting
  —kVp and mA; adjusts if necessary
  —Focal spot/filament size

	Procedure		Repeat		Competency	
28. Exposes the cassette/receptor after telling the patient to hold still and after giving the patient proper breathing instructions (AP—quiet breathing; Y—expiration) *for each projection.*	☐	☐	☐	☐	☐	☐
29. Provides each radiograph with the proper identification (flash) and/or processes each cassette (image) without difficulty (regardless of technology—film, CR, or DR).	▨	▨	▨	▨	☐	☐
30. Properly completes the examination by filling out all necessary paperwork, entering the examination in the computer, having the images checked by the appropriate staff members, and informing the patient that he or she is finished.	▨	▨	▨	▨	☐	☐
31. Exhibits the ability to adapt to new and difficult situations if and when necessary.	▨	▨	▨	▨	☐	☐
32. Accepts constructive criticism and uses it to his or her advantage.	☐	☐	☐	☐	☐	☐
33. Leaves the radiographic room neat and clean for the next examination.	▨	▨	▨	▨	☐	☐
34. Completes the examination within a reasonable time frame.	☐	☐	☐	☐	☐	☐

Comments:

_____

_____

(continued)

RADIOGRAPHIC IMAGE QUALITY
The student is able to critique his or her radiographs as to whether they demonstrate:

	Procedure		Repeat		Competency	
	Yes	No	Yes	No	Yes	No
35. Proper technique/optimal density	☐	☐	☐	☐	☐	☐
36. Enhanced detail, without evidence of motion and without any visible artifacts	☐	☐	☐	☐	☐	☐
37. Proper positioning (all anatomy included, evidence of proper centering/alignment, etc.)	☐	☐	☐	☐	☐	☐
38. Proper marker placement	☐	☐	☐	☐	☐	☐
39. Evidence of proper collimation and radiation protection	☐	☐	☐	☐	☐	☐
40. Long vs. short scale of contrast	☐	☐	☐	☐	☐	☐

Comments:

_____

_____

SCAPULA ANATOMY
The student is able to identify:

	Procedure		Repeat		Competency	
	Yes	No	Yes	No	Yes	No
41. Glenoid fossa	☐	☐	☐	☐	☐	☐
42. Acromion process	☐	☐	☐	☐	☐	☐
43. Clavicle	☐	☐	☐	☐	☐	☐
44. Coracoid process	☐	☐	☐	☐	☐	☐
45. Axillary and vertebral borders of the scapula	☐	☐	☐	☐	☐	☐
46. Inferior angle of the scapula	☐	☐	☐	☐	☐	☐
47. AC articulation	☐	☐	☐	☐	☐	☐
48. Humerus	☐	☐	☐	☐	☐	☐
49. Obvious pathology	☐	☐	☐	☐	☐	☐

Comments:

_____

_____

_____   _____   _____
Procedure Evaluator Signature   Repeat Evaluator Signature   Competency Evaluator Signature

_____   _____   _____
Date   Date   Date

END SCAPULA (AP AND SCAPULAR Y) EVALUATION

The objective of this evaluation is to determine the student's competency level when performing specific radiographic examinations.

Student Name:_____

	Procedure Grade	Repeat Grade	Competency Grade

PATIENT INFORMATION OR SIMULATED PROCEDURE *(circle if simulated)*

	Procedure	Repeat	Competency
Age			
Medical Record No.			
Ability to Cooperate			
Condition/Pathology			
Technical Factors Used			
Exposure Index			

FACILITY PREPARATION
The student:

	Procedure Yes No	Repeat Yes No	Competency Yes No
1. Examines the radiographic room and cleans/straightens it before escorting the patient in.	☐ ☐	☐ ☐	☐ ☐
2. Has all equipment and supplies (patient gown, pillow, markers, lead blockers, etc.) readily available before escorting the patient in.	☐ ☐	☐ ☐	☐ ☐
3. Is able to manipulate all radiographic equipment with ease, and centers the central ray to the cassette/receptor *for all projections*.	☐ ☐	☐ ☐	☐ ☐
4. Adjusts the tube to the proper SID *for each projection*.	☐ ☐	☐ ☐	☐ ☐
5. Selects cassettes/receptor of the appropriate sizes *for all projections*, according to the patient's size and examination.	☐ ☐	☐ ☐	☐ ☐

Comments:

_____

_____

PATIENT PREPARATION
The student:

	Procedure Yes No	Repeat Yes No	Competency Yes No
6. Identifies the correct patient and examination according to the requisition while establishing a good rapport with him or her.	☐ ☐	☐ ☐	☐ ☐
7. Obtains and documents the patient's history before the examination.	▦ ▦	▦ ▦	☐ ☐
8. Explains the examination in terms the patient fully understands, and properly communicates with the patient throughout the examination.	☐ ☐	☐ ☐	☐ ☐
9. Asks female patients of childbearing age the date of their last menstrual period and documents this; inquires about the possibility of pregnancy and has them sign pregnancy consent forms.	☐ ☐	☐ ☐	☐ ☐
10. Removes all obscuring objects (snaps, zippers, belt, etc.) so as *not* to produce radiographic artifacts.	☐ ☐	☐ ☐	☐ ☐

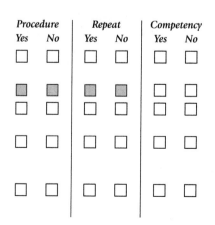

(continued)

	Procedure		Repeat		Competency	
	Yes	No	Yes	No	Yes	No
11. Respects the patient's modesty and provides ample comfort for him or her.	☐	☐	☐	☐	☐	☐

Comments:

_____

_____

PATIENT POSITIONING FOR A CLAVICLE
AP or PA
The student:

	Procedure		Repeat		Competency	
	Yes	No	Yes	No	Yes	No
12. Places the patient in the AP position, or in the PA position against the receptor.	☐	☐	☐	☐	☐	☐
13. Selects the appropriate receptor or places cassette crosswise in the Bucky. For conventional cassettes, the flash must be away from any anatomy.	☐	☐	☐	☐	☐	☐
14. Centers the clavicle from end to end to the center of the cassette/receptor, including both the acromioclavicular joint and the sternoclavicular joint.	☐	☐	☐	☐	☐	☐
15. Centers the central ray perpendicularly to the midshaft of the clavicle, at the level of the coracoid process.	☐	☐	☐	☐	☐	☐

AP Lordotic
The student:

	Procedure		Repeat		Competency	
	Yes	No	Yes	No	Yes	No
16. Places the patient in the AP position approximately 1 foot away from the Bucky/receptor.	☐	☐	☐	☐	☐	☐
17. Centers the clavicle from end to the center of the cassette/receptor, including both joints.	☐	☐	☐	☐	☐	☐
18. Placing one hand on the patient's lumbar region, assists the patient as he or she leans back into the lordotic position.	☐	☐	☐	☐	☐	☐
19. Centers the central ray perpendicularly to the midshaft of the clavicle (angling the central ray 0–30° cephalad, depending the patient's flexibility).	☐	☐	☐	☐	☐	☐

Or
PA Axial
The student:

	Procedure		Repeat		Competency	
	Yes	No	Yes	No	Yes	No
20. Places the patient in the PA position against the Bucky/receptor.	☐	☐	☐	☐	☐	☐
21. Centers the clavicle from the end to the center of the cassette/receptor, including both joints.	☐	☐	☐	☐	☐	☐
22. Centers the central ray perpendicularly to the midshaft of the clavicle (angling the central ray 15–30° caudad).	☐	☐	☐	☐	☐	☐

Comments:

_____

_____

IMPORTANT DETAILS
The student:

	Procedure		Repeat		Competency	
	Yes	No	Yes	No	Yes	No
23. Instills confidence in the patient by exhibiting self-confidence throughout the examination.	☐	☐	☐	☐	☐	☐

	Procedure		Repeat		Competency	
	Yes	No	Yes	No	Yes	No
24. Places a lead marker in the appropriate area of the cassette/receptor (top/bottom/anteriorly/laterally), where it will be visualized on the finished radiograph, on the proper anatomical side (right/left), and in the appropriate position (face up/face down), depending on the patient's position.	☐	☐	☐	☐	☐	☐
25. Provides radiation protection (shield) for the patient, self, and others (closes doors).	☐	☐	☐	☐	☐	☐
26. Applies proper collimation and makes adjustments as necessary.	☐	☐	☐	☐	☐	☐
27. Properly measures the patient along the course of the central ray *for each projection.*	☐	☐	☐	☐	☐	☐
28. Sets the proper exposure techniques:	☐	☐	☐	☐	☐	☐

28. Sets the proper exposure techniques:

Conventional systems
- Sets the proper kVp, mA, and time, and makes adjustments as necessary.

or

CR or DR systems
- Identifies the patient on the work-list (or manually types the patient information into the system).
- Selects appropriate body region, specific body part, and accurate view/projection.
- Double-checks preset parameters:
  —Adult vs. pediatric patients
    ○ Small, medium, or large
  —Bucky/receptor (upright vs. table) *or* non-Bucky
  —AEC vs. fixed
    ○ If AEC, checks ion chambers
    ○ Density setting
  —kVp and mA; adjusts if necessary
  —Focal spot/filament size

	Procedure		Repeat		Competency	
	Yes	No	Yes	No	Yes	No
29. Exposes the cassette/receptor after telling the patient to hold still and after giving the patient proper breathing instructions (expiration) *for each projection.*	☐	☐	☐	☐	☐	☐
30. Provides each radiograph with the proper identification (flash) and/or processes each cassette (image) without difficulty (regardless of technology—film, CR, or DR).	▣	▣	▣	▣	☐	☐
31. Properly completes the examination by filling out all necessary paperwork, entering the examination in the computer, having the images checked by the appropriate staff members, and informing the patient that he or she is finished.	▣	▣	▣	▣	☐	☐
32. Exhibits the ability to adapt to new and difficult situations if and when necessary.	▣	▣	▣	▣	☐	☐
33. Accepts constructive criticism and uses it to his or her advantage.	☐	☐	☐	☐	☐	☐
34. Leaves the radiographic room neat and clean for the next examination.	▣	▣	▣	▣	☐	☐
35. Completes the examination within a reasonable time frame.	☐	☐	☐	☐	☐	☐

Comments:

_____

_____

_____

(continued)

RADIOGRAPHIC IMAGE QUALITY
The student is able to critique his or her radiographs as to whether they demonstrate:

	Procedure Yes	Procedure No	Repeat Yes	Repeat No	Competency Yes	Competency No
36. Proper technique/optimal density	☐	☐	☐	☐	☐	☐
37. Enhanced detail, without evidence of motion and without any visible artifacts	☐	☐	☐	☐	☐	☐
38. Proper positioning (all anatomy included, evidence of proper centering/ alignment, etc.)	☐	☐	☐	☐	☐	☐
39. Proper marker placement	☐	☐	☐	☐	☐	☐
40. Evidence of proper collimation and radiation protection	☐	☐	☐	☐	☐	☐
41. Long vs. short scale of contrast	☐	☐	☐	☐	☐	☐

Comments:

_____

_____

CLAVICLE ANATOMY
The student is able to identify:

	Procedure Yes	Procedure No	Repeat Yes	Repeat No	Competency Yes	Competency No
42. Clavicle	☐	☐	☐	☐	☐	☐
43. Acromion process	☐	☐	☐	☐	☐	☐
44. Coracoid process	☐	☐	☐	☐	☐	☐
45. Acromioclavicular joint	☐	☐	☐	☐	☐	☐
46. Sternoclavicular joint	☐	☐	☐	☐	☐	☐
47. Obvious pathology	☐	☐	☐	☐	☐	☐

Comments:

_____

_____

_____ _____ _____
Procedure Evaluator Signature   Repeat Evaluator Signature   Competency Evaluator Signature

_____ _____ _____
Date   Date   Date

END CLAVICLE EVALUATION

The objective of this evaluation is to determine the student's competency level when performing specific radiographic examinations.

Student Name:_____

Procedure Grade	Repeat Grade	Competency Grade

PATIENT INFORMATION OR SIMULATED PROCEDURE *(circle if simulated)*

	Procedure	Repeat	Competency
Age			
Medical Record No.			
Ability to Cooperate			
Condition/Pathology			
Technical Factors Used			
Exposure Index			

FACILITY PREPARATION
The student:

	Procedure Yes	Procedure No	Repeat Yes	Repeat No	Competency Yes	Competency No
1. Examines the radiographic room and cleans/straightens it before escorting the patient in.	☐	☐	☐	☐	☐	☐
2. Has all equipment and supplies (patient gown, pillow, markers, lead blockers, etc.) readily available before escorting the patient in.	☐	☐	☐	☐	☐	☐
3. Is able to manipulate all radiographic equipment with ease, and centers the central ray to the cassette/receptor *for all projections.*	☐	☐	☐	☐	☐	☐
4. Adjusts the tube to the proper SID *for each projection.*	☐	☐	☐	☐	☐	☐
5. Selects cassettes/receptor of the appropriate sizes *for all projections,* according to the patient's size and examination.	☐	☐	☐	☐	☐	☐

Comments:

_____

_____

PATIENT PREPARATION
The student:

	Procedure Yes	Procedure No	Repeat Yes	Repeat No	Competency Yes	Competency No
6. Identifies the correct patient and examination according to the requisition while establishing a good rapport with him or her.	☐	☐	☐	☐	☐	☐
7. Obtains and documents the patient's history before the examination.	▨	▨	▨	▨	☐	☐
8. Explains the examination in terms the patient fully understands, and properly communicates with the patient throughout the examination.	☐	☐	☐	☐	☐	☐
9. Asks female patients of childbearing age the date of their last menstrual period and documents this; inquires about the possibility of pregnancy and has them sign pregnancy consent forms.	☐	☐	☐	☐	☐	☐
10. Removes all obscuring objects (snaps, zippers, belt, etc.) so as *not* to produce radiographic artifacts.	☐	☐	☐	☐	☐	☐

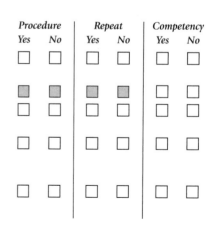

(continued)

147

	Procedure		Repeat		Competency	
	Yes	No	Yes	No	Yes	No
11. Respects the patient's modesty and provides ample comfort for him or her.	☐	☐	☐	☐	☐	☐

Comments:

PATIENT POSITIONING FOR BILATERAL ACROMIOCLAVICULAR JOINTS
AP Without Weights
The student:

	Procedure		Repeat		Competency	
	Yes	No	Yes	No	Yes	No
12. Places the patient in the erect position, with his or her back in contact with the erect Bucky/receptor and with his or her weight evenly distributed.	☐	☐	☐	☐	☐	☐
13. Selects the appropriate receptor or places cassette crosswise in the Bucky. For conventional cassettes, the flash must be high or low enough that it does not obscure any anatomy.	☐	☐	☐	☐	☐	☐
14. With the patient's arms hanging by his or her sides, adjusts the shoulders so that they lie in the same transverse plane.	☐	☐	☐	☐	☐	☐
15. Centers the central ray to the midsagittal plane, making sure both acromioclavicular joints will be demonstrated on the finished radiograph.	☐	☐	☐	☐	☐	☐
16. Centers the central ray perpendicularly at the level of the acromioclavicular joints.	☐	☐	☐	☐	☐	☐

AP With Weights
The student:

	Procedure		Repeat		Competency	
	Yes	No	Yes	No	Yes	No
17. Places the patient in the erect position, with his or her back in contact with the erect Bucky/receptor and with his or her weight evenly distributed.	☐	☐	☐	☐	☐	☐
18. With the patient's arms hanging by his or her sides, simultaneously hands the patient sandbags/weights of equal weight.	☐	☐	☐	☐	☐	☐
19. Centers the central ray to the midsagittal plane, making sure both acromioclavicular joints will be demonstrated on the finished radiograph.	☐	☐	☐	☐	☐	☐
20. Centers the central ray perpendicularly at the level of the acromioclavicular joints.	☐	☐	☐	☐	☐	☐

Comments:

IMPORTANT DETAILS
The student:

	Procedure		Repeat		Competency	
	Yes	No	Yes	No	Yes	No
21. Instills confidence in the patient by exhibiting self-confidence throughout the examination.	☐	☐	☐	☐	☐	☐
22. Places a lead marker in the appropriate area of the cassette/receptor (top/bottom/anteriorly/laterally), where it will be visualized on the finished radiograph, on the proper anatomical side (right/left), and in the appropriate position (face up/face down), depending on the patient's position.	☐	☐	☐	☐	☐	☐
23. Provides radiation protection (shield) for the patient, self, and others (closes doors).	☐	☐	☐	☐	☐	☐

	Procedure		Repeat		Competency	
	Yes	No	Yes	No	Yes	No
24. Applies proper collimation and makes adjustments as necessary.	☐	☐	☐	☐	☐	☐
25. Properly measures the patient along the course of the central ray *for each projection.*	☐	☐	☐	☐	☐	☐
26. Sets the proper exposure techniques:	☐	☐	☐	☐	☐	☐

Conventional systems
- Sets the proper kVp, mA, and time, and makes adjustments as necessary.

or

CR or DR systems
- Identifies the patient on the work-list (or manually types the patient information into the system).
- Selects appropriate body region, specific body part, and accurate view/projection.
- Double-checks preset parameters:
  —Adult vs. pediatric patients
    ○ Small, medium, or large
  —Bucky/receptor (upright vs. table) *or* non-Bucky
  —AEC vs. fixed
    ○ If AEC, checks ion chambers
    ○ Density setting
  —kVp and mA; adjusts if necessary
  —Focal spot/filament size

	Procedure		Repeat		Competency	
	Yes	No	Yes	No	Yes	No
27. Exposes the cassette/receptor after telling the patient to hold still and after giving the patient proper breathing instructions (expiration) *for each projection.*	☐	☐	☐	☐	☐	☐
28. Provides each radiograph with the proper identification (flash) and/or processes each cassette (image) without difficulty (regardless of technology—film, CR, or DR).	▣	▣	▣	▣	☐	☐
29. Properly completes the examination by filling out all necessary paperwork, entering the examination in the computer, having the images checked by the appropriate staff members, and informing the patient that he or she is finished.	▣	▣	▣	▣	☐	☐
30. Exhibits the ability to adapt to new and difficult situations if and when necessary.	▣	▣	▣	▣	☐	☐
31. Accepts constructive criticism and uses it to his or her advantage.	☐	☐	☐	☐	☐	☐
32. Leaves the radiographic room neat and clean for the next examination.	▣	▣	▣	▣	☐	☐
33. Completes the examination within a reasonable time frame.	☐	☐	☐	☐	☐	☐

Comments:

RADIOGRAPHIC IMAGE QUALITY
The student is able to critique his or her radiographs as to whether they demonstrate:

	Procedure		Repeat		Competency	
	Yes	No	Yes	No	Yes	No
34. Proper technique/optimal density	▣	▣	▣	▣	☐	☐
35. Enhanced detail, without evidence of motion and without any visible artifacts	▣	▣	▣	▣	☐	☐
36. Proper positioning (all anatomy included, evidence of proper centering/alignment, etc.)	▣	▣	▣	▣	☐	☐
37. Proper marker placement	▣	▣	▣	▣	☐	☐
38. Evidence of proper collimation and radiation protection	▣	▣	▣	▣	☐	☐

(continued)

	Procedure		Repeat		Competency	
	Yes	No	Yes	No	Yes	No
39. Long vs. short scale of contrast	☐	☐	☐	☐	☐	☐

Comments:

_____

_____

AC JOINTS ANATOMY
The student is able to identify:

	Procedure		Repeat		Competency	
	Yes	No	Yes	No	Yes	No
40. Coracoid process	☐	☐	☐	☐	☐	☐
41. Clavicle	☐	☐	☐	☐	☐	☐
42. Acromioclavicular joint	☐	☐	☐	☐	☐	☐
43. Acromion process	☐	☐	☐	☐	☐	☐
44. Scapula	☐	☐	☐	☐	☐	☐
45. Humerus	☐	☐	☐	☐	☐	☐
46. Sternoclavicular joint	☐	☐	☐	☐	☐	☐
47. Obvious pathology	☐	☐	☐	☐	☐	☐

Comments:

_____

_____

_____ | _____ | _____
Procedure Evaluator Signature | Repeat Evaluator Signature | Competency Evaluator Signature

_____ | _____ | _____
Date | Date | Date

END AC JOINTS EVALUATION

Student Name:_____

Procedure Grade	Repeat Grade	Competency Grade

PATIENT INFORMATION OR SIMULATED PROCEDURE *(circle if simulated)*

	Procedure	Repeat	Competency
Age			
Medical Record No.			
Ability to Cooperate			
Condition/Pathology			
Technical Factors Used			
Exposure Index			

FACILITY PREPARATION
The student:

	Procedure Yes No	Repeat Yes No	Competency Yes No
1. Examines the radiographic room and cleans/straightens it before escorting the patient in.	☐ ☐	☐ ☐	☐ ☐
2. Has all equipment and supplies (patient gown, pillow, markers, lead blockers, etc.) readily available before escorting the patient in.	☐ ☐	☐ ☐	☐ ☐
3. Is able to manipulate all radiographic equipment with ease, and centers the central ray to the cassette/receptor *for all projections*.	☐ ☐	☐ ☐	☐ ☐
4. Adjusts the tube to the proper SID *for each projection*.	☐ ☐	☐ ☐	☐ ☐
5. Selects cassettes/receptor of the appropriate sizes *for all projections*, according to the patient's size and examination.	☐ ☐	☐ ☐	☐ ☐

Comments:

_____

_____

PATIENT PREPARATION
The student:

	Procedure Yes No	Repeat Yes No	Competency Yes No
6. Identifies the correct patient and examination according to the requisition while establishing a good rapport with him or her.	☐ ☐	☐ ☐	☐ ☐
7. Obtains and documents the patient's history before the examination.	▦ ▦	▦ ▦	☐ ☐
8. Explains the examination in terms the patient fully understands, and properly communicates with the patient throughout the examination.	☐ ☐	☐ ☐	☐ ☐
9. Asks female patients of childbearing age the date of their last menstrual period and documents this; inquires about the possibility of pregnancy and has them sign pregnancy consent forms.	☐ ☐	☐ ☐	☐ ☐
10. Removes all obscuring objects (snaps, zippers, belt, etc.) so as *not* to produce radiographic artifacts.	☐ ☐	☐ ☐	☐ ☐

(continued)

151

	Procedure		Repeat		Competency	
	Yes	No	Yes	No	Yes	No
11. Respects the patient's modesty and provides ample comfort for him or her.	☐	☐	☐	☐	☐	☐

Comments:

_____

_____

PATIENT POSITIONING FOR TRAUMA OF THE UPPER EXTREMITY
AP or PA
The student:

	Procedure		Repeat		Competency	
	Yes	No	Yes	No	Yes	No
12. Places the patient in the truest AP or PA position possible.	☐	☐	☐	☐	☐	☐
13. Selects the appropriate receptor or places cassette appropriately. For conventional cassettes, the flash must be high or low enough that it does not obscure any anatomy.	☐	☐	☐	☐	☐	☐
14. Centers the central ray to the midline of the affected area, making sure both the proximal and distal joints will be demonstrated on the finished radiograph (if required).	☐	☐	☐	☐	☐	☐
15. Centers the central ray perpendicularly or with the appropriate angle relative to the part being radiographed.	☐	☐	☐	☐	☐	☐

Lateral
The student:

	Procedure		Repeat		Competency	
	Yes	No	Yes	No	Yes	No
16. Places the patient in the truest lateral position possible, or prepares the patient for a shoot-through radiograph.	☐	☐	☐	☐	☐	☐
17. Selects the appropriate receptor or places cassette appropriately. For conventional cassettes, the flash must be high or low enough that it does not obscure any anatomy.	☐	☐	☐	☐	☐	☐
18. Centers the central ray to the midline of the affected area, making sure both the proximal and distal joints will be demonstrated on the finished radiograph (if required).	☐	☐	☐	☐	☐	☐
19. Centers the central ray perpendicularly or with the appropriate angle relative to the part being radiographed.	☐	☐	☐	☐	☐	☐

Comments:

_____

_____

IMPORTANT DETAILS
The student:

	Procedure		Repeat		Competency	
	Yes	No	Yes	No	Yes	No
20. Instills confidence in the patient by exhibiting self-confidence throughout the examination.	☐	☐	☐	☐	☐	☐
21. Places a lead marker in the appropriate area of the cassette/receptor (top/bottom/anteriorly/laterally), where it will be visualized on the finished radiograph, on the proper anatomical side (right/left), and in the appropriate position (face up/face down), depending on the patient's position.	☐	☐	☐	☐	☐	☐
22. Provides radiation protection (shield) for the patient, self, and others (closes doors).	☐	☐	☐	☐	☐	☐
23. Applies proper collimation and makes adjustments as necessary.	☐	☐	☐	☐	☐	☐
24. Properly measures the patient along the course of the central ray *for each projection.*	☐	☐	☐	☐	☐	☐

	Procedure		Repeat		Competency	
	Yes	No	Yes	No	Yes	No
25. Sets the proper exposure techniques:	☐	☐	☐	☐	☐	☐

Conventional systems
- Sets the proper kVp, mA, and time, and makes adjustments as necessary.

or

CR or DR systems
- Identifies the patient on the work-list (or manually types the patient information into the system).
- Selects appropriate body region, specific body part, and accurate view/projection.
- Double-checks preset parameters:
  —Adult vs. pediatric patients
    ○ Small, medium, or large
  —Bucky/receptor (upright vs. table) *or* non-Bucky
  —AEC vs. fixed
    ○ If AEC, checks ion chambers
    ○ Density setting
  —kVp and mA; adjusts if necessary
  —Focal spot/filament size

	Procedure		Repeat		Competency	
26. Exposes the cassette/receptor after telling the patient to hold still and supporting and/or immobilizing the area of interest if necessary *for each projection.*	☐	☐	☐	☐	☐	☐
27. Provides each radiograph with the proper identification (flash) and/or processes each cassette (image) without difficulty (regardless of technology—film, CR, or DR).	☐	☐	☐	☐	☐	☐
28. Properly completes the examination by filling out all necessary paperwork, entering the examination in the computer, having the images checked by the appropriate staff members, and informing the patient that he or she is finished.	☐	☐	☐	☐	☐	☐
29. Exhibits the ability to adapt to new and difficult situations if and when necessary.	☐	☐	☐	☐	☐	☐
30. Accepts constructive criticism and uses it to his or her advantage.	☐	☐	☐	☐	☐	☐
31. Leaves the radiographic room neat and clean for the next examination.	☐	☐	☐	☐	☐	☐
32. Completes the examination within a reasonable time frame.	☐	☐	☐	☐	☐	☐

Comments:

_____

_____

RADIOGRAPHIC IMAGE QUALITY

The student is able to critique his or her radiographs as to whether they demonstrate:

	Procedure		Repeat		Competency	
	Yes	No	Yes	No	Yes	No
33. Proper technique/optimal density	☐	☐	☐	☐	☐	☐
34. Enhanced detail, without evidence of motion and without any visible artifacts	☐	☐	☐	☐	☐	☐
35. Proper positioning (all anatomy included, evidence of proper centering/alignment, etc.)	☐	☐	☐	☐	☐	☐
36. Proper marker placement	☐	☐	☐	☐	☐	☐
37. Evidence of proper collimation and radiation protection	☐	☐	☐	☐	☐	☐
38. Long vs. short scale of contrast	☐	☐	☐	☐	☐	☐

(continued)

Comments:

_____

_____

TRAUMA UPPER EXTREMITY ANATOMY
The student is able to identify:

	Procedure		Repeat		Competency	
	Yes	No	Yes	No	Yes	No
39. _____	☐	☐	☐	☐	☐	☐
40. _____	☐	☐	☐	☐	☐	☐
41. _____	☐	☐	☐	☐	☐	☐
42. _____	☐	☐	☐	☐	☐	☐
43. _____	☐	☐	☐	☐	☐	☐
44. _____	☐	☐	☐	☐	☐	☐
45. _____	☐	☐	☐	☐	☐	☐
46. Obvious pathology	☐	☐	☐	☐	☐	☐

Comments:

_____

_____

_____   _____   _____
Procedure Evaluator Signature   Repeat Evaluator Signature   Competency Evaluator Signature

_____   _____   _____
Date   Date   Date

END TRAUMA UPPER EXTREMITY (NONSHOULDER) EVALUATION

specific radiographic examinations.

Student Name:_____

Procedure Grade	Repeat Grade	Competency Grade

PATIENT INFORMATION OR SIMULATED PROCEDURE *(circle if simulated)*

	Procedure	Repeat	Competency
Age			
Medical Record No.			
Ability to Cooperate			
Condition/Pathology			
Technical Factors Used			
Exposure Index			

FACILITY PREPARATION
The student:

	Procedure Yes No	Repeat Yes No	Competency Yes No
1. Examines the radiographic room and cleans/straightens it before escorting the patient in.	☐ ☐	☐ ☐	☐ ☐
2. Has all equipment and supplies (patient gown, pillow, markers, lead blockers, etc.) readily available before escorting the patient in.	☐ ☐	☐ ☐	☐ ☐
3. Is able to manipulate all radiographic equipment with ease, and centers the central ray to the cassette/receptor *for all projections*.	☐ ☐	☐ ☐	☐ ☐
4. Adjusts the tube to the proper SID *for each projection*.	☐ ☐	☐ ☐	☐ ☐
5. Selects cassettes/receptor of the appropriate sizes *for all projections*, according to the patient's size and examination.	☐ ☐	☐ ☐	☐ ☐

Comments:

_____

_____

PATIENT PREPARATION
The student:

	Procedure Yes No	Repeat Yes No	Competency Yes No
6. Identifies the correct patient and examination according to the requisition while establishing a good rapport.	☐ ☐	☐ ☐	☐ ☐
7. Obtains and documents the patient's history before the examination.	▨ ▨	▨ ▨	☐ ☐
8. Explains the examination in terms the parent/guardian fully understands, and properly communicates with the patient and parent/guardian throughout the examination.	☐ ☐	☐ ☐	☐ ☐
9. If she intends to stay in the room during the exposure, asks the patient's mother/female guardian of childbearing age the date of her last menstrual period and documents this; inquires about the possibility of pregnancy and has her sign a pregnancy consent form.	☐ ☐	☐ ☐	☐ ☐

(continued)

	Procedure		Repeat		Competency	
	Yes	No	Yes	No	Yes	No
10. Removes all obscuring objects (snaps, zippers, jewelry, etc.) so as *not* to produce radiographic artifacts.	☐	☐	☐	☐	☐	☐
11. Respects the patient's modesty and provides ample comfort for the patient.	☐	☐	☐	☐	☐	☐

Comments:

_____

_____

PATIENT POSITIONING FOR A PEDIATRIC UPPER EXTREMITY
AP or PA
The student:

	Procedure		Repeat		Competency	
	Yes	No	Yes	No	Yes	No
12. Places the patient in the supine or prone position on the radiographic table, without rotation.	☐	☐	☐	☐	☐	☐
13. Selects the appropriate receptor or places the cassette appropriately in the Bucky drawer. For conventional cassettes, the flash must be away from any anatomy.	☐	☐	☐	☐	☐	☐
14. Centers the central ray to the midline (between the lateral surfaces) of the affected extremity.	☐	☐	☐	☐	☐	☐
15. Directs the central ray perpendicularly.	☐	☐	☐	☐	☐	☐

Lateral
The student:

	Procedure		Repeat		Competency	
	Yes	No	Yes	No	Yes	No
16. Places the patient in the true lateral position, without rotation.	☐	☐	☐	☐	☐	☐
17. Selects the appropriate receptor or places the cassette appropriately in the Bucky drawer. For conventional cassettes, the flash must be away from any anatomy.	☐	☐	☐	☐	☐	☐
18. Centers the central ray midway between the anterior and posterior surfaces of the affected extremity.	☐	☐	☐	☐	☐	☐
19. Directs the central ray perpendicularly.	☐	☐	☐	☐	☐	☐

Comments:

_____

_____

IMPORTANT DETAILS
The student:

	Procedure		Repeat		Competency	
	Yes	No	Yes	No	Yes	No
20. Instills confidence in the patient by exhibiting self-confidence throughout the examination.	☐	☐	☐	☐	☐	☐
21. Places a lead marker in the appropriate area of the cassette/receptor (top/bottom/anteriorly/laterally), where it will be visualized on the finished radiograph, on the proper anatomical side (right/left), and in the appropriate position (face up/face down), depending on the patient's position.	☐	☐	☐	☐	☐	☐
22. Provides radiation protection (shield) for the patient, self, and others (closes doors).	☐	☐	☐	☐	☐	☐
23. Applies proper collimation and makes adjustments as necessary.	☐	☐	☐	☐	☐	☐
24. Properly measures the patient along the course of the central ray *for each projection.*	☐	☐	☐	☐	☐	☐

	Procedure		Repeat		Competency	
	Yes	No	Yes	No	Yes	No
25. Sets the proper exposure techniques:	☐	☐	☐	☐	☐	☐

Conventional systems
- Sets the proper kVp, mA, and time, and makes adjustments as necessary.

or

CR or DR systems
- Identifies the patient on the work-list (or manually types the patient information into the system).
- Selects appropriate body region, specific body part, and accurate view/ projection.
- Double-checks preset parameters:
  —Adult vs. pediatric patients
    ◦ Small, medium, or large
  —Bucky/receptor (upright vs. table) *or* non-Bucky
  —AEC vs. fixed
    ◦ If AEC, checks ion chambers
    ◦ Density setting
  —kVp and mA; adjusts if necessary
  —Focal spot/filament size

	Procedure		Repeat		Competency	
26. Exposes the cassette/receptor after telling the patient to hold still and after giving the patient proper breathing instructions (if necessary) *for each projection.*	☐	☐	☐	☐	☐	☐
27. Provides each radiograph with the proper identification (flash) and/or processes each cassette (image) without difficulty (regardless of technology—film, CR, or DR).	■	■	■	■	☐	☐
28. Properly completes the examination by filling out all necessary paperwork, entering the examination in the computer, having the images checked by the appropriate staff members, and informing the patient that he or she is finished.	■	■	■	■	☐	☐
29. Exhibits the ability to adapt to new and difficult situations if and when necessary.	■	■	■	■	☐	☐
30. Accepts constructive criticism and uses it to his or her advantage.	☐	☐	☐	☐	☐	☐
31. Leaves the radiographic room neat and clean for the next examination.	■	■	■	■	☐	☐
32. Completes the examination within a reasonable time frame.	☐	☐	☐	☐	☐	☐

Comments:

_____

_____

RADIOGRAPHIC IMAGE QUALITY
The student is able to critique his or her radiographs as to whether they demonstrate:

	Procedure		Repeat		Competency	
	Yes	No	Yes	No	Yes	No
33. Proper technique/optimal density	■	■	■	■	☐	☐
34. Enhanced detail, without evidence of motion and without any visible artifacts	■	■	■	■	☐	☐
35. Proper positioning (all anatomy included, evidence of proper centering/ alignment, etc.)	■	■	■	■	☐	☐
36. Proper marker placement	■	■	■	■	☐	☐
37. Evidence of proper collimation and radiation protection	■	■	■	■	☐	☐
38. Long vs. short scale of contrast	■	■	■	■	☐	☐

(continued)

Comments:

_____

_____

PEDIATRIC UPPER EXTREMITY ANATOMY
The student is able to identify:

	Procedure		Repeat		Competency	
	Yes	No	Yes	No	Yes	No
39. _____	☐	☐	☐	☐	☐	☐
40. _____	☐	☐	☐	☐	☐	☐
41. _____	☐	☐	☐	☐	☐	☐
42. _____	☐	☐	☐	☐	☐	☐
43. _____	☐	☐	☐	☐	☐	☐
44. _____	☐	☐	☐	☐	☐	☐
45. _____	☐	☐	☐	☐	☐	☐
46. Obvious pathology	☐	☐	☐	☐	☐	☐

Comments:

_____

_____

_____ _____ _____
Procedure Evaluator Signature   Repeat Evaluator Signature   Competency Evaluator Signature

_____ _____ _____
Date   Date   Date

END PEDIATRIC UPPER EXTREMITY (AGE 6 OR YOUNGER) EVALUATION

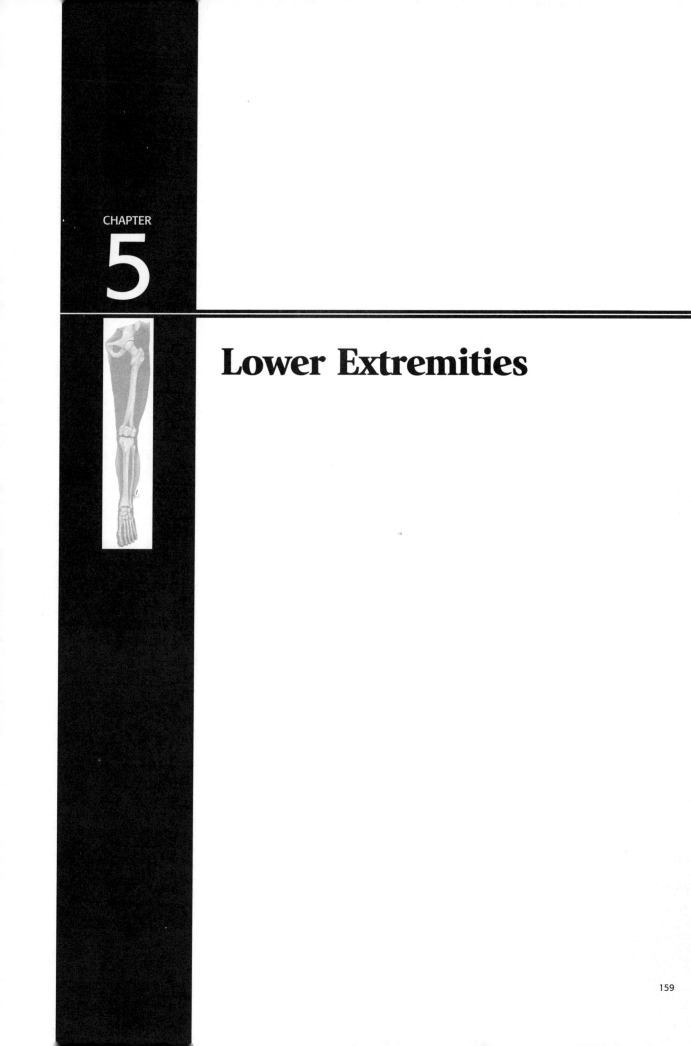

CHAPTER

5

Lower Extremities

159

Toe

The objective of this evaluation is to determine the student's competency level when performing specific radiographic examinations.

Student Name:_____

Procedure Grade	Repeat Grade	Competency Grade

PATIENT INFORMATION OR SIMULATED PROCEDURE *(circle if simulated)*

	Procedure	Repeat	Competency
Age			
Medical Record No.			
Ability to Cooperate			
Condition/Pathology			
Technical Factors Used			
Exposure Index			

FACILITY PREPARATION
The student:

	Procedure Yes	No	Repeat Yes	No	Competency Yes	No
1. Examines the radiographic room and cleans/straightens it before escorting the patient in.	☐	☐	☐	☐	☐	☐
2. Has all equipment and supplies (patient gown, shield, markers, lead blockers, etc.) readily available before escorting the patient in.	☐	☐	☐	☐	☐	☐
3. Is able to manipulate all radiographic equipment with ease, and centers the central ray to cassette/receptor *for all projections.*	☐	☐	☐	☐	☐	☐
4. Adjusts the tube to the proper SID *for each projection.*	☐	☐	☐	☐	☐	☐
5. Selects cassette/receptor of the appropriate sizes *for all projections,* according to patient size and examination.	☐	☐	☐	☐	☐	☐

Comments:

_____

_____

PATIENT PREPARATION
The student:

	Procedure Yes	No	Repeat Yes	No	Competency Yes	No
6. Identifies the correct patient and examination according to the requisition while establishing a good rapport with him or her.	☐	☐	☐	☐	☐	☐
7. Obtains and documents the patient's history before the examination.	☐	☐	☐	☐	☐	☐
8. Explains the examination in terms the patient fully understands and properly communicates with the patient throughout the examination.	☐	☐	☐	☐	☐	☐
9. Asks female patients of childbearing age the date of their last menstrual period and documents this; inquires about the possibility of pregnancy and has them sign pregnancy consent forms.	☐	☐	☐	☐	☐	☐
10. Removes all obscuring objects (shoes, zippers, belts, etc.) so as *not* to produce radiographic artifacts.	☐	☐	☐	☐	☐	☐

(continued)

	Procedure		Repeat		Competency	
	Yes	No	Yes	No	Yes	No
11. Respects the patient's modesty and provides ample comfort for him or her.	☐	☐	☐	☐	☐	☐

Comments:

_____

_____

PATIENT POSITIONING FOR A TOE

Anteroposterior
The student:

	Procedure		Repeat		Competency	
	Yes	No	Yes	No	Yes	No
12. If using conventional film, divides the cassette into appropriate sections with lead blockers.	☐	☐	☐	☐	☐	☐
13. Instructs the patient to flex his or her knee and flatten his or her foot as much as possible.	☐	☐	☐	☐	☐	☐
14. Places the sole of the foot on the appropriate area of the cassette/receptor.	☐	☐	☐	☐	☐	☐
15. Centers the anatomy of interest to the center of the cassette/receptor.	☐	☐	☐	☐	☐	☐
16. Centers the central ray perpendicularly to the metatarsophalangeal joint or to open the joint space, angles the central ray 15° cephalad/posteriorly.	☐	☐	☐	☐	☐	☐

Oblique
The student:

	Procedure		Repeat		Competency	
	Yes	No	Yes	No	Yes	No
17. If using conventional film, adjusts the lead blockers to divide the cassette appropriately.	☐	☐	☐	☐	☐	☐
18. Instructs the patient to keep his or her foot as straight and flat as possible.	☐	☐	☐	☐	☐	☐
19. Using a wedge sponge and immobilization devices if necessary, rotates the foot internally or externally 30°, as appropriate, on the appropriate area of the cassette/receptor.	☐	☐	☐	☐	☐	☐
20. Centers the anatomy of interest to the center of the cassette/receptor.	☐	☐	☐	☐	☐	☐
21. Centers the central ray perpendicularly to the metatarsophalangeal joint.	☐	☐	☐	☐	☐	☐

Lateral
The student:

	Procedure		Repeat		Competency	
	Yes	No	Yes	No	Yes	No
22. If using conventional film, adjusts the lead blockers to divide the cassette appropriately.	☐	☐	☐	☐	☐	☐
23. Instructs the patient to keep his or her foot as straight as possible and immobilizes other toes out of the way of the toe of interest.	☐	☐	☐	☐	☐	☐
24. Rotates the foot 90°, or until it is in the true lateral position on the appropriate area of the cassette/receptor, keeping it parallel with the cassette/receptor.	☐	☐	☐	☐	☐	☐
25. Centers the anatomy of interest to the center of the cassette/receptor.	☐	☐	☐	☐	☐	☐
26. Centers the central ray perpendicularly to the proximal interphalangeal (PIP) joint (or the metatarsophalangeal joint, for the great toe).	☐	☐	☐	☐	☐	☐

Comments:

_____

_____

IMPORTANT DETAILS
The student:

	Procedure		Repeat		Competency	
	Yes	No	Yes	No	Yes	No
27. Instills confidence in the patient by exhibiting self-confidence throughout the examination.	☐	☐	☐	☐	☐	☐
28. Places a lead marker in the appropriate area of the cassette/receptor (top/bottom/anteriorly/laterally), where it will be visualized on the finished radiograph, on the proper anatomical side (right/left), and in the appropriate position (face up/face down), depending on the patient's position.	☐	☐	☐	☐	☐	☐
29. Provides radiation protection (shield) for the patient, self, and others (closes doors).	☐	☐	☐	☐	☐	☐
30. Applies proper collimation and makes adjustments as necessary.	☐	☐	☐	☐	☐	☐
31. Properly measures the patient along the course of the central ray *for each projection.*	☐	☐	☐	☐	☐	☐
32. Sets the proper exposure techniques:	☐	☐	☐	☐	☐	☐

Conventional systems
- Sets the proper kVp, mA, and time, and makes adjustments as necessary.

or

CR or DR systems
- Identifies the patient on the work-list (or manually types the patient information into the system).
- Selects appropriate body region, specific body part, and accurate view/ projection.
- Double-checks preset parameters:
  —Adult vs. pediatric patients
    ◦ Small, medium, or large
  —Bucky/receptor (upright vs. table) *or* non-Bucky
  —AEC vs. fixed
    ◦ If AEC, checks ion chambers
    ◦ Density setting
  —kVp and mA; adjusts if necessary
  —Focal spot/filament size

	Procedure		Repeat		Competency	
33. Exposes the cassette/receptor after telling the patient to hold still *for each projection.*	☐	☐	☐	☐	☐	☐
34. Provides each radiograph with the proper identification (flash) and/or processes each cassette (image) without difficulty (regardless of technology—film, CR, or DR).	▦	▦	▦	▦	☐	☐
35. Properly completes the examination by filling out all necessary paperwork, entering the examination in the computer, having the images checked by the appropriate staff members, answering any last-minute questions, and informing the patient that he or she is finished.	▦	▦	▦	▦	☐	☐
36. Exhibits the ability to adapt to new and difficult situations if and when necessary.	▦	▦	▦	▦	☐	☐
37. Accepts constructive criticism and uses it to his or her advantage.	☐	☐	☐	☐	☐	☐
38. Leaves the radiographic room neat and clean for the next examination.	▦	▦	▦	▦	☐	☐
39. Completes the examination within a reasonable time frame.	☐	☐	☐	☐	☐	☐

Comments:

_____

_____

(continued)

RADIOGRAPHIC IMAGE QUALITY
The student is able to critique his or her radiographs as to whether they demonstrate:

	Procedure		Repeat		Competency	
	Yes	No	Yes	No	Yes	No
40. Proper technique/optimal density	☐	☐	☐	☐	☐	☐
41. Enhanced detail, without evidence of motion and without any visible artifacts	☐	☐	☐	☐	☐	☐
42. Proper positioning (all anatomy included, evidence of proper centering/alignment, etc.)	☐	☐	☐	☐	☐	☐
43. Proper marker placement	☐	☐	☐	☐	☐	☐
44. Evidence of proper collimation and radiation protection	☐	☐	☐	☐	☐	☐
45. Long vs. short scale of contrast	☐	☐	☐	☐	☐	☐

Comments:

_____

_____

TOE ANATOMY
The student is able to identify:

	Procedure		Repeat		Competency	
	Yes	No	Yes	No	Yes	No
46. Distal phalanx	☐	☐	☐	☐	☐	☐
47. Medial phalanx	☐	☐	☐	☐	☐	☐
48. Proximal phalanx	☐	☐	☐	☐	☐	☐
49. Distal interphalangeal joint	☐	☐	☐	☐	☐	☐
50. PIP joint	☐	☐	☐	☐	☐	☐
51. Metatarsophalangeal joint	☐	☐	☐	☐	☐	☐
52. Obvious pathology	☐	☐	☐	☐	☐	☐

Comments:

_____

_____

Procedure Evaluator Signature	Repeat Evaluator Signature	Competency Evaluator Signature
Date	Date	Date

END TOE EVALUATION

Sesamoids

The objective of this evaluation is to determine the student's competency level when performing specific radiographic examinations.

Student Name:_____

Procedure Grade	Repeat Grade	Competency Grade

PATIENT INFORMATION OR SIMULATED PROCEDURE *(circle if simulated)*

	Procedure	Repeat	Competency
Age			
Medical Record No.			
Ability to Cooperate			
Condition/Pathology			
Technical Factors Used			
Exposure Index			

FACILITY PREPARATION
The student:

	Procedure Yes No	Repeat Yes No	Competency Yes No
1. Examines the radiographic room and cleans/straightens it before escorting the patient in.	☐ ☐	☐ ☐	☐ ☐
2. Has all equipment and supplies (patient gown, shield, markers, lead blockers, etc.) readily available before escorting the patient in.	☐ ☐	☐ ☐	☐ ☐
3. Is able to manipulate all radiographic equipment with ease, and centers the central ray to cassette/receptor.	☐ ☐	☐ ☐	☐ ☐
4. Adjusts the tube to the proper SID.	☐ ☐	☐ ☐	☐ ☐
5. Selects a cassette/receptor of the appropriate size.	☐ ☐	☐ ☐	☐ ☐

Comments:

_____

_____

PATIENT PREPARATION
The student:

	Procedure Yes No	Repeat Yes No	Competency Yes No
6. Identifies the correct patient and examination according to the requisition while establishing a good rapport with him or her.	☐ ☐	☐ ☐	☐ ☐
7. Obtains and documents the patient's history before the examination.	☐ ☐	☐ ☐	☐ ☐
8. Explains the examination in terms the patient fully understands and properly communicates with the patient throughout the examination.	☐ ☐	☐ ☐	☐ ☐
9. Asks female patients of childbearing age the date of their last menstrual period and documents this; inquires about the possibility of pregnancy and has them sign pregnancy consent forms.	☐ ☐	☐ ☐	☐ ☐
10. Removes all obscuring objects (shoes, zippers, belts, etc.) so as *not* to produce radiographic artifacts.	☐ ☐	☐ ☐	☐ ☐
11. Respects the patient's modesty and provides ample comfort for him or her.	☐ ☐	☐ ☐	☐ ☐

(continued)

Comments:

_____

_____

PATIENT POSITIONING FOR THE SESAMOID BONES OF A FOOT, USING A TANGENTIAL PROJECTION/THE LEWIS METHOD

The student:

	Procedure		Repeat		Competency	
	Yes	No	Yes	No	Yes	No
12. Places the patient in the prone position on the radiographic table.	☐	☐	☐	☐	☐	☐
13. Asks the patient to rest his or her great toe on the table in a dorsiflexed position so that the ball of the foot is perpendicular to the table.	☐	☐	☐	☐	☐	☐
14. Adjusts the position to avoid added rotation of the entire foot.	☐	☐	☐	☐	☐	☐
15. Centers the second metatarsal to the center of the cassette/receptor.	☐	☐	☐	☐	☐	☐
16. Centers the central ray to the second metatarsophalangeal joint.	☐	☐	☐	☐	☐	☐

Comments:

_____

_____

IMPORTANT DETAILS

The student:

	Procedure		Repeat		Competency	
	Yes	No	Yes	No	Yes	No
17. Instills confidence in the patient by exhibiting self-confidence throughout the examination.	☐	☐	☐	☐	☐	☐
18. Places a lead marker in the appropriate area of the cassette/receptor (top/bottom/anteriorly/laterally), where it will be visualized on the finished radiograph, on the proper anatomical side (right/left), and in the appropriate position (face up/face down), depending on the patient's position.	☐	☐	☐	☐	☐	☐
19. Provides radiation protection (shield) for the patient (when appropriate), self, and others (closes doors).	☐	☐	☐	☐	☐	☐
20. Applies proper collimation and makes adjustments as necessary.	☐	☐	☐	☐	☐	☐
21. Properly measures the patient along the course of the central ray.	☐	☐	☐	☐	☐	☐
22. Sets the proper exposure techniques:	☐	☐	☐	☐	☐	☐

Conventional systems
- Sets the proper kVp, mA, and time, and makes adjustments as necessary.

or

CR or DR systems
- Identifies the patient on the work-list (or manually types the patient information into the system).
- Selects appropriate body region, specific body part, and accurate view/projection.
- Double-checks preset parameters:
  —Adult vs. pediatric patients
   ○ Small, medium, or large
  —Bucky/receptor (upright vs. table) *or* non-Bucky
  —AEC vs. fixed
   ○ If AEC, checks ion chambers
   ○ Density setting
  —kVp and mA; adjusts if necessary
  —Focal spot/filament size

23. Exposes the cassette/receptor after telling the patient to hold still *for each projection.*	☐	☐	☐	☐	☐	☐

	Procedure		Repeat		Competency	
	Yes	No	Yes	No	Yes	No
24. Provides each radiograph with the proper identification (flash) and/or processes each cassette (image) without difficulty (regardless of technology—film, CR, or DR).	■	■	■	■	☐	☐
25. Properly completes the examination by filling out all necessary paperwork, entering the examination in the computer, having the images checked by the appropriate staff members, answering any last-minute questions, and informing the patient that he or she is finished.	■	■	■	■	☐	☐
26. Exhibits the ability to adapt to new and difficult situations if and when necessary.	■	■	■	■	☐	☐
27. Accepts constructive criticism and uses it to his or her advantage.	☐	☐	☐	☐	☐	☐
28. Leaves the radiographic room neat and clean for the next examination.	■	■	■	■	☐	☐
29. Completes the examination within a reasonable time frame.	☐	☐	☐	☐	☐	☐

Comments:

_____

_____

RADIOGRAPHIC IMAGE QUALITY
The student is able to critique his or her radiographs as to whether they demonstrate:

	Procedure		Repeat		Competency	
	Yes	No	Yes	No	Yes	No
30. Proper technique/optimal density	■	■	■	■	☐	☐
31. Enhanced detail, without evidence of motion and without any visible artifacts	■	■	■	■	☐	☐
32. Proper positioning (all anatomy included, evidence of proper centering/ alignment, etc.)	■	■	■	■	☐	☐
33. Proper marker placement	■	■	■	■	☐	☐
34. Evidence of proper collimation and radiation protection	■	■	■	■	☐	☐
35. Long vs. short scale of contrast	■	■	■	■	☐	☐

Comments:

_____

_____

SESAMOID ANATOMY
The student is able to identify:

	Procedure		Repeat		Competency	
	Yes	No	Yes	No	Yes	No
36. Proximal phalanx	■	■	■	■	☐	☐
37. Metatarsal head	■	■	■	■	☐	☐
38. Sesamoids	■	■	■	■	☐	☐
39. Obvious pathology	■	■	■	■	☐	☐

Comments:

_____

_____

_____

Procedure Evaluator Signature Repeat Evaluator Signature Competency Evaluator Signature

_____

Date Date Date

END SESAMOIDS EVALUATION

specific radiographic examinations.

Student Name:_____

Procedure Grade	Repeat Grade	Competency Grade

PATIENT INFORMATION OR SIMULATED PROCEDURE *(circle if simulated)*

	Procedure	Repeat	Competency
Age			
Medical Record No.			
Ability to Cooperate			
Condition/Pathology			
Technical Factors Used			
Exposure Index			

FACILITY PREPARATION
The student:

	Procedure Yes / No	Repeat Yes / No	Competency Yes / No
1. Examines the radiographic room and cleans/straightens it before escorting the patient in.	☐ ☐	☐ ☐	☐ ☐
2. Has all equipment and supplies (patient gown, shield, markers, lead blockers, etc.) readily available before escorting the patient in.	☐ ☐	☐ ☐	☐ ☐
3. Is able to manipulate all radiographic equipment with ease, and centers the central ray to cassette/receptor *for all projections.*	☐ ☐	☐ ☐	☐ ☐
4. Adjusts the tube to the proper SID *for each projection.*	☐ ☐	☐ ☐	☐ ☐
5. Selects cassettes/receptor of the appropriate sizes *for all projections,* . according to patient size and examination.	☐ ☐	☐ ☐	☐ ☐

Comments:

_____

_____

PATIENT PREPARATION
The student:

	Procedure Yes / No	Repeat Yes / No	Competency Yes / No
6. Identifies the correct patient and examination according to the requisition while establishing a good rapport with him or her.	☐ ☐	☐ ☐	☐ ☐
7. Obtains and documents the patient's history before the examination.	▦ ▦	▦ ▦	☐ ☐
8. Explains the examination in terms the patient fully understands and properly communicates with the patient throughout the examination.	☐ ☐	☐ ☐	☐ ☐
9. Asks female patients of childbearing age the date of their last menstrual period and documents this; inquires about the possibility of pregnancy and has them sign pregnancy consent forms.	☐ ☐	☐ ☐	☐ ☐
10. Removes all obscuring objects (shoes, zippers, belts, etc.) so as *not* to produce radiographic artifacts.	☐ ☐	☐ ☐	☐ ☐
11. Respects the patient's modesty and provides ample comfort for him or her.	☐ ☐	☐ ☐	☐ ☐

(continued)

Comments:

_____

_____

PATIENT POSITIONING FOR A FOOT
Anteroposterior
The student:

	Procedure		Repeat		Competency	
	Yes	No	Yes	No	Yes	No
12. If using conventional film, divides the cassette into appropriate sections with lead blockers.	☐	☐	☐	☐	☐	☐
13. Instructs the patient to flex his or her knee and flatten his or her foot as much as possible.	☐	☐	☐	☐	☐	☐
14. Places the sole of the foot on the appropriate area of the cassette/receptor (for conventional cassettes, the flash must be away from any anatomy at the heel).	☐	☐	☐	☐	☐	☐
15. Centers the anatomy of interest to the center of the cassette/receptor.	☐	☐	☐	☐	☐	☐
16. Directs the central ray 0–10° cephalad/posteriorly to the base of the third metatarsal.	☐	☐	☐	☐	☐	☐

Medial Oblique
The student:

	Procedure		Repeat		Competency	
	Yes	No	Yes	No	Yes	No
17. If using conventional film, adjusts the lead blockers to divide the cassette appropriately.	☐	☐	☐	☐	☐	☐
18. Instructs the patient to keep his or her foot as straight and flat as possible.	☐	☐	☐	☐	☐	☐
19. Using a wedge sponge and immobilization devices if necessary, rotates the foot internally 30° on the appropriate area of the cassette/receptor.	☐	☐	☐	☐	☐	☐
20. Centers the anatomy of interest to the center of the cassette/receptor.	☐	☐	☐	☐	☐	☐
21. Centers the central ray perpendicularly to the base of the third metatarsal.	☐	☐	☐	☐	☐	☐

Lateral
The student:

	Procedure		Repeat		Competency	
	Yes	No	Yes	No	Yes	No
22. Selects a new cassette/receptor.	☐	☐	☐	☐	☐	☐
23. While instructing the patient to dorsiflex the foot, reminds the patient to keep his or her foot as straight as possible over the appropriate area of the cassette/receptor.	☐	☐	☐	☐	☐	☐
24. Rotates the foot laterally 90°, or until the plantar surface is perpendicular to the cassette/receptor, while supporting the knee to avoid overrotation.	☐	☐	☐	☐	☐	☐
25. Centers the anatomy of interest to the center of the cassette/receptor.	☐	☐	☐	☐	☐	☐
26. Centers the central ray perpendicularly to the base of the proximal metatarsals.	☐	☐	☐	☐	☐	☐

Comments:

_____

_____

IMPORTANT DETAILS
The student:

	Procedure		Repeat		Competency	
	Yes	No	Yes	No	Yes	No
27. Instills confidence in the patient by exhibiting self-confidence throughout the examination.	☐	☐	☐	☐	☐	☐

	Procedure		Repeat		Competency	
	Yes	No	Yes	No	Yes	No
28. Places a lead marker in the appropriate area of the cassette/receptor (top/bottom/anteriorly/laterally), where it will be visualized on the finished radiograph, on the proper anatomical side (right/left), and in the appropriate position (face up/face down), depending on the patient's position.	☐	☐	☐	☐	☐	☐
29. Provides radiation protection (shield) for the patient (when appropriate), self, and others (closes doors).	☐	☐	☐	☐	☐	☐
30. Applies proper collimation and makes adjustments as necessary.	☐	☐	☐	☐	☐	☐
31. Properly measures the patient along the course of the central ray *for each projection.*	☐	☐	☐	☐	☐	☐
32. Sets the proper exposure techniques:	☐	☐	☐	☐	☐	☐

Conventional systems
- Sets the proper kVp, mA, and time, and makes adjustments as necessary.

or

CR or DR systems
- Identifies the patient on the work-list (or manually types the patient information into the system).
- Selects appropriate body region, specific body part, and accurate view/projection.
- Double-checks preset parameters:
  —Adult vs. pediatric patients
   ◦ Small, medium, or large
  —Bucky/receptor (upright vs. table) *or* non-Bucky
  —AEC vs. fixed
   ◦ If AEC, checks ion chambers
   ◦ Density setting
  —kVp and mA; adjusts if necessary
  —Focal spot/filament size

	Procedure		Repeat		Competency	
33. Exposes the cassette/receptor after telling the patient to hold still *for each projection.*	☐	☐	☐	☐	☐	☐
34. Provides each radiograph with the proper identification (flash) and/or processes each cassette (image) without difficulty (regardless of technology—film, CR, or DR).	▨	▨	▨	▨	☐	☐
35. Properly completes the examination by filling out all necessary paperwork, entering the examination in the computer, having the images checked by the appropriate staff members, answering any last-minute questions, and informing the patient that he or she is finished.	▨	▨	▨	▨	☐	☐
36. Exhibits the ability to adapt to new and difficult situations if and when necessary.	▨	▨	▨	▨	☐	☐
37. Accepts constructive criticism and uses it to his or her advantage.	☐	☐	☐	☐	☐	☐
38. Leaves the radiographic room neat and clean for the next examination.	▨	▨	▨	▨	☐	☐
39. Completes the examination within a reasonable time frame.	☐	☐	☐	☐	☐	☐

Comments:

_____

_____

RADIOGRAPHIC IMAGE QUALITY
The student is able to critique his or her radiographs as to whether they demonstrate:

	Procedure		Repeat		Competency	
	Yes	No	Yes	No	Yes	No
40. Proper technique/optimal density	▨	▨	▨	▨	☐	☐

(continued)

	Procedure		Repeat		Competency	
	Yes	No	Yes	No	Yes	No
41. Enhanced detail, without evidence of motion and without any visible artifacts	☐	☐	☐	☐	☐	☐
42. Proper positioning (all anatomy included, evidence of proper centering/ alignment, etc.)	☐	☐	☐	☐	☐	☐
43. Proper marker placement	☐	☐	☐	☐	☐	☐
44. Evidence of proper collimation and radiation protection	☐	☐	☐	☐	☐	☐
45. Long vs. short scale of contrast	☐	☐	☐	☐	☐	☐

Comments:

_____

_____

FOOT ANATOMY
The student is able to identify:

	Procedure		Repeat		Competency	
	Yes	No	Yes	No	Yes	No
46. Sesamoid bones	☐	☐	☐	☐	☐	☐
47. Distal phalanx	☐	☐	☐	☐	☐	☐
48. Medial phalanx	☐	☐	☐	☐	☐	☐
49. Proximal phalanx	☐	☐	☐	☐	☐	☐
50. Distal interphalangeal joint	☐	☐	☐	☐	☐	☐
51. PIP joint	☐	☐	☐	☐	☐	☐
52. Metatarsals (head vs. base)	☐	☐	☐	☐	☐	☐
53. Metatarsophalangeal joint	☐	☐	☐	☐	☐	☐
54. Tarsometatarsal joint	☐	☐	☐	☐	☐	☐
55. Talus/astragalus	☐	☐	☐	☐	☐	☐
56. Calcaneus/os calcis	☐	☐	☐	☐	☐	☐
57. Navicular/scaphoid	☐	☐	☐	☐	☐	☐
58. Sinus tarsi	☐	☐	☐	☐	☐	☐
59. Cuboid	☐	☐	☐	☐	☐	☐
60. First/internal, middle/second, and external/third cuneiforms	☐	☐	☐	☐	☐	☐
61. Obvious pathology	☐	☐	☐	☐	☐	☐

Comments:

_____

_____

_____
Procedure Evaluator Signature   Repeat Evaluator Signature   Competency Evaluator Signature

_____
Date   Date   Date

END FOOT EVALUATION

Student Name:_____

Procedure Grade	Repeat Grade	Competency Grade

PATIENT INFORMATION OR SIMULATED PROCEDURE *(circle if simulated)*

	Procedure	Repeat	Competency
Age			
Medical Record No.			
Ability to Cooperate			
Condition/Pathology			
Technical Factors Used			
Exposure Index			

FACILITY PREPARATION
The student:

	Procedure Yes No	Repeat Yes No	Competency Yes No
1. Examines the radiographic room and cleans/straightens it before escorting the patient in.	☐ ☐	☐ ☐	☐ ☐
2. Has all equipment and supplies (patient gown, shield, markers, lead blockers, etc.) readily available before escorting the patient in.	☐ ☐	☐ ☐	☐ ☐
3. Is able to manipulate all radiographic equipment with ease, and centers the central ray to cassette/receptor *for both projections.*	☐ ☐	☐ ☐	☐ ☐
4. Adjusts the tube to the proper SID *for each projection.*	☐ ☐	☐ ☐	☐ ☐
5. Selects cassettes/receptor of the appropriate sizes *for both projections, .* according to patient size and examination.	☐ ☐	☐ ☐	☐ ☐

Comments:

_____

_____

PATIENT PREPARATION
The student:

	Procedure Yes No	Repeat Yes No	Competency Yes No
6. Identifies the correct patient and examination according to the requisition while establishing a good rapport with him or her.	☐ ☐	☐ ☐	☐ ☐
7. Obtains and documents the patient's history before the examination.	▣ ▣	▣ ▣	☐ ☐
8. Explains the examination in terms the patient fully understands and properly communicates with the patient throughout the examination.	☐ ☐	☐ ☐	☐ ☐
9. Asks female patients of childbearing age the date of their last menstrual period and documents this; inquires about the possibility of pregnancy and has them sign pregnancy consent forms.	☐ ☐	☐ ☐	☐ ☐
10. Removes all obscuring objects (shoes, zippers, belts, etc.) so as *not* to produce radiographic artifacts.	☐ ☐	☐ ☐	☐ ☐
11. Respects the patient's modesty and provides ample comfort for him or her.	☐ ☐	☐ ☐	☐ ☐

Comments:

(continued)

	Procedure		Repeat		Competency	
	Yes	No	Yes	No	Yes	No

PATIENT POSITIONING FOR A WEIGHT-BEARING AXIAL FOOT
First Exposure for the Forefoot
The student:

	Procedure		Repeat		Competency	
	Yes	No	Yes	No	Yes	No
12. Instructs the patient to stand with the affected foot on the cassette/receptor and with the unaffected foot one step backward, to avoid superimposition of the leg.	☐	☐	☐	☐	☐	☐
13. Centers the anatomy of interest to the center of the cassette/receptor.	☐	☐	☐	☐	☐	☐
14. Directs the central ray from the toes toward the ankle at a 15° angle, centered to the scaphoid/navicular.	☐	☐	☐	☐	☐	☐
15. Before taking the exposure, cautions the patient not to move his or her affected foot until directed to do so.	☐	☐	☐	☐	☐	☐
16. Obtains and documents the appropriate technique for a foot, but to produce good radiographic density, cuts the technique in half since the second projection (with the same factors) will double-expose the cassette (if using conventional film).	☐	☐	☐	☐	☐	☐

Second Exposure for the Calcaneus/Os Calcis
The student:

	Procedure		Repeat		Competency	
	Yes	No	Yes	No	Yes	No
17. Instructs the patient to step forward with the unaffected foot, while keeping the affected foot centered and as still as possible.	☐	☐	☐	☐	☐	☐
18. Directs the central ray from the heel toward the toes at a 25° angle, centered to the posterior surface of the ankle, emerging at the lateral malleolus.	☐	☐	☐	☐	☐	☐

Comments:

IMPORTANT DETAILS
The student:

	Procedure		Repeat		Competency	
	Yes	No	Yes	No	Yes	No
19. Instills confidence in the patient by exhibiting self-confidence throughout the examination.	☐	☐	☐	☐	☐	☐
20. Places a lead marker in the appropriate area of the cassette/receptor (top/bottom/anteriorly/laterally), where it will be visualized on the finished radiograph, on the proper anatomical side (right/left), and in the appropriate position (face up/face down), depending on the patient's position.	☐	☐	☐	☐	☐	☐
21. Provides radiation protection (shield) for the patient (when appropriate), self, and others (closes doors).	☐	☐	☐	☐	☐	☐
22. Applies proper collimation and makes adjustments as necessary.	☐	☐	☐	☐	☐	☐
23. Properly measures the patient along the course of the central ray *for each projection.*	☐	☐	☐	☐	☐	☐
24. Sets the proper exposure techniques:	☐	☐	☐	☐	☐	☐

Conventional systems
• Sets the proper kVp, mA, and time, and makes adjustments as necessary.

or

CR or DR systems

	Procedure		Repeat		Competency	
	Yes	No	Yes	No	Yes	No

- Identifies the patient on the work-list (or manually types the patient information into the system).
- Selects appropriate body region, specific body part, and accurate view/projection.
- Double-checks preset parameters:
  - —Adult vs. pediatric patients
    - ○ Small, medium, or large
  - —Bucky/receptor (upright vs. table) *or* non-Bucky
  - —AEC vs. fixed
    - ○ If AEC, checks ion chambers
    - ○ Density setting
  - —kVp and mA; adjusts if necessary
  - —Focal spot/filament size

	Procedure Yes	Procedure No	Repeat Yes	Repeat No	Competency Yes	Competency No
25. Exposes the cassette/receptor after telling the patient to hold still *for each projection.*	☐	☐	☐	☐	☐	☐
26. Provides each radiograph with the proper identification (flash) and/or processes each cassette (image) without difficulty (regardless of technology—film, CR, or DR).	▨	▨	▨	▨	☐	☐
27. Properly completes the examination by filling out all necessary paperwork, entering the examination in the computer, having the images checked by the appropriate staff members, answering any last-minute questions, and informing the patient that he or she is finished, and showing the patient how to exit.	▨	▨	▨	▨	☐	☐
28. Exhibits the ability to adapt to new and difficult situations if and when necessary.	▨	▨	▨	▨	☐	☐
29. Accepts constructive criticism and uses it to his or her advantage.	☐	☐	☐	☐	☐	☐
30. Leaves the radiographic room neat and clean for the next examination.	▨	▨	▨	▨	☐	☐
31. Completes the examination within a reasonable time frame.	☐	☐	☐	☐	☐	☐

Comments:

RADIOGRAPHIC IMAGE QUALITY

The student is able to critique his or her radiographs as to whether they demonstrate:

	Procedure Yes	Procedure No	Repeat Yes	Repeat No	Competency Yes	Competency No
32. Proper technique/optimal density	▨	▨	▨	▨	☐	☐
33. Enhanced detail, without evidence of motion and without any visible artifacts	▨	▨	▨	▨	☐	☐
34. Proper positioning (all anatomy included, evidence of proper centering/alignment, etc.)	▨	▨	▨	▨	☐	☐
35. Proper marker placement	▨	▨	▨	▨	☐	☐
36. Evidence of proper collimation and radiation protection	▨	▨	▨	▨	☐	☐
37. Long vs. short scale of contrast	▨	▨	▨	▨	☐	☐

Comments:

FOOT ANATOMY

Procedure	Repeat	Competency

(continued)

The student is able to identify:

	Yes	No	Yes	No	Yes	No
38. Sesamoids	☐	☐	☐	☐	☐	☐
39. Distal phalanx	☐	☐	☐	☐	☐	☐
40. Medial phalanx	☐	☐	☐	☐	☐	☐
41. Proximal phalanx	☐	☐	☐	☐	☐	☐
42. Distal interphalangeal joint	☐	☐	☐	☐	☐	☐
43. PIP joint	☐	☐	☐	☐	☐	☐
44. Metatarsals (head vs. base)	☐	☐	☐	☐	☐	☐
45. Metatarsophalangeal joint	☐	☐	☐	☐	☐	☐
46. Tarsometatarsal joint	☐	☐	☐	☐	☐	☐
47. Talus/astragalus	☐	☐	☐	☐	☐	☐
48. Calcaneus/os calcis	☐	☐	☐	☐	☐	☐
49. Navicular/scaphoid	☐	☐	☐	☐	☐	☐
50. Cuboid	☐	☐	☐	☐	☐	☐
51. First/internal, middle/second, and external/third cuneiforms	☐	☐	☐	☐	☐	☐
52. Obvious pathology	☐	☐	☐	☐	☐	☐

Comments:

_____

_____

Procedure Evaluator Signature	Repeat Evaluator Signature	Competency Evaluator Signature
Date	Date	Date

END WEIGHT-BEARING AXIAL FOOT EVALUATION

Student Name:_____

Procedure Grade	Repeat Grade	Competency Grade

PATIENT INFORMATION OR SIMULATED PROCEDURE *(circle if simulated)*

	Procedure	Repeat	Competency
Age			
Medical Record No.			
Ability to Cooperate			
Condition/Pathology			
Technical Factors Used			
Exposure Index			

FACILITY PREPARATION
The student:

	Procedure Yes	No	Repeat Yes	No	Competency Yes	No
1. Examines the radiographic room and cleans/straightens it before escorting the patient in.	☐	☐	☐	☐	☐	☐
2. Has all equipment and supplies (patient gown, shield, markers, lead blockers, etc.) readily available before escorting the patient in.	☐	☐	☐	☐	☐	☐
3. Is able to manipulate all radiographic equipment with ease, and centers the central ray to cassette/receptor.	☐	☐	☐	☐	☐	☐
4. Adjusts the tube to the proper SID.	☐	☐	☐	☐	☐	☐
5. Selects a cassette/receptor of the appropriate size.	☐	☐	☐	☐	☐	☐

Comments:

_____

_____

PATIENT PREPARATION
The student:

	Procedure Yes	No	Repeat Yes	No	Competency Yes	No
6. Identifies the correct patient and examination according to the requisition while establishing a good rapport with him or her.	☐	☐	☐	☐	☐	☐
7. Obtains and documents the patient's history before the examination.	■	■	■	■	☐	☐
8. Explains the examination in terms the patient fully understands and properly communicates with the patient throughout the examination.	☐	☐	☐	☐	☐	☐
9. Asks female patients of childbearing age the date of their last menstrual period and documents this; inquires about the possibility of pregnancy and has them sign pregnancy consent forms.	☐	☐	☐	☐	☐	☐
10. Removes all obscuring objects (shoes, zippers, belts, etc.) so as *not* to produce radiographic artifacts.	☐	☐	☐	☐	☐	☐
11. Respects the patient's modesty and provides ample comfort for him or her.	☐	☐	☐	☐	☐	☐

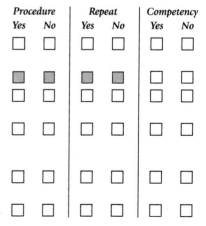

(continued)

Comments:

_____

_____

PATIENT POSITIONING FOR A WEIGHT-BEARING LATERAL FOOT FOR A LONGITUDINAL ARCH
The student:

	Procedure		Repeat		Competency	
	Yes	No	Yes	No	Yes	No
12. Instructs the patient to stand with his or her weight evenly distributed and with cassette/receptor below the plantar surface of the affected foot.	☐	☐	☐	☐	☐	☐
13. Places the cassette/receptor in a vertical position next to the medial surface of the foot.	☐	☐	☐	☐	☐	☐
14. Centers the foot to the appropriate area of the cassette/receptor.	☐	☐	☐	☐	☐	☐
15. Directs the central ray perpendicularly to a point just above the base of the fifth metatarsal.	☐	☐	☐	☐	☐	☐

Comments:

_____

_____

IMPORTANT DETAILS
The student:

	Procedure		Repeat		Competency	
	Yes	No	Yes	No	Yes	No
16. Instills confidence in the patient by exhibiting self-confidence throughout the examination.	☐	☐	☐	☐	☐	☐
17. Places a lead marker in the appropriate area of the cassette/receptor (top/bottom/anteriorly/laterally), where it will be visualized on the finished radiograph, on the proper anatomical side (right/left), and in the appropriate position (face up/face down), depending on the patient's position.	☐	☐	☐	☐	☐	☐
18. Provides radiation protection (shield) for the patient (when appropriate), self, and others (closes doors).	☐	☐	☐	☐	☐	☐
19. Applies proper collimation and makes adjustments as necessary.	☐	☐	☐	☐	☐	☐
20. Properly measures the patient along the course of the central ray.	☐	☐	☐	☐	☐	☐
21. Sets the proper exposure techniques:	☐	☐	☐	☐	☐	☐

Conventional systems
- Sets the proper kVp, mA, and time, and makes adjustments as necessary.

or

CR or DR systems
- Identifies the patient on the work-list (or manually types the patient information into the system).
- Selects appropriate body region, specific body part, and accurate view/projection.
- Double-checks preset parameters:
  —Adult vs. pediatric patients
    ○ Small, medium, or large
  —Bucky/receptor (upright vs. table) *or* non-Bucky
  —AEC vs. fixed
    ○ If AEC, checks ion chambers
    ○ Density setting
  —kVp and mA; adjusts if necessary
  —Focal spot/filament size

	Procedure		Repeat		Competency	
22. Exposes the cassette/receptor after telling the patient to hold still *for each projection.*	☐	☐	☐	☐	☐	☐

	Procedure		Repeat		Competency	
	Yes	No	Yes	No	Yes	No
23. Provides each radiograph with the proper identification (flash) and/or processes each cassette (image) without difficulty (regardless of technology—film, CR, or DR).	☐	☐	☐	☐	☐	☐
24. Properly completes the examination by filling out all necessary paperwork, entering the examination in the computer, having the images checked by the appropriate staff members, answering any last-minute questions, and informing the patient that he or she is finished, and showing the patient how to exit.	☐	☐	☐	☐	☐	☐
25. Exhibits the ability to adapt to new and difficult situations if and when necessary.	☐	☐	☐	☐	☐	☐
26. Accepts constructive criticism and uses it to his or her advantage.	☐	☐	☐	☐	☐	☐
27. Leaves the radiographic room neat and clean for the next examination.	☐	☐	☐	☐	☐	☐
28. Completes the examination within a reasonable time frame.	☐	☐	☐	☐	☐	☐

Comments:

_____

_____

RADIOGRAPHIC IMAGE QUALITY

The student is able to critique his or her radiographs as to whether they demonstrate:

	Procedure		Repeat		Competency	
	Yes	No	Yes	No	Yes	No
29. Proper technique/optimal density	☐	☐	☐	☐	☐	☐
30. Enhanced detail, without evidence of motion and without any visible artifacts	☐	☐	☐	☐	☐	☐
31. Proper positioning (all anatomy included, evidence of proper centering/ alignment, etc.)	☐	☐	☐	☐	☐	☐
32. Proper marker placement	☐	☐	☐	☐	☐	☐
33. Evidence of proper collimation and radiation protection	☐	☐	☐	☐	☐	☐
34. Long vs. short scale of contrast	☐	☐	☐	☐	☐	☐

Comments:

_____

FOOT ANATOMY

The student is able to identify:

	Procedure		Repeat		Competency	
	Yes	No	Yes	No	Yes	No
35. Distal phalanx	☐	☐	☐	☐	☐	☐
36. Proximal phalanx	☐	☐	☐	☐	☐	☐
37. Distal interphalangeal joint	☐	☐	☐	☐	☐	☐
38. PIP joint	☐	☐	☐	☐	☐	☐
39. Metatarsals (base vs. head)	☐	☐	☐	☐	☐	☐
40. Metatarsophalangeal joint	☐	☐	☐	☐	☐	☐
41. Tarsometatarsal joint	☐	☐	☐	☐	☐	☐
42. Navicular/scaphoid	☐	☐	☐	☐	☐	☐
43. Talus/astragalus	☐	☐	☐	☐	☐	☐
44. Calcaneus/os calcis	☐	☐	☐	☐	☐	☐
45. Sinus tarsi	☐	☐	☐	☐	☐	☐
46. Superimposed cuneiforms	☐	☐	☐	☐	☐	☐

(continued)

	Procedure		Repeat		Competency	
	Yes	No	Yes	No	Yes	No
47. Longitudinal arch	☐	☐	☐	☐	☐	☐
48. Obvious pathology	☐	☐	☐	☐	☐	☐

Comments:

_____

_____

_____   _____   _____
Procedure Evaluator Signature   Repeat Evaluator Signature   Competency Evaluator Signature

_____   _____   _____
Date   Date   Date

END WEIGHT-BEARING LATERAL FOOT EVALUATION

Student Name:_____

Procedure Grade	Repeat Grade	Competency Grade

PATIENT INFORMATION OR SIMULATED PROCEDURE *(circle if simulated)*

	Procedure	Repeat	Competency
Age			
Medical Record No.			
Ability to Cooperate			
Condition/Pathology			
Technical Factors Used			
Exposure Index			

FACILITY PREPARATION
The student:

	Procedure Yes No	Repeat Yes No	Competency Yes No
1. Examines the radiographic room and cleans/straightens it before escorting the patient in.	☐ ☐	☐ ☐	☐ ☐
2. Has all equipment and supplies (patient gown, shield, markers, lead blockers, etc.) readily available before escorting the patient in.	☐ ☐	☐ ☐	☐ ☐
3. Is able to manipulate all radiographic equipment with ease, and centers the central ray to cassette/receptor *for both projections.*	☐ ☐	☐ ☐	☐ ☐
4. Adjusts the tube to the proper SID *for each projection.*	☐ ☐	☐ ☐	☐ ☐
5. Selects cassettes/receptor of the appropriate sizes *for both projections,* according to patient size and examination.	☐ ☐	☐ ☐	☐ ☐

Comments:

_____

_____

PATIENT PREPARATION
The student:

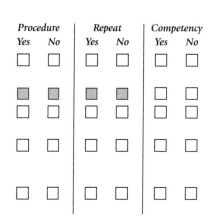

	Procedure Yes No	Repeat Yes No	Competency Yes No
6. Identifies the correct patient and examination according to the requisition while establishing a good rapport with him or her.	☐ ☐	☐ ☐	☐ ☐
7. Obtains and documents the patient's history before the examination.	▨ ▨	▨ ▨	☐ ☐
8. Explains the examination in terms the patient fully understands and properly communicates with the patient throughout the examination.	☐ ☐	☐ ☐	☐ ☐
9. Asks female patients of childbearing age the date of their last menstrual period and documents this; inquires about the possibility of pregnancy and has them sign pregnancy consent forms.	☐ ☐	☐ ☐	☐ ☐
10. Removes all obscuring objects (shoes, zippers, belts, etc.) so as *not* to produce radiographic artifacts.	☐ ☐	☐ ☐	☐ ☐

(continued)

	Procedure		Repeat		Competency	
	Yes	No	Yes	No	Yes	No
11. Respects the patient's modesty and provides ample comfort for him or her.	☐	☐	☐	☐	☐	☐

Comments:

_____

_____

PATIENT POSITIONING FOR AN OS CALCIS
Axial/Plantodorsal
The student:

	Procedure		Repeat		Competency	
	Yes	No	Yes	No	Yes	No
12. If using conventional film, divides the cassette into appropriate sections with lead blockers.	☐	☐	☐	☐	☐	☐
13. Instructs the patient to extend the knees and places the posterior surface of the heel on the appropriate area of the cassette/receptor.	☐	☐	☐	☐	☐	☐
14. Dorsiflexes the foot and places the plantar surface of the foot perpendicular to the cassette/receptor, without rotation, using immobilization devices if necessary.	☐	☐	☐	☐	☐	☐
15. Centers the anatomy of interest to the center of the cassette/receptor.	☐	☐	☐	☐	☐	☐
16. Directs the central ray at an angle of 40° cephalad, entering the base of the third metatarsal and exiting just proximal to the ankle joint.	☐	☐	☐	☐	☐	☐

Lateral
The student:

	Procedure		Repeat		Competency	
	Yes	No	Yes	No	Yes	No
17. If using conventional film, adjusts the lead blockers to divide the cassette appropriately.	☐	☐	☐	☐	☐	☐
18. While keeping the foot dorsiflexed, reminds the patient to keep his or her foot as straight as possible over the appropriate area of the cassette/receptor.	☐	☐	☐	☐	☐	☐
19. While flexing the patient's knee, rotates the ankle laterally 90°, or until the plantar surface of the foot is perpendicular to the cassette/receptor, while supporting the knee to avoid overrotation.	☐	☐	☐	☐	☐	☐
20. Centers the anatomy of interest to the center of the cassette/receptor.	☐	☐	☐	☐	☐	☐
21. Centers the central ray perpendicularly to the mid-os calcis/calcaneus, including the ankle joint and adjacent tarsal bones.	☐	☐	☐	☐	☐	☐

Comments:

_____

_____

IMPORTANT DETAILS
The student:

	Procedure		Repeat		Competency	
	Yes	No	Yes	No	Yes	No
22. Instills confidence in the patient by exhibiting self-confidence throughout the examination.	☐	☐	☐	☐	☐	☐
23. Places a lead marker in the appropriate area of the cassette/receptor (top/bottom/anteriorly/laterally), where it will be visualized on the finished radiograph, on the proper anatomical side (right/left), and in the appropriate position (face up/face down), depending on the patient's position.	☐	☐	☐	☐	☐	☐
24. Provides radiation protection (shield) for the patient (when appropriate), self, and others (closes doors).	☐	☐	☐	☐	☐	☐
25. Applies proper collimation and makes adjustments as necessary.	☐	☐	☐	☐	☐	☐

	Procedure		Repeat		Competency	
	Yes	No	Yes	No	Yes	No
26. Properly measures the patient along the course of the central ray *for each projection.*	☐	☐	☐	☐	☐	☐
27. Sets the proper exposure techniques:	☐	☐	☐	☐	☐	☐

Conventional systems
- Sets the proper kVp, mA, and time, and makes adjustments as necessary.

or

CR or DR systems
- Identifies the patient on the work-list (or manually types the patient information into the system).
- Selects appropriate body region, specific body part, and accurate view/projection.
- Double-checks preset parameters:
  —Adult vs. pediatric patients
  ○ Small, medium, or large
  —Bucky/receptor (upright vs. table) *or* non-Bucky
  —AEC vs. fixed
  ○ If AEC, checks ion chambers
  ○ Density setting
  —kVp and mA; adjusts if necessary
  —Focal spot/filament size

	Procedure		Repeat		Competency	
28. Exposes the cassette/receptor after telling the patient to hold still *for each projection.*	☐	☐	☐	☐	☐	☐
29. Provides each radiograph with the proper identification (flash) and/or processes each cassette (image) without difficulty (regardless of technology—film, CR, or DR).	▣	▣	▣	▣	☐	☐
30. Properly completes the examination by filling out all necessary paperwork, entering the examination in the computer, having the images checked by the appropriate staff members, answering any last-minute questions, and informing the patient that he or she is finished, and showing the patient how to exit.	▣	▣	▣	▣	☐	☐
31. Exhibits the ability to adapt to new and difficult situations if and when necessary.	▣	▣	▣	▣	☐	☐
32. Accepts constructive criticism and uses it to his or her advantage.	☐	☐	☐	☐	☐	☐
33. Leaves the radiographic room neat and clean for the next examination.	▣	▣	▣	▣	☐	☐
34. Completes the examination within a reasonable time frame.	☐	☐	☐	☐	☐	☐

Comments:

_____

_____

RADIOGRAPHIC IMAGE QUALITY

The student is able to critique his or her radiographs as to whether they demonstrate:

	Procedure		Repeat		Competency	
	Yes	No	Yes	No	Yes	No
35. Proper technique/optimal density	▣	▣	▣	▣	☐	☐
36. Enhanced detail, without evidence of motion and without any visible artifacts	▣	▣	▣	▣	☐	☐
37. Proper positioning (all anatomy included, evidence of proper centering/alignment, etc.)	▣	▣	▣	▣	☐	☐
38. Proper marker placement	▣	▣	▣	▣	☐	☐
39. Evidence of proper collimation and radiation protection	▣	▣	▣	▣	☐	☐
40. Long vs. short scale of contrast	▣	▣	▣	▣	☐	☐

(continued)

Comments:

_____

_____

OS CALCIS ANATOMY
The student is able to identify:

	Procedure		Repeat		Competency	
	Yes	No	Yes	No	Yes	No
41. Sustentaculum tali	☐	☐	☐	☐	☐	☐
42. Trochlear process	☐	☐	☐	☐	☐	☐
43. Lateral process	☐	☐	☐	☐	☐	☐
44. Tuberosity	☐	☐	☐	☐	☐	☐
45. Sinus tarsi	☐	☐	☐	☐	☐	☐
46. Talus/astragalus	☐	☐	☐	☐	☐	☐
47. Navicular/scaphoid	☐	☐	☐	☐	☐	☐
48. Obvious pathology	☐	☐	☐	☐	☐	☐

Comments:

_____

_____

Procedure Evaluator Signature	Repeat Evaluator Signature	Competency Evaluator Signature

Date	Date	Date

END CALCANEUS (OS CALCIS) EVALUATION

Student Name:_____

Procedure Grade	Repeat Grade	Competency Grade

PATIENT INFORMATION OR SIMULATED PROCEDURE *(circle if simulated)*

	Procedure	Repeat	Competency
Age			
Medical Record No.			
Ability to Cooperate			
Condition/Pathology			
Technical Factors Used			
Exposure Index			

FACILITY PREPARATION
The student:

	Procedure		Repeat		Competency	
	Yes	No	Yes	No	Yes	No
1. Examines the radiographic room and cleans/straightens it before escorting the patient in.	☐	☐	☐	☐	☐	☐
2. Has all equipment and supplies (patient gown, shield, markers, lead blockers, etc.) readily available before escorting the patient in.	☐	☐	☐	☐	☐	☐
3. Is able to manipulate all radiographic equipment with ease, and centers the central ray to cassette/receptor *for all projections.*	☐	☐		☐	☐	☐
4. Adjusts the tube to the proper SID *for each projection.*	☐	☐	☐	☐	☐	☐
5. Selects cassettes/receptor of the appropriate sizes *for all projections,* according to patient size and examination.	☐	☐	☐	☐	☐	☐

Comments:

_____

_____

PATIENT PREPARATION
The student:

	Procedure		Repeat		Competency	
	Yes	No	Yes	No	Yes	No
6. Identifies the correct patient and examination according to the requisition while establishing a good rapport with him or her.	☐	☐	☐	☐	☐	☐
7. Obtains and documents the patient's history before the examination.	▣	▣	▣	▣	☐	☐
8. Explains the examination in terms the patient fully understands and properly communicates with the patient throughout the examination.	☐	☐	☐	☐	☐	☐
9. Asks female patients of childbearing age the date of their last menstrual period and documents this; inquires about the possibility of pregnancy and has them sign pregnancy consent forms.	☐	☐	☐	☐	☐	☐
10. Removes all obscuring objects (shoes, zippers, belts, etc.) so as *not* to produce radiographic artifacts.	☐	☐	☐	☐	☐	☐

(continued)

	Procedure		Repeat		Competency	
	Yes	No	Yes	No	Yes	No
11. Respects the patient's modesty and provides ample comfort for him or her.	☐	☐	☐	☐	☐	☐

Comments:

_____

_____

PATIENT POSITIONING FOR AN ANKLE
Anteroposterior
The student:

	Procedure		Repeat		Competency	
	Yes	No	Yes	No	Yes	No
12. If using conventional film, divides the cassette into appropriate sections with lead blockers.	☐	☐	☐	☐	☐	☐
13. Instructs the patient to extend the knees and places the posterior surface of the ankle on the appropriate area of the cassette/receptor.	☐	☐	☐	☐	☐	☐
14. Places the posterior surface of the ankle against the cassette/receptor and dorsiflexes the foot while internally rotating the leg 5-7°.	☐	☐	☐	☐	☐	☐
15. Centers the anatomy of interest to the center of the cassette/receptor.	☐	☐	☐	☐	☐	☐
16. Centers the central ray perpendicularly to the ankle joint (between the malleoli).	☐	☐	☐	☐	☐	☐

Lateral
The student:

	Procedure		Repeat		Competency	
	Yes	No	Yes	No	Yes	No
17. If using conventional film, adjusts the lead blockers to divide the cassette appropriately.	☐	☐	☐	☐	☐	☐
18. While keeping the foot dorsiflexed, reminds the patient to keep his or her foot as straight as possible over the appropriate area of the cassette/receptor.	☐	☐	☐	☐	☐	☐
19. Rotates the leg 90°, or until the plantar surface of the foot is perpendicular to the cassette/receptor, while supporting the knee to avoid overrotation.	☐	☐	☐	☐	☐	☐
20. Centers the anatomy of interest to the center of the cassette/receptor.	☐	☐	☐	☐	☐	☐
21. Centers the central ray perpendicularly to the medial malleolus.	☐	☐	☐	☐	☐	☐

Medial/Internal Oblique
The student:

	Procedure		Repeat		Competency	
	Yes	No	Yes	No	Yes	No
22. If using conventional film, selects a new cassette and divides it into appropriate sections with lead blockers.	☐	☐	☐	☐	☐	☐
23. Rotates the entire leg 45° medially/internally on the appropriate area of the cassette/receptor (or 15–20° specifically for the ankle mortise).	☐	☐	☐	☐	☐	☐
24. Centers the anatomy of interest to the center of the cassette/receptor.	☐	☐	☐	☐	☐	☐
25. Centers the central ray perpendicularly to the ankle joint.	☐	☐	☐	☐	☐	☐

Lateral/External Oblique
The student:

	Procedure		Repeat		Competency	
	Yes	No	Yes	No	Yes	No
26. If using conventional film, adjusts the lead blockers to divide the cassette appropriately.	☐	☐	☐	☐	☐	☐
27. Rotates the entire leg 45° laterally/externally on the appropriate area of the cassette/receptor.	☐	☐	☐	☐	☐	☐
28. Centers the anatomy of interest to the center of the cassette/receptor.	☐	☐	☐	☐	☐	☐
29. Centers the central ray perpendicularly to the ankle joint.	☐	☐	☐	☐	☐	☐

Comments:

_____

_____

IMPORTANT DETAILS
The student:

	Procedure		Repeat		Competency	
	Yes	No	Yes	No	Yes	No
30. Instills confidence in the patient by exhibiting self-confidence throughout the examination.	☐	☐	☐	☐	☐	☐
31. Places a lead marker in the appropriate area of the cassette/receptor (top/bottom/anteriorly/laterally), where it will be visualized on the finished radiograph, on the proper anatomical side (right/left), and in the appropriate position (face up/face down), depending on the patient's position.	☐	☐	☐	☐	☐	☐
32. Provides radiation protection (shield) for the patient (when appropriate), self, and others (closes doors).	☐	☐	☐	☐	☐	☐
33. Applies proper collimation and makes adjustments as necessary.	☐	☐	☐	☐	☐	☐
34. Properly measures the patient along the course of the central ray *for each projection.*	☐	☐	☐	☐	☐	☐
35. Sets the proper exposure techniques:	☐	☐	☐	☐	☐	☐

Conventional systems
- Sets the proper kVp, mA, and time, and makes adjustments as necessary.

or

CR or DR systems
- Identifies the patient on the work-list (or manually types the patient information into the system).
- Selects appropriate body region, specific body part, and accurate view/projection.
- Double-checks preset parameters:
  —Adult vs. pediatric patients
  ○ Small, medium, or large
  —Bucky/receptor (upright vs. table) *or* non-Bucky
  —AEC vs. fixed
  ○ If AEC, checks ion chambers
  ○ Density setting
  —kVp and mA; adjusts if necessary
  —Focal spot/filament size

	Procedure		Repeat		Competency	
36. Exposes the cassette/receptor after telling the patient to hold still *for each projection.*	☐	☐	☐	☐	☐	☐
37. Provides each radiograph with the proper identification (flash) and/or processes each cassette (image) without difficulty (regardless of technology—film, CR, or DR).	▣	▣	▣	▣	☐	☐
38. Properly completes the examination by filling out all necessary paperwork, entering the examination in the computer, having the images checked by the appropriate staff members, answering any last-minute questions, and informing the patient that he or she is finished.	▣	▣	▣	▣	☐	☐
39. Exhibits the ability to adapt to new and difficult situations if and when necessary.	▣	▣	▣	▣	☐	☐
40. Accepts constructive criticism and uses it to his or her advantage.	☐	☐	☐	☐	☐	☐
41. Leaves the radiographic room neat and clean for the next examination.	▣	▣	▣	▣	☐	☐
42. Completes the examination within a reasonable time frame.	☐	☐	☐	☐	☐	☐

(continued)

Comments:

_____

_____

RADIOGRAPHIC IMAGE QUALITY

The student is able to critique his or her radiographs as to whether they demonstrate:

	Procedure		Repeat		Competency	
	Yes	No	Yes	No	Yes	No
43. Proper technique/optimal density	☐	☐	☐	☐	☐	☐
44. Enhanced detail, without evidence of motion and without any visible artifacts	☐	☐	☐	☐	☐	☐
45. Proper positioning (all anatomy included, evidence of proper centering/ alignment, etc.)	☐	☐	☐	☐	☐	☐
46. Proper marker placement	☐	☐	☐	☐	☐	☐
47. Evidence of proper collimation and radiation protection	☐	☐	☐	☐	☐	☐
48. Long vs. short scale of contrast	☐	☐	☐	☐	☐	☐

Comments:

_____

_____

ANKLE ANATOMY

The student is able to identify:

	Procedure		Repeat		Competency	
	Yes	No	Yes	No	Yes	No
49. Distal fibula	☐	☐	☐	☐	☐	☐
50. Distal tibia	☐	☐	☐	☐	☐	☐
51. Lateral malleolus	☐	☐	☐	☐	☐	☐
52. Medial malleolus	☐	☐	☐	☐	☐	☐
53. Talus	☐	☐	☐	☐	☐	☐
54. Mortise	☐	☐	☐	☐	☐	☐
55. Calcaneus/os calcis	☐	☐	☐	☐	☐	☐
56. Navicular/scaphoid	☐	☐	☐	☐	☐	☐
57. Cuboid	☐	☐	☐	☐	☐	☐
58. Obvious pathology	☐	☐	☐	☐	☐	☐

Comments:

_____

_____

_____   _____   _____
Procedure Evaluator Signature   Repeat Evaluator Signature   Competency Evaluator Signature

_____   _____   _____
Date   Date   Date

END ANKLE EVALUATION

Student Name:_____

Procedure Grade	Repeat Grade	Competency Grade

PATIENT INFORMATION OR SIMULATED PROCEDURE *(circle if simulated)*

	Procedure	Repeat	Competency
Age			
Medical Record No.			
Ability to Cooperate			
Condition/Pathology			
Technical Factors Used			
Exposure Index			

FACILITY PREPARATION
The student:

	Procedure Yes	No	Repeat Yes	No	Competency Yes	No
1. Examines the radiographic room and cleans/straightens it before escorting the patient in.	☐	☐	☐	☐	☐	☐
2. Has all equipment and supplies (patient gown, shield, markers, lead blockers, etc.) readily available before escorting the patient in.	☐	☐	☐	☐	☐	☐
3. Is able to manipulate all radiographic equipment with ease, and centers the central ray to the cassette/receptor *for both projections*.	☐	☐	☐	☐	☐	☐
4. Adjusts the tube to the proper SID *for each projection*.	☐	☐	☐	☐	☐	☐
5. Selects cassettes/receptor of the appropriate sizes *for both projections*, according to patient size and examination.	☐	☐	☐	☐	☐	☐

Comments:

_____

_____

PATIENT PREPARATION
The student:

	Procedure Yes	No	Repeat Yes	No	Competency Yes	No
6. Identifies the correct patient and examination according to the requisition while establishing a good rapport with him or her.	☐	☐	☐	☐	☐	☐
7. Obtains and documents the patient's history before the examination.	■	■	■	■	☐	☐
8. Explains the examination in terms the patient fully understands and properly communicates with the patient throughout the examination.	☐	☐	☐	☐	☐	☐
9. Asks female patients of childbearing age the date of their last menstrual period and documents this; inquires about the possibility of pregnancy and has them sign pregnancy consent forms.	☐	☐	☐	☐	☐	☐
10. Removes all obscuring objects (shoes, zippers, belts, etc.) so as *not* to produce radiographic artifacts.	☐	☐	☐	☐	☐	☐

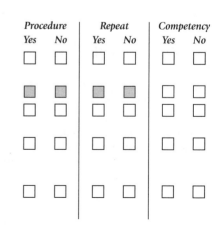

(continued)

	Procedure		Repeat		Competency	
	Yes	No	Yes	No	Yes	No
11. Respects the patient's modesty and provides ample comfort for him or her.	☐	☐	☐	☐	☐	☐

Comments:

_____

_____

PATIENT POSITIONING FOR A TIBIA AND FIBULA
Anteroposterior
The student:

	Procedure		Repeat		Competency	
	Yes	No	Yes	No	Yes	No
12. If using conventional film, divides cassette the into appropriate sections with lead blockers, if appropriate.	☐	☐	☐	☐	☐	☐
13. Instructs the patient to extend the knee and places the posterior surface of the leg on the appropriate area of the cassette/receptor.	☐	☐	☐	☐	☐	☐
14. Places the posterior surface of the lower leg against the cassette/receptor and inverts the foot slightly while checking that the femoral epicondyles are parallel with the cassette/receptor.	☐	☐	☐	☐	☐	☐
15. Centers the anatomy of interest to the center of the cassette/receptor, including both joints.	☐	☐	☐	☐	☐	☐
16. Centers the central ray perpendicularly to the midtibial/midfibular area, at the center of the cassette/receptor.	☐	☐	☐	☐	☐	☐

Lateral
The student:

	Procedure		Repeat		Competency	
	Yes	No	Yes	No	Yes	No
17. If using conventional film, adjusts the lead blockers to divide the cassette appropriately.	☐	☐	☐	☐	☐	☐
18. While instructing the patient to flex his or her knee and roll laterally onto his or her affected side, positions the patient until the patella and femoral epicondyles are perpendicular to the cassette/receptor.	☐	☐	☐	☐	☐	☐
19. Ensures that the plantar surface of the foot is perpendicular to the cassette/receptor and supports the foot/ankle to avoid rotation.	☐	☐	☐	☐	☐	☐
20. Centers the anatomy of interest to the center of the cassette/receptor, including both joints.	☐	☐	☐	☐	☐	☐
21. Centers the central ray perpendicularly to the midtibial/midfibular area.	☐	☐	☐	☐	☐	☐

Comments:

_____

_____

IMPORTANT DETAILS
The student:

	Procedure		Repeat		Competency	
	Yes	No	Yes	No	Yes	No
22. Instills confidence in the patient by exhibiting self-confidence throughout the examination.	☐	☐	☐	☐	☐	☐
23. Places a lead marker in the appropriate area of the cassette/receptor (top/bottom/anteriorly/laterally), where it will be visualized on the finished radiograph, on the proper anatomical side (right/left), and in the appropriate position (face up/face down), depending on the patient's position.	☐	☐	☐	☐	☐	☐
24. Provides radiation protection (shield) for the patient (when appropriate), self, and others (closes doors).	☐	☐	☐	☐	☐	☐
25. Applies proper collimation and makes adjustments as necessary.	☐	☐	☐	☐	☐	☐

	Procedure		Repeat		Competency	
	Yes	No	Yes	No	Yes	No
26. Properly measures the patient along the course of the central ray *for each projection.*	☐	☐	☐	☐	☐	☐
27. Sets the proper exposure techniques:	☐	☐	☐	☐	☐	☐

Conventional systems
- Sets the proper kVp, mA, and time, and makes adjustments as necessary.

or

CR or DR systems
- Identifies the patient on the work-list (or manually types the patient information into the system).
- Selects appropriate body region, specific body part, and accurate view/projection.
- Double-checks preset parameters:
  —Adult vs. pediatric patients
    ○ Small, medium, or large
  —Bucky/receptor (upright vs. table) *or* non-Bucky
  —AEC vs. fixed
    ○ If AEC, checks ion chambers
    ○ Density setting
  —kVp and mA; adjusts if necessary
  —Focal spot/filament size

	Procedure		Repeat		Competency	
28. Exposes the cassette/receptor after telling the patient to hold still *for each projection.*	☐	☐	☐	☐	☐	☐
29. Provides each radiograph with the proper identification (flash) and/or processes each cassette (image) without difficulty (regardless of technology—film, CR, or DR).	▨	▨	▨	▨	☐	☐
30. Properly completes the examination by filling out all necessary paperwork, entering the examination in the computer, having the images checked by the appropriate staff members, answering any last-minute questions, and informing the patient that he or she is finished.	▨	▨	▨	▨	☐	☐
31. Exhibits the ability to adapt to new and difficult situations if and when necessary.	▨	▨	▨	▨	☐	☐
32. Accepts constructive criticism and uses it to his or her advantage.	☐	☐	☐	☐	☐	☐
33. Leaves the radiographic room neat and clean for the next examination.	▨	▨	▨	▨	☐	☐
34. Completes the examination within a reasonable time frame.	☐	☐	☐	☐	☐	☐

Comments:

_____

RADIOGRAPHIC IMAGE QUALITY
The student is able to critique his or her radiographs as to whether they demonstrate:

	Procedure		Repeat		Competency	
	Yes	No	Yes	No	Yes	No
35. Proper technique/optimal density	▨	▨	▨	▨	☐	☐
36. Enhanced detail, without evidence of motion and without any visible artifacts	▨	▨	▨	▨	☐	☐
37. Proper positioning (all anatomy included, evidence of proper centering/alignment, etc.)	▨	▨	▨	▨	☐	☐
38. Proper marker placement	▨	▨	▨	▨	☐	☐
39. Evidence of proper collimation and radiation protection	▨	▨	▨	▨	☐	☐
40. Long vs. short scale of contrast	▨	▨	▨	▨	☐	☐

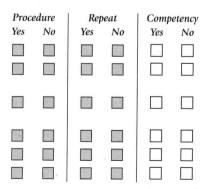

(continued)

Comments:

_____

_____

TIBIA AND FIBULA ANATOMY
The student is able to identify:

	Procedure		Repeat		Competency	
	Yes	No	Yes	No	Yes	No
41. Distal fibula	☐	☐	☐	☐	☐	☐
42. Distal tibia	☐	☐	☐	☐	☐	☐
43. Lateral malleolus	☐	☐	☐	☐	☐	☐
44. Medial malleolus	☐	☐	☐	☐	☐	☐
45. Talus	☐	☐	☐	☐	☐	☐
46. Femoral condyles	☐	☐	☐	☐	☐	☐
47. Knee joint	☐	☐	☐	☐	☐	☐
48. Intercondylar eminence	☐	☐	☐	☐	☐	☐
49. Tibial condyles	☐	☐	☐	☐	☐	☐
50. Tibial tuberosity	☐	☐	☐	☐	☐	☐
51. Tibial plateau	☐	☐	☐	☐	☐	☐
52. Fibular head	☐	☐	☐	☐	☐	☐
53. Patella	☐	☐	☐	☐	☐	☐
54. Obvious pathology	☐	☐	☐	☐	☐	☐

Comments:

_____

_____

_____   _____   _____
Procedure Evaluator Signature   Repeat Evaluator Signature   Competency Evaluator Signature

_____   _____   _____
Date   Date   Date

END TIBIA-FIBULA EVALUATION

Student Name:_____

PATIENT INFORMATION OR SIMULATED PROCEDURE *(circle if simulated)*

	Procedure	*Repeat*	*Competency*
Age			
Medical Record No.			
Ability to Cooperate			
Condition/Pathology			
Technical Factors Used			
Exposure Index			

FACILITY PREPARATION
The student:

	Procedure Yes No	Repeat Yes No	Competency Yes No
1. Examines the radiographic room and cleans/straightens it before escorting the patient in.	☐ ☐	☐ ☐	☐ ☐
2. Has all equipment and supplies (patient gown, shield, markers, lead blockers, etc.) readily available before escorting the patient in.	☐ ☐	☐ ☐	☐ ☐
3. Is able to manipulate all radiographic equipment with ease, and centers the central ray to the cassette/receptor *for all projections.*	☐ ☐	☐ ☐	☐ ☐
4. Adjusts the tube to the proper SID *for each projection.*	☐ ☐	☐ ☐	☐ ☐
5. Selects cassettes/receptor of the appropriate sizes *for all projections,* according to patient size and examination.	☐ ☐	☐ ☐	☐ ☐

Comments:

_____

_____

PATIENT PREPARATION
The student:

	Procedure Yes No	Repeat Yes No	Competency Yes No
6. Identifies the correct patient and examination according to the requisition while establishing a good rapport with him or her.	☐ ☐	☐ ☐	☐ ☐
7. Obtains and documents the patient's history before the examination.	▣ ▣	▣ ▣	☐ ☐
8. Explains the examination in terms the patient fully understands and properly communicates with the patient throughout the examination.	☐ ☐	☐ ☐	☐ ☐
9. Asks female patients of childbearing age the date of their last menstrual period and documents this; inquires about the possibility of pregnancy and has them sign pregnancy consent forms.	☐ ☐	☐ ☐	☐ ☐
10. Removes all obscuring objects (shoes, zippers, belts, etc.) so as *not to* produce radiographic artifacts.	☐ ☐	☐ ☐	☐ ☐

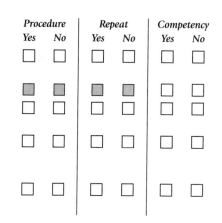

(continued)

	Procedure		Repeat		Competency	
	Yes	No	Yes	No	Yes	No
11. Respects the patient's modesty and provides ample comfort for him or her.	☐	☐	☐	☐	☐	☐

Comments:

_____

_____

PATIENT POSITIONING FOR A KNEE
Anteroposterior
The student:

	Procedure		Repeat		Competency	
	Yes	No	Yes	No	Yes	No
12. Instructs the patient to extend the knee as much as possible.	☐	☐	☐	☐	☐	☐
13. Places the posterior surface of the knee in contact with the radiographic table and internally rotates the leg while checking that the femoral epicondyles are parallel to the cassette/receptor.	☐	☐	☐	☐	☐	☐
14. Centers the anatomy of interest to the center of the cassette/receptor.	☐	☐	☐	☐	☐	☐
15. Centers the central ray perpendicularly (or angles it 5–7° cephalad) to a point approximately 1/2 inch below the patellar apex.	☐	☐	☐	☐	☐	☐

Lateral
The student:

	Procedure		Repeat		Competency	
	Yes	No	Yes	No	Yes	No
16. While instructing the patient to flex his or her knee 30°, rolls him or her laterally onto his or her affected side until the patella and femoral epicondyles are perpendicular to the cassette/receptor.	☐	☐	☐	☐	☐	☐
17. Centers the anatomy of interest to the center of the cassette/receptor.	☐	☐	☐	☐	☐	☐
18. Centers the central ray perpendicularly to a point 1/2 inch below the femoral condyles.	☐	☐	☐	☐	☐	☐

Medial/Internal Oblique
The student:

	Procedure		Repeat		Competency	
	Yes	No	Yes	No	Yes	No
19. Rotates the entire leg 45° medially/internally.	☐	☐	☐	☐	☐	☐
20. Elevates and supports the affected hip.	☐	☐	☐	☐	☐	☐
21. Centers the anatomy of interest to the center of the cassette/receptor.	☐	☐	☐	☐	☐	☐
22. Centers the central ray perpendicularly to the knee joint at a point approximately 1/2 inch below the patellar apex.	☐	☐	☐	☐	☐	☐

Lateral/External Oblique
The student:

	Procedure		Repeat		Competency	
	Yes	No	Yes	No	Yes	No
23. Rotates the entire leg 45° laterally/externally.	☐	☐	☐	☐	☐	☐
24. Elevates and supports the unaffected hip.	☐	☐	☐	☐	☐	☐
25. Centers the anatomy of interest to the center of the cassette/receptor.	☐	☐	☐	☐	☐	☐
26. Centers the central ray perpendicularly to the knee joint at a point approximately 1/2 inch below the patellar apex.	☐	☐	☐	☐	☐	☐

Comments:

_____

_____

IMPORTANT DETAILS
The student:

	Procedure		Repeat		Competency	
	Yes	No	Yes	No	Yes	No
27. Instills confidence in the patient by exhibiting self-confidence throughout the examination.	☐	☐	☐	☐	☐	☐
28. Places a lead marker in the appropriate area of the cassette/receptor (top/bottom/anteriorly/laterally), where it will be visualized on the finished radiograph, on the proper anatomical side (right/left), and in the appropriate position (face up/face down), depending on the patient's position.	☐	☐	☐	☐	☐	☐
29. Provides radiation protection (shield) for the patient (when appropriate), self, and others (closes doors).	☐	☐	☐	☐	☐	☐
30. Applies proper collimation and makes adjustments as necessary.	☐	☐	☐	☐	☐	☐
31. Properly measures the patient along the course of the central ray *for each projection.*	☐	☐	☐	☐	☐	☐
32. Sets the proper exposure techniques:	☐	☐	☐	☐	☐	☐

32. Sets the proper exposure techniques:

Conventional systems
- Sets the proper kVp, mA, and time, and makes adjustments as necessary.

or

CR or DR systems
- Identifies the patient on the work-list (or manually types the patient information into the system).
- Selects appropriate body region, specific body part, and accurate view/ projection.
- Double-checks preset parameters:
  —Adult vs. pediatric patients
  ◦ Small, medium, or large
  —Bucky/receptor (upright vs. table) *or* non-Bucky
  —AEC vs. fixed
  ◦ If AEC, checks ion chambers
  ◦ Density setting
  —kVp and mA; adjusts if necessary
  —Focal spot/filament size

	Procedure		Repeat		Competency	
33. Exposes the cassette/receptor after telling the patient to hold still *for each projection.*	☐	☐	☐	☐	☐	☐
34. Provides each radiograph with the proper identification (flash) and/or processes each cassette (image) without difficulty (regardless of technology—film, CR, or DR).	▨	▨	▨	▨	☐	☐
35. Properly completes the examination by filling out all necessary paperwork, entering the examination in the computer, having the images checked by the appropriate staff members, answering any last-minute questions, and informing the patient that he or she is finished.	▨	☐	▨	☐	☐	☐
36. Exhibits the ability to adapt to new and difficult situations if and when necessary.	▨	▨	▨	▨	☐	☐
37. Accepts constructive criticism and uses it to his or her advantage.	☐	☐	☐	☐	☐	☐
38. Leaves the radiographic room neat and clean for the next examination.	▨	▨	▨	▨	☐	☐
39. Completes the examination within a reasonable time frame.	☐	☐	☐	☐	☐	☐

Comments:

_____

_____

(continued)

RADIOGRAPHIC IMAGE QUALITY

The student is able to critique his or her radiographs as to whether they demonstrate:

	Procedure		Repeat		Competency	
	Yes	No	Yes	No	Yes	No
40. Proper technique/optimal density	☐	☐	☐	☐	☐	☐
41. Enhanced detail, without evidence of motion and without any visible artifacts	☐	☐	☐	☐	☐	☐
42. Proper positioning (all anatomy included, evidence of proper centering/alignment, etc.)	☐	☐	☐	☐	☐	☐
43. Proper marker placement	☐	☐	☐	☐	☐	☐
44. Evidence of proper collimation and radiation protection	☐	☐	☐	☐	☐	☐
45. Long vs. short scale of contrast	☐	☐	☐	☐	☐	☐

Comments:

_____

_____

KNEE ANATOMY

The student is able to identify:

	Procedure		Repeat		Competency	
	Yes	No	Yes	No	Yes	No
46. Proximal fibula (head)	☐	☐	☐	☐	☐	☐
47. Proximal tibia	☐	☐	☐	☐	☐	☐
48. Medial and lateral tibial condyles	☐	☐	☐	☐	☐	☐
49. Intercondylar eminence	☐	☐	☐	☐	☐	☐
50. Tibial plateau	☐	☐	☐	☐	☐	☐
51. Tibial spines	☐	☐	☐	☐	☐	☐
52. Tibial tuberosity	☐	☐	☐	☐	☐	☐
53. Medial and lateral femoral condyles	☐	☐	☐	☐	☐	☐
54. Medial and lateral femoral epicondyles	☐	☐	☐	☐	☐	☐
55. Femur	☐	☐	☐	☐	☐	☐
56. Patellar apex	☐	☐	☐	☐	☐	☐
57. Patellar base	☐	☐	☐	☐	☐	☐
58. Obvious pathology	☐	☐	☐	☐	☐	☐

Comments:

_____

_____

_____
Procedure Evaluator Signature

_____
Repeat Evaluator Signature

_____
Competency Evaluator Signature

_____
Date

_____
Date

_____
Date

END KNEE EVALUATION

Student Name:_____

	Procedure Grade	Repeat Grade	Competency Grade

PATIENT INFORMATION OR SIMULATED PROCEDURE *(circle if simulated)*

	Procedure	Repeat	Competency
Age			
Medical Record No.			
Ability to Cooperate			
Condition/Pathology			
Technical Factors Used			
Exposure Index			

FACILITY PREPARATION
The student:

	Procedure		Repeat		Competency	
	Yes	No	Yes	No	Yes	No
1. Examines the radiographic room and cleans/straightens it before escorting the patient in.	☐	☐	☐	☐	☐	☐
2. Has all equipment and supplies (patient gown, shield, markers, lead blockers, etc.) readily available before escorting the patient in.	☐	☐	☐	☐	☐	☐
3. Is able to manipulate all radiographic equipment with ease, and centers the central ray to the cassette/receptor.	☐	☐	☐	☐	☐	☐
4. Adjusts the tube to the proper SID.	☐	☐	☐	☐	☐	☐
5. Selects a cassette/receptor of the appropriate size.	☐	☐	☐	☐	☐	☐

Comments:

_____

_____

PATIENT PREPARATION
The student:

	Procedure		Repeat		Competency	
	Yes	No	Yes	No	Yes	No
6. Identifies the correct patient and examination according to the requisition while establishing a good rapport with him or her.	☐	☐	☐	☐	☐	☐
7. Obtains and documents the patient's history before the examination.	▨	▨	▨	▨	☐	☐
8. Explains the examination in terms the patient fully understands and properly communicates with the patient throughout the examination.	☐	☐	☐	☐	☐	☐
9. Asks female patients of childbearing age the date of their last menstrual period and documents this; inquires about the possibility of pregnancy and has them sign pregnancy consent forms.	☐	☐	☐	☐	☐	☐
10. Removes all obscuring objects (shoes, zippers, belts, etc.) so as *not* to produce radiographic artifacts.	☐	☐	☐	☐	☐	☐

(continued)

	Procedure		Repeat		Competency	
	Yes	No	Yes	No	Yes	No
11. Respects the patient's modesty and provides ample comfort for him or her.	☐	☐	☐	☐	☐	☐

Comments:

_____

_____

PATIENT POSITIONING FOR A WEIGHT-BEARING KNEE
The student:

	Procedure		Repeat		Competency	
	Yes	No	Yes	No	Yes	No
12. Places the patient in the erect position with the posterior surface of both knees in contact with the upright Bucky/receptor.	☐	☐	☐	☐	☐	☐
13. Instructs the patient to distribute his or her weight evenly on both feet, with toes pointed straight ahead and feet slightly separated.	☐	☐	☐	☐	☐	☐
14. Centers the anatomy of interest to the center of the cassette/receptor.	☐	☐	☐	☐	☐	☐
15. Using a horizontal beam, directs the central ray perpendicularly to a point 1/2 inch below the apices of both patellae.	☐	☐	☐	☐	☐	☐

Comments:

_____

_____

IMPORTANT DETAILS
The student:

	Procedure		Repeat		Competency	
	Yes	No	Yes	No	Yes	No
16. Instills confidence in the patient by exhibiting self-confidence throughout the examination.	☐	☐	☐	☐	☐	☐
17. Places a lead marker in the appropriate area of the cassette/receptor (top/bottom/anteriorly/laterally), where it will be visualized on the finished radiograph, on the proper anatomical side (right/left), and in the appropriate position (face up/face down), depending on the patient's position.	☐	☐	☐	☐	☐	☐
18. Provides radiation protection (shield) for the patient (when appropriate), self, and others (closes doors).	☐	☐	☐	☐	☐	☐
19. Applies proper collimation and makes adjustments as necessary.	☐	☐	☐	☐	☐	☐
20. Properly measures the patient along the course of the central ray *for each projection.*	☐	☐	☐	☐	☐	☐
21. Sets the proper exposure techniques:	☐	☐	☐	☐	☐	☐

Conventional systems
- Sets the proper kVp, mA, and time, and makes adjustments as necessary.

or

CR or DR systems
- Identifies the patient on the work-list (or manually types the patient information into the system).
- Selects appropriate body region, specific body part, and accurate view/ projection.
- Double-checks preset parameters:
  —Adult vs. pediatric patients
    ○ Small, medium, or large
  —Bucky/receptor (upright vs. table) *or* non-Bucky
  —AEC vs. fixed
    ○ If AEC, checks ion chambers
    ○ Density setting
  —kVp and mA; adjusts if necessary
  —Focal spot/filament size

	Procedure		Repeat		Competency	
	Yes	No	Yes	No	Yes	No
22. Exposes the cassette/receptor after telling the patient to hold still *for each projection.*	☐	☐	☐	☐	☐	☐
23. Provides each radiograph with the proper identification (flash) and/or processes each cassette (image) without difficulty (regardless of technology—film, CR, or DR).	▣	▣	▣	▣	☐	☐
24. Properly completes the examination by filling out all necessary paperwork, entering the examination in the computer, having the images checked by the appropriate staff members, answering any last-minute questions, and informing the patient that he or she is finished.	▣	▣	▣	▣	☐	☐
25. Exhibits the ability to adapt to new and difficult situations if and when necessary.	▣	▣	▣	▣	☐	☐
26. Accepts constructive criticism and uses it to his or her advantage.	☐	☐	☐	☐	☐	☐
27. Leaves the radiographic room neat and clean for the next examination.	▣	▣	▣	▣	☐	☐
28. Completes the examination within a reasonable time frame.	☐	☐	☐	☐	☐	☐

Comments:

RADIOGRAPHIC IMAGE QUALITY

The student is able to critique his or her radiographs as to whether they demonstrate:

	Procedure		Repeat		Competency	
	Yes	No	Yes	No	Yes	No
29. Proper technique/optimal density	▣	▣	▣	▣	☐	☐
30. Enhanced detail, without evidence of motion and without any visible artifacts	▣	▣	▣	▣	☐	☐
31. Proper positioning (all anatomy included, evidence of proper centering/alignment, etc.)	▣	▣	▣	▣	☐	☐
32. Proper marker placement	▣	▣	▣	▣	☐	☐
33. Evidence of proper collimation and radiation protection	▣	▣	▣	▣	☐	☐
34. Long vs. short scale of contrast	▣	▣	▣	▣	☐	☐

Comments:

KNEE ANATOMY

The student is able to identify:

	Procedure		Repeat		Competency	
	Yes	No	Yes	No	Yes	No
34. Proximal fibula (head)	▣	▣	▣	▣	☐	☐
35. Proximal tibia	▣	▣	▣	▣	☐	☐
36. Medial and lateral tibial condyles	▣	▣	▣	▣	☐	☐
37. Intercondylar eminence	▣	▣	▣	▣	☐	☐
38. Tibial plateau	▣	▣	▣	▣	☐	☐
39. Tibial spines	▣	▣	▣	▣	☐	☐
40. Medial and lateral femoral condyles	▣	▣	▣	▣	☐	☐
41. Medial and lateral femoral epicondyles	▣	▣	▣	▣	☐	☐
42. Femur	▣	▣	▣	▣	☐	☐

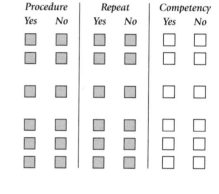

(continued)

	Procedure		Repeat		Competency	
	Yes	No	Yes	No	Yes	No
43. Patellar apex	☐	☐	☐	☐	☐	☐
44. Patellar base	☐	☐	☐	☐	☐	☐
45. Obvious pathology	☐	☐	☐	☐	☐	☐

Comments:

_____

_____

_____   _____   _____
Procedure Evaluator Signature   Repeat Evaluator Signature   Competency Evaluator Signature

_____   _____   _____
Date   Date   Date

END WEIGHT-BEARING KNEE EVALUATION

The objective of this evaluation is to determine the student's competency level when performing specific radiographic examinations.

Student Name:_____

Procedure Grade	Repeat Grade	Competency Grade

PATIENT INFORMATION OR SIMULATED PROCEDURE *(circle if simulated)*

	Procedure	Repeat	Competency
Age			
Medical Record No.			
Ability to Cooperate			
Condition/Pathology			
Technical Factors Used			
Exposure Index			

FACILITY PREPARATION
The student:

	Procedure Yes	No	Repeat Yes	No	Competency Yes	No
1. Examines the radiographic room and cleans/straightens it before escorting the patient in.	☐	☐	☐	☐	☐	☐
2. Has all equipment and supplies (patient gown, shield, markers, lead blockers, etc.) readily available before escorting the patient in.	☐	☐	☐	☐	☐	☐
3. Is able to manipulate all radiographic equipment with ease, and centers the central ray to the cassette/receptor *for all projections*.	☐	☐	☐	☐	☐	☐
4. Adjusts the tube to the proper SID *for each projection*.	☐	☐	☐	☐	☐	☐
5. Selects cassettes/receptor of the appropriate sizes *for all projections*, according to patient size and examination.	☐	☐	☐	☐	☐	☐

Comments:

_____

_____

PATIENT PREPARATION
The student:

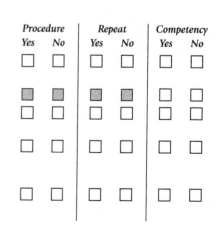

	Procedure Yes	No	Repeat Yes	No	Competency Yes	No
6. Identifies the correct patient and examination according to the requisition while establishing a good rapport with him or her.	☐	☐	☐	☐	☐	☐
7. Obtains and documents the patient's history before the examination.	☐	☐	☐	☐	☐	☐
8. Explains the examination in terms the patient fully understands and properly communicates with the patient throughout the examination.	☐	☐	☐	☐	☐	☐
9. Asks female patients of childbearing age the date of their last menstrual period and documents this; inquires about the possibility of pregnancy and has them sign pregnancy consent forms.	☐	☐	☐	☐	☐	☐
10. Removes all obscuring objects (shoes, zippers, belts, etc.) so as *not* to produce radiographic artifacts.	☐	☐	☐	☐	☐	☐

(continued)

	Procedure		Repeat		Competency	
	Yes	No	Yes	No	Yes	No
11. Respects the patient's modesty and provides ample comfort for him or her.	☐	☐	☐	☐	☐	☐

Comments:

_____

_____

PATIENT POSITIONING FOR A PATELLA
Posteroanterior
The student:

	Procedure		Repeat		Competency	
	Yes	No	Yes	No	Yes	No
12. Places the patient in the prone position on the radiographic table.	☐	☐	☐	☐	☐	☐
13. Rotates the heel 5–10° laterally so that the patella is parallel to the cassette/receptor, and if the knee is tender, places supports under the thigh and leg to relieve pressure.	☐	☐	☐	☐	☐	☐
14. Centers the area of interest to the center of the cassette/receptor.	☐	☐	☐	☐	☐	☐
15. Centers the central ray perpendicularly to the midpopliteal region (exiting the patella).	☐	☐	☐	☐	☐	☐

Lateral
The student:

	Procedure		Repeat		Competency	
	Yes	No	Yes	No	Yes	No
16. Instructs the patient to flex the affected hip as he or she rolls laterally onto the affected side and places the unaffected foot in front of the affected limb.	☐	☐	☐	☐	☐	☐
17. Instructs the patient to gently flex the affected knee 5–10°.	☐	☐	☐	☐	☐	☐
18. Checks that the affected patella and femoral epicondyles are perpendicular to the cassette/receptor.	☐	☐	☐	☐	☐	☐
19. Centers the anatomy of interest to the center of the cassette/receptor.	☐	☐	☐	☐	☐	☐
20. Centers the central ray perpendicularly to the midpatellofemoral joint.	☐	☐	☐	☐	☐	☐

Tangential/Settegast/Sunrise/Skyline (After the Lateral View Clears the Patient of Suspected Transverse Patellar Fracture)
The student:

	Procedure		Repeat		Competency	
	Yes	No	Yes	No	Yes	No
21. Places the patient in the prone position on the radiographic table.	☐	☐	☐	☐	☐	☐
22. Slowly flexes the knee as much as possible (placing the lower leg vertical to the table), or until the patella is perpendicular to the cassette/receptor.	☐	☐	☐	☐	☐	☐
23. Centers the anatomy of interest to the center of the cassette/receptor.	☐	☐	☐	☐	☐	☐
24. Centers the central ray perpendicular to the joint space between the patella and the femoral condyles, angling the central ray when necessary.	☐	☐	☐	☐	☐	☐

Comments:

_____

_____

IMPORTANT DETAILS
The student:

	Procedure		Repeat		Competency	
	Yes	No	Yes	No	Yes	No
25. Instills confidence in the patient by exhibiting self-confidence throughout the examination.	☐	☐	☐	☐	☐	☐

	Procedure		Repeat		Competency	
	Yes	No	Yes	No	Yes	No
26. Places a lead marker in the appropriate area of the cassette/receptor (top/bottom/anteriorly/laterally), where it will be visualized on the finished radiograph, on the proper anatomical side (right/left), and in the appropriate position (face up/face down), depending on the patient's position.	☐	☐	☐	☐	☐	☐
27. Provides radiation protection (shield) for the patient (when appropriate), self, and others (closes doors).	☐	☐	☐	☐	☐	☐
28. Applies proper collimation and makes adjustments as necessary.	☐	☐	☐	☐	☐	☐
29. Properly measures the patient along the course of the central ray *for each projection.*	☐	☐	☐	☐	☐	☐
30. Sets the proper exposure techniques:	☐	☐	☐	☐	☐	☐

30. Sets the proper exposure techniques:

Conventional systems
- Sets the proper kVp, mA, and time, and makes adjustments as necessary.

or

CR or DR systems
- Identifies the patient on the work-list (or manually types the patient information into the system).
- Selects appropriate body region, specific body part, and accurate view/ projection.
- Double-checks preset parameters:
  —Adult vs. pediatric patients
    ○ Small, medium, or large
  —Bucky/receptor (upright vs. table) *or* non-Bucky
  —AEC vs. fixed
    ○ If AEC, checks ion chambers
    ○ Density setting
  —kVp and mA; adjusts if necessary
  —Focal spot/filament size

	Procedure		Repeat		Competency	
31. Exposes the cassette/receptor after telling the patient to hold still *for each projection.*	☐	☐	☐	☐	☐	☐
32. Provides each radiograph with the proper identification (flash) and/or processes each cassette (image) without difficulty (regardless of technology—film, CR, or DR).	▣	▣	▣	▣	☐	☐
33. Properly completes the examination by filling out all necessary paperwork, entering the examination in the computer, having the images checked by the appropriate staff members, answering any last-minute questions, and informing the patient that he or she is finished.	▣	▣	▣	▣	☐	☐
34. Exhibits the ability to adapt to new and difficult situations if and when necessary.	▣	▣	▣	▣	☐	☐
35. Accepts constructive criticism and uses it to his or her advantage.	☐	☐	☐	☐	☐	☐
36. Leaves the radiographic room neat and clean for the next examination.	▣	▣	▣	▣	☐	☐
37. Completes the examination within a reasonable time frame.	☐	☐	☐	☐	☐	☐

Comments:

_____

_____

RADIOGRAPHIC IMAGE QUALITY
The student is able to critique his or her radiographs as to whether they demonstrate:

	Procedure		Repeat		Competency	
	Yes	No	Yes	No	Yes	No
38. Proper technique/optimal density	▣	▣	▣	▣	☐	☐

(continued)

	Procedure		Repeat		Competency	
	Yes	No	Yes	No	Yes	No
39. Enhanced detail, without evidence of motion and without any visible artifacts	☐	☐	☐	☐	☐	☐
40. Proper positioning (all anatomy included, evidence of proper centering/alignment, etc.)	☐	☐	☐	☐	☐	☐
41. Proper marker placement	☐	☐	☐	☐	☐	☐
42. Evidence of proper collimation and radiation protection	☐	☐	☐	☐	☐	☐
43. Long vs. short scale of contrast	☐	☐	☐	☐	☐	☐

Comments:

_____

_____

KNEE ANATOMY
The student is able to identify:

	Procedure		Repeat		Competency	
	Yes	No	Yes	No	Yes	No
44. Femoropatellar articulation	☐	☐	☐	☐	☐	☐
45. Fibula	☐	☐	☐	☐	☐	☐
46. Medial and lateral femoral condyles	☐	☐	☐	☐	☐	☐
47. Patella	☐	☐	☐	☐	☐	☐
48. Obvious pathology	☐	☐	☐	☐	☐	☐

Comments:

_____

_____

_____ _____ _____
Procedure Evaluator Signature   Repeat Evaluator Signature   Competency Evaluator Signature

_____ _____ _____
Date   Date   Date

END PATELLA EVALUATION

Intercondylar Fossa (Camp-Coventry)

The objective of this evaluation is to determine the student's competency level when performing specific radiographic examinations.

Student Name:_____

Procedure Grade	Repeat Grade	Competency Grade

PATIENT INFORMATION OR SIMULATED PROCEDURE *(circle if simulated)*

	Procedure	Repeat	Competency
Age			
Medical Record No.			
Ability to Cooperate			
Condition/Pathology			
Technical Factors Used			
Exposure Index			

FACILITY PREPARATION
The student:

	Procedure Yes No	Repeat Yes No	Competency Yes No
1. Examines the radiographic room and cleans/straightens it before escorting the patient in.	☐ ☐	☐ ☐	☐ ☐
2. Has all equipment and supplies (patient gown, shield, markers, lead blockers, etc.) readily available before escorting the patient in.	☐ ☐	☐ ☐	☐ ☐
3. Is able to manipulate all radiographic equipment with ease, and centers the central ray to the cassette/receptor.	☐ ☐	☐ ☐	☐ ☐
4. Adjusts the tube to the proper SID.	☐ ☐	☐ ☐	☐ ☐
5. Selects a cassette/receptor of the appropriate size.	☐ ☐	☐ ☐	☐ ☐

Comments:

_____

_____

PATIENT PREPARATION
The student:

	Procedure Yes No	Repeat Yes No	Competency Yes No
6. Identifies the correct patient and examination according to the requisition while establishing a good rapport with him or her.	☐ ☐	☐ ☐	☐ ☐
7. Obtains and documents the patient's history before the examination.	▦ ▦	▦ ▦	☐ ☐
8. Explains the examination in terms the patient fully understands and properly communicates with the patient throughout the examination.	☐ ☐	☐ ☐	☐ ☐
9. Asks female patients of childbearing age the date of their last menstrual period and documents this; inquires about the possibility of pregnancy and has them sign pregnancy consent forms.	☐ ☐	☐ ☐	☐ ☐
10. Removes all obscuring objects (shoes, zippers, belts, etc.) so as *not* to produce radiographic artifacts.	☐ ☐	☐ ☐	☐ ☐
11. Respects the patient's modesty and provides ample comfort for him or her.	☐ ☐	☐ ☐	☐ ☐

(continued)

Comments:

_____

_____

PATIENT POSITIONING FOR AN INTERCONDYLAR FOSSA, USING A PA AXIAL PROJECTION (THE CAMP-COVENTRY METHOD)

The student:

	Procedure		Repeat		Competency	
	Yes	No	Yes	No	Yes	No
12. Places the patient in the prone position on the radiographic table.	☐	☐	☐	☐	☐	☐
13. Slowly flexes the knee until the lower leg forms approximately a 40° angle with the table and rests the foot on a suitable support.	☐	☐	☐	☐	☐	☐
14. Ensures that there is no medial or lateral rotation of the knee/leg.	☐	☐	☐	☐	☐	☐
15. Centers the anatomy of interest to the center of the cassette/receptor.	☐	☐	☐	☐	☐	☐
16. Centers the central ray to the knee joint space at an angle that places the central ray perpendicular to the lower leg.	☐	☐	☐	☐	☐	☐

Comments:

_____

_____

IMPORTANT DETAILS

The student:

	Procedure		Repeat		Competency	
	Yes	No	Yes	No	Yes	No
17. Instills confidence in the patient by exhibiting self-confidence throughout the examination.	☐	☐	☐	☐	☐	☐
18. Places a lead marker in the appropriate area of the cassette/receptor (top/bottom/anteriorly/laterally), where it will be visualized on the finished radiograph, on the proper anatomical side (right/left), and in the appropriate position (face up/face down), depending on the patient's position.	☐	☐	☐	☐	☐	☐
19. Provides radiation protection (shield) for the patient (when appropriate), self, and others (closes doors).	☐	☐	☐	☐	☐	☐
20. Applies proper collimation and makes adjustments as necessary.	☐	☐	☐	☐	☐	☐
21. Properly measures the patient along the course of the central ray *for each projection.*	☐	☐	☐	☐	☐	☐
22. Sets the proper exposure techniques:	☐	☐	☐	☐	☐	☐

22. Sets the proper exposure techniques:

Conventional systems
- Sets the proper kVp, mA, and time, and makes adjustments as necessary.

or

CR or DR systems
- Identifies the patient on the work-list (or manually types the patient information into the system).
- Selects appropriate body region, specific body part, and accurate view/ projection.
- Double-checks preset parameters:
  —Adult vs. pediatric patients
  ○ Small, medium, or large
  —Bucky/receptor (upright vs. table) *or* non-Bucky
  —AEC vs. fixed
  ○ If AEC, checks ion chambers
  ○ Density setting
  —kVp and mA; adjusts if necessary
  —Focal spot/filament size

23. Exposes the cassette/receptor after telling the patient to hold still *for each projection.*	☐	☐	☐	☐	☐	☐

	Procedure		Repeat		Competency	
	Yes	No	Yes	No	Yes	No
24. Provides each radiograph with the proper identification (flash) and/or processes each cassette (image) without difficulty (regardless of technology—film, CR, or DR).	☐	☐	☐	☐	☐	☐
25. Properly completes the examination by filling out all necessary paperwork, entering the examination in the computer, having the images checked by the appropriate staff members, answering any last-minute questions, and informing the patient that he or she is finished.	☐	☐	☐	☐	☐	☐
26. Exhibits the ability to adapt to new and difficult situations if and when necessary.	☐	☐	☐	☐	☐	☐
27. Accepts constructive criticism and uses it to his or her advantage.	☐	☐	☐	☐	☐	☐
28. Leaves the radiographic room neat and clean for the next examination.	☐	☐	☐	☐	☐	☐
29. Completes the examination within a reasonable time frame.	☐	☐	☐	☐	☐	☐

Comments:

_____

_____

RADIOGRAPHIC IMAGE QUALITY
The student is able to critique his or her radiographs as to whether they demonstrate:

	Procedure		Repeat		Competency	
	Yes	No	Yes	No	Yes	No
30. Proper technique/optimal density	☐	☐	☐	☐	☐	☐
31. Enhanced detail, without evidence of motion and without any visible artifacts	☐	☐	☐	☐	☐	☐
32. Proper positioning (all anatomy included, evidence of proper centering/alignment, etc.)	☐	☐	☐	☐	☐	☐
33. Proper marker placement	☐	☐	☐	☐	☐	☐
34. Evidence of proper collimation and radiation protection	☐	☐	☐	☐	☐	☐
35. Long vs. short scale of contrast	☐	☐	☐	☐	☐	☐

Comments:

_____

_____

KNEE ANATOMY
The student is able to identify:

	Procedure		Repeat		Competency	
	Yes	No	Yes	No	Yes	No
36. Intercondylar fossa	☐	☐	☐	☐	☐	☐
37. Fibula	☐	☐	☐	☐	☐	☐
38. Medial and lateral condyles	☐	☐	☐	☐	☐	☐
39. Patella	☐	☐	☐	☐	☐	☐
40. Tibial spines	☐	☐	☐	☐	☐	☐
41. Obvious pathology	☐	☐	☐	☐	☐	☐

Comments:

_____

_____

Procedure Evaluator Signature	Repeat Evaluator Signature	Competency Evaluator Signature
Date	Date	Date

END INTERCONDYLAR FOSSA (CAMP-COVENTRY) EVALUATION

The objective of this evaluation is to determine the student's competency level when performing specific radiographic examinations.

Student Name:_____

Procedure Grade	Repeat Grade	Competency Grade

PATIENT INFORMATION OR SIMULATED PROCEDURE *(circle if simulated)*

	Procedure	Repeat	Competency
Age			
Medical Record No.			
Ability to Cooperate			
Condition/Pathology			
Technical Factors Used			
Exposure Index			

FACILITY PREPARATION
The student:

	Procedure Yes No	Repeat Yes No	Competency Yes No
1. Examines the radiographic room and cleans/straightens it before escorting the patient in.	☐ ☐	☐ ☐	☐ ☐
2. Has all equipment and supplies (patient gown, shield, markers, lead blockers, etc.) readily available before escorting the patient in.	☐ ☐	☐ ☐	☐ ☐
3. Is able to manipulate all radiographic equipment with ease, and centers the central ray to the cassette/receptor *for both projections.*	☐ ☐	☐ ☐	☐ ☐
4. Adjusts the tube to the proper SID *for each projection.*	☐ ☐	☐ ☐	☐ ☐
5. Selects cassettes/receptor of the appropriate sizes *for both projections,* according to patient size and examination.	☐ ☐	☐ ☐	☐ ☐

Comments:

_____

_____

PATIENT PREPARATION
The student:

	Procedure Yes No	Repeat Yes No	Competency Yes No
6. Identifies the correct patient and examination according to the requisition while establishing a good rapport with him or her.	☐ ☐	☐ ☐	☐ ☐
7. Obtains and documents the patient's history before the examination.	▩ ▩	▩ ▩	☐ ☐
8. Explains the examination in terms the patient fully understands and properly communicates with the patient throughout the examination.	☐ ☐	☐ ☐	☐ ☐
9. Asks female patients of childbearing age the date of their last menstrual period and documents this; inquires about the possibility of pregnancy and has them sign pregnancy consent forms.	☐ ☐	☐ ☐	☐ ☐
10. Removes all obscuring objects (shoes, zippers, belts, etc.) so as *not* to produce radiographic artifacts.	☐ ☐	☐ ☐	☐ ☐

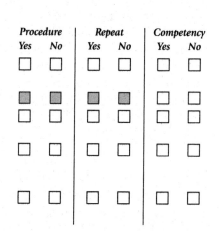

(continued)

	Procedure Yes	No	Repeat Yes	No	Competency Yes	No
11. Respects the patient's modesty and provides ample comfort for him or her.	☐	☐	☐	☐	☐	☐

Comments:

_____

_____

PATIENT POSITIONING FOR A FEMUR
Anteroposterior
The student:

	Procedure Yes	No	Repeat Yes	No	Competency Yes	No
12. Instructs the patient to extend the knee, and places the posterior surface of the leg on the appropriate area of the table.	☐	☐	☐	☐	☐	☐
13. Places the posterior surface of the femur in contact with the radiographic table and rotates the leg medially while ensuring that the femoral epicondyles are parallel with the table.	☐	☐	☐	☐	☐	☐
14. Centers the anatomy of interest to the center of the cassette/receptor, including the appropriate joint.	☐	☐	☐	☐	☐	☐
15. Centers the central ray perpendicularly to the midfemur area, at the center of the cassette/receptor.	☐	☐	☐	☐	☐	☐

Lateral
The student:

	Procedure Yes	No	Repeat Yes	No	Competency Yes	No
16. While instructing the patient to flex his or her knee approximately 30°, instructs the patient to roll laterally toward his or her affected side, and does one of the following:	☐	☐	☐	☐	☐	☐
a. For the knee joint, positions the patient until the pelvis, patella, and femoral epicondyles are perpendicular to the cassette/receptor by bringing the unaffected leg up toward the pelvis.						
b. For the hip joint, positions the patient with the unaffected leg drawn posteriorly and the pelvis tilted just enough to avoid superimposition.						
17. Centers the anatomy of interest to the center of the cassette/receptor, including the appropriate joint.	☐	☐	☐	☐	☐	☐

Comments:

_____

_____

IMPORTANT DETAILS
The student:

	Procedure Yes	No	Repeat Yes	No	Competency Yes	No
18. Instills confidence in the patient by exhibiting self-confidence throughout the examination.	☐	☐	☐	☐	☐	☐
19. Places a lead marker in the appropriate area of the cassette/receptor (top/bottom/anteriorly/laterally), where it will be visualized on the finished radiograph, on the proper anatomical side (right/left), and in the appropriate position (face up/face down), depending on the patient's position.	☐	☐	☐	☐	☐	☐
20. Provides radiation protection (shield) for the patient (when appropriate), self, and others (closes doors).	☐	☐	☐	☐	☐	☐
21. Applies proper collimation and makes adjustments as necessary.	☐	☐	☐	☐	☐	☐
22. Properly measures the patient along the course of the central ray *for each projection.*	☐	☐	☐	☐	☐	☐

	Procedure		Repeat		Competency	
	Yes	No	Yes	No	Yes	No
23. Sets the proper exposure techniques:	☐	☐	☐	☐	☐	☐

Conventional systems
- Sets the proper kVp, mA, and time, and makes adjustments as necessary.

or

CR or DR systems
- Identifies the patient on the work-list (or manually types the patient information into the system).
- Selects appropriate body region, specific body part, and accurate view/ projection.
- Double-checks preset parameters:
  —Adult vs. pediatric patients
    ○ Small, medium, or large
  —Bucky/receptor (upright vs. table) *or* non-Bucky
  —AEC vs. fixed
    ○ If AEC, checks ion chambers
    ○ Density setting
  —kVp and mA; adjusts if necessary
  —Focal spot/filament size

	Procedure		Repeat		Competency	
	Yes	No	Yes	No	Yes	No
24. Exposes the cassette/receptor after telling the patient to hold still *for each projection*.	☐	☐	☐	☐	☐	☐
25. Provides each radiograph with the proper identification (flash) and/or processes each cassette (image) without difficulty (regardless of technology—film, CR, or DR).	☒	☒	☒	☒	☐	☐
26. Properly completes the examination by filling out all necessary paperwork, entering the examination in the computer, having the images checked by the appropriate staff members, answering any last-minute questions, and informing the patient that he or she is finished.	☒	☒	☒	☒	☐	☐
27. Exhibits the ability to adapt to new and difficult situations if and when necessary.	☒	☒	☒	☒	☐	☐
28. Accepts constructive criticism and uses it to his or her advantage.	☐	☐	☐	☐	☐	☐
29. Leaves the radiographic room neat and clean for the next examination.	☒	☒	☒	☒	☐	☐
30. Completes the examination within a reasonable time frame.	☐	☐	☐	☐	☐	☐

Comments:

_____

_____

RADIOGRAPHIC IMAGE QUALITY
The student is able to critique his or her radiographs as to whether they demonstrate:

	Procedure		Repeat		Competency	
	Yes	No	Yes	No	Yes	No
31. Proper technique/optimal density	☒	☒	☒	☒	☐	☐
32. Enhanced detail, without evidence of motion and without any visible artifacts	☒	☒	☒	☒	☐	☐
33. Proper positioning (all anatomy included, evidence of proper centering/alignment, etc.)	☒	☒	☒	☒	☐	☐
34. Proper marker placement	☒	☒	☒	☒	☐	☐
35. Evidence of proper collimation and radiation protection	☒	☒	☒	☒	☐	☐
36. Long vs. short scale of contrast	☒	☒	☒	☒	☐	☐

(continued)

Comments:

_____

_____

FEMUR ANATOMY
The student is able to identify:

	Procedure		Repeat		Competency	
	Yes	No	Yes	No	Yes	No
37. Acetabulum	☐	☐	☐	☐	☐	☐
38. Femoral head	☐	☐	☐	☐	☐	☐
39. Greater and lesser trochanters	☐	☐	☐	☐	☐	☐
40. Femoral neck	☐	☐	☐	☐	☐	☐
41. Ischial tuberosity	☐	☐	☐	☐	☐	☐
42. Medial and lateral femoral condyles	☐	☐	☐	☐	☐	☐
43. Medial and lateral femoral epicondyles	☐	☐	☐	☐	☐	☐
44. Knee joint	☐	☐	☐	☐	☐	☐
45. Proximal fibula and tibia	☐	☐	☐	☐	☐	☐
46. Patella	☐	☐	☐	☐	☐	☐
47. Obvious pathology	☐	☐	☐	☐	☐	☐

Comments:

_____

_____

_____ _____ _____
Procedure Evaluator Signature   Repeat Evaluator Signature   Competency Evaluator Signature

_____ _____ _____
Date   Date   Date

END FEMUR EVALUATION

Student Name:_____

	Procedure Grade	Repeat Grade	Competency Grade

PATIENT INFORMATION OR SIMULATED PROCEDURE *(circle if simulated)*

	Procedure	Repeat	Competency
Age			
Medical Record No.			
Ability to Cooperate			
Condition/Pathology			
Technical Factors Used			
Exposure Index			

FACILITY PREPARATION
The student:

	Procedure Yes No	Repeat Yes No	Competency Yes No
1. Examines the radiographic room and cleans/straightens it before escorting the patient in.	☐ ☐	☐ ☐	☐ ☐
2. Has all equipment and supplies (patient gown, shield, markers, lead blockers, etc.) readily available before escorting the patient in.	☐ ☐	☐ ☐	☐ ☐
3. Is able to manipulate all radiographic equipment with ease, and centers the central ray to the cassette/receptor *for both projections.*	☐ ☐	☐ ☐	☐ ☐
4. Adjusts the tube to the proper SID *for each projection.*	☐ ☐	☐ ☐	☐ ☐
5. Selects cassettes/receptor of the appropriate sizes *for both projections,* according to patient size and examination.	☐ ☐	☐ ☐	☐ ☐

Comments:

_____

_____

PATIENT PREPARATION
The student:

	Procedure Yes No	Repeat Yes No	Competency Yes No
6. Identifies the correct patient and examination according to the requisition while establishing a good rapport with him or her.	☐ ☐	☐ ☐	☐ ☐
7. Obtains and documents the patient's history before the examination.	▨ ▨	▨ ▨	☐ ☐
8. Explains the examination in terms the patient fully understands and properly communicates with the patient throughout the examination.	☐ ☐	☐ ☐	☐ ☐
9. Asks female patients of childbearing age the date of their last menstrual period and documents this; inquires about the possibility of pregnancy and has them sign pregnancy consent forms.	☐ ☐	☐ ☐	☐ ☐
10. Removes all obscuring objects (shoes, zippers, belts, etc.) so as *not* to produce radiographic artifacts.	☐ ☐	☐ ☐	☐ ☐

(continued)

	Procedure		Repeat		Competency	
	Yes	No	Yes	No	Yes	No
11. Respects the patient's modesty and provides ample comfort for him or her.	☐	☐	☐	☐	☐	☐

Comments:

_____

_____

PATIENT POSITIONING FOR A HIP
Anteroposterior
The student:

	Procedure		Repeat		Competency	
	Yes	No	Yes	No	Yes	No
12. Places the patient in the supine position on the radiographic table, with the affected hip over the appropriate area of the Bucky/receptor, without rotation.	☐	☐	☐	☐	☐	☐
13. Rotates the leg internally, approximately 15°.	☐	☐	☐	☐	☐	☐
14. Centers the hip to the center of the cassette/receptor, or for bilateral hips, centers along the midsagittal plane.	☐	☐	☐	☐	☐	☐
15. Centers the central ray perpendicularly to the hip joint at the level just above the greater trochanter (between the anterosuperior iliac spine [ASIS] and the symphysis).	☐	☐	☐	☐	☐	☐

Lateral
The student:

	Procedure		Repeat		Competency	
	Yes	No	Yes	No	Yes	No
16. Positions the patient for one of the following:	☐	☐	☐	☐	☐	☐
a. For frog-leg lateral, instructs the patient to flex the affected hip and knee by bringing the sole of the affected foot up to the opposite knee, and then abducts the affected thigh, if possible, 40° from vertical (for bilateral hips, places the soles of the feet together and abducts both thighs evenly).						
b. For roll-up lateral, instructs the patient to roll laterally toward his or her affected side, and adjusts the position so that the unaffected hip lies posteriorly enough to prevent superimposition.						
17. Centers the hip to the center of the cassette/receptor.	☐	☐	☐	☐	☐	☐
18. Centers the central ray perpendicularly to the hip joint, between the ASIS and the symphysis.	☐	☐	☐	☐	☐	☐

Comments:

_____

_____

IMPORTANT DETAILS
The student:

	Procedure		Repeat		Competency	
	Yes	No	Yes	No	Yes	No
19. Instills confidence in the patient by exhibiting self-confidence throughout the examination.	☐	☐	☐	☐	☐	☐
20. Places a lead marker in the appropriate area of the cassette/receptor (top/bottom/anteriorly/laterally), where it will be visualized on the finished radiograph, on the proper anatomical side (right/left), and in the appropriate position (face up/face down), depending on the patient's position.	☐	☐	☐	☐	☐	☐
21. Provides radiation protection (shield) for the patient (when appropriate), self, and others (closes doors).	☐	☐	☐	☐	☐	☐
22. Applies proper collimation and makes adjustments as necessary.	☐	☐	☐	☐	☐	☐

	Procedure		Repeat		Competency	
	Yes	No	Yes	No	Yes	No
23. Properly measures the patient along the course of the central ray *for each projection*.	☐	☐	☐	☐	☐	☐

24. Sets the proper exposure techniques:
 	
Conventional systems
• Sets the proper kVp, mA, and time, and makes adjustments as necessary.
or
CR or DR systems
• Identifies the patient on the work-list (or manually types the patient information into the system).
• Selects appropriate body region, specific body part, and accurate view/projection.
• Double-checks preset parameters:
  —Adult vs. pediatric patients
    ○ Small, medium, or large
  —Bucky/receptor (upright vs. table) *or* non-Bucky
  —AEC vs. fixed
    ○ If AEC, checks ion chambers
    ○ Density setting
  —kVp and mA; adjusts if necessary
  —Focal spot/filament size
	☐	☐	☐	☐	☐	☐

25. Exposes the cassette/receptor after telling the patient to hold still and after giving the patient proper breathing instructions (expiration) *for each projection*.	☐	☐	☐	☐	☐	☐
26. Provides each radiograph with the proper identification (flash) and/or processes each cassette (image) without difficulty (regardless of technology—film, CR, or DR).	■	■	■	■	☐	☐
27. Properly completes the examination by filling out all necessary paperwork, entering the examination in the computer, having the images checked by the appropriate staff members, answering any last-minute questions, and informing the patient that he or she is finished.	■	■	■	■	☐	☐
28. Exhibits the ability to adapt to new and difficult situations if and when necessary.	■	■	■	■	☐	☐
29. Accepts constructive criticism and uses it to his or her advantage.	☐	☐	☐	☐	☐	☐
30. Leaves the radiographic room neat and clean for the next examination.	■	■	■	■	☐	☐
31. Completes the examination within a reasonable time frame.	☐	☐	☐	☐	☐	☐

Comments:

_____

_____

RADIOGRAPHIC IMAGE QUALITY

The student is able to critique his or her radiographs as to whether they demonstrate:

	Procedure		Repeat		Competency	
	Yes	No	Yes	No	Yes	No
32. Proper technique/optimal density	■	■	■	■	☐	☐
33. Enhanced detail, without evidence of motion and without any visible artifacts	■	■	■	■	☐	☐
34. Proper positioning (all anatomy included, evidence of proper centering/alignment, etc.)	■	■	■	■	☐	☐
35. Proper marker placement	■	■	■	■	☐	☐
36. Evidence of proper collimation and radiation protection	■	■	■	■	☐	☐
37. Long vs. short scale of contrast	■	■	■	■	☐	☐

(continued)

Comments:

_____

_____

HIP ANATOMY
The student is able to identify:

	Procedure		Repeat		Competency	
	Yes	No	Yes	No	Yes	No
38. Acetabulum	☐	☐	☐	☐	☐	☐
39. Femoral head	☐	☐	☐	☐	☐	☐
40. Greater and lesser trochanters	☐	☐	☐	☐	☐	☐
41. Femoral neck	☐	☐	☐	☐	☐	☐
42. Ischial tuberosity	☐	☐	☐	☐	☐	☐
43. Ilium	☐	☐	☐	☐	☐	☐
44. Public symphysis	☐	☐	☐	☐	☐	☐
45. Obturator foramen	☐	☐	☐	☐	☐	☐
46. Obvious pathology	☐	☐	☐	☐	☐	☐

Comments:

_____

_____

_____   _____   _____
Procedure Evaluator Signature   Repeat Evaluator Signature   Competency Evaluator Signature

_____   _____   _____
Date   Date   Date

END HIP EVALUATION

Student Name:_____

Procedure Grade	Repeat Grade	Competency Grade

PATIENT INFORMATION OR SIMULATED PROCEDURE *(circle if simulated)*

	Procedure	Repeat	Competency
Age			
Medical Record No.			
Ability to Cooperate			
Condition/Pathology			
Technical Factors Used			
Exposure Index			

FACILITY PREPARATION
The student:

	Procedure Yes No	Repeat Yes No	Competency Yes No
1. Examines the radiographic room and cleans/straightens it before escorting the patient in.	☐ ☐	☐ ☐	☐ ☐
2. Has all equipment and supplies (patient gown, shield, markers, lead blockers, etc.) readily available before escorting the patient in.	☐ ☐	☐ ☐	☐ ☐
3. Is able to manipulate all radiographic equipment with ease, and centers the central ray to the cassette/receptor *for both projections*.	☐ ☐	☐ ☐	☐ ☐
4. Adjusts the tube to the proper SID *for each projection*.	☐ ☐	☐ ☐	☐ ☐
5. Selects cassettes/receptor of the appropriate sizes *for both projections*, according to patient size and examination.	☐ ☐	☐ ☐	☐ ☐

Comments:

_____

_____

PATIENT PREPARATION
The student:

	Procedure Yes No	Repeat Yes No	Competency Yes No
6. Identifies the correct patient and examination according to the requisition while establishing a good rapport with him or her.	☐ ☐	☐ ☐	☐ ☐
7. Obtains and documents the patient's history before the examination.	▨ ▨	▨ ▨	☐ ☐
8. Explains the examination in terms the patient fully understands and properly communicates with the patient throughout the examination.	☐ ☐	☐ ☐	☐ ☐
9. Asks female patients of childbearing age the date of their last menstrual period and documents this; inquires about the possibility of pregnancy and has them sign pregnancy consent forms.	☐ ☐	☐ ☐	☐ ☐
10. Removes all obscuring objects (shoes, zippers, belts, etc.) so as *not* to produce radiographic artifacts.	☐ ☐	☐ ☐	☐ ☐

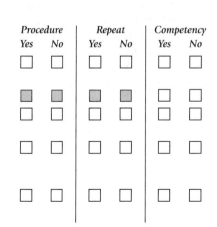

(continued)

	Procedure		Repeat		Competency	
	Yes	No	Yes	No	Yes	No
11. Respects the patient's modesty and provides ample comfort for him or her.	☐	☐	☐	☐	☐	☐

Comments:

_____

_____

PATIENT POSITIONING FOR A TRAUMA HIP
Anteroposterior
The student:

	Procedure		Repeat		Competency	
	Yes	No	Yes	No	Yes	No
12. Places the patient in the supine position on the radiographic table, with the affected hip over the appropriate area of the Bucky/receptor, without rotation.	☐	☐	☐	☐	☐	☐
13. If possible, rotates the leg internally approximately 15°.	☐	☐	☐	☐	☐	☐
14. Centers the hip to the center of the cassette/receptor.	☐	☐	☐	☐	☐	☐
15. Centers the central ray perpendicularly to the hip joint at a level just above the greater trochanter (between the ASIS and the symphysis).	☐	☐	☐	☐	☐	☐

Axiolateral Projection (Danelius-Miller Modification of Lorenz Method)
The student:

	Procedure		Repeat		Competency	
	Yes	No	Yes	No	Yes	No
16. Places a grided cassette/receptor vertically at the crease at the top of the iliac crest so that it is centered and parallel to the femoral neck.	☐	☐	☐	☐	☐	☐
17. Flexes the patient's unaffected hip and knee, and rests the knee on an elevated support high enough so that it does not interfere with the projection of the central ray.	☐	☐	☐	☐	☐	☐
18. Horizontally centers the central ray perpendicularly to the hip joint/femoral neck.	☐	☐	☐	☐	☐	☐

Comments:

_____

_____

IMPORTANT DETAILS
The student:

	Procedure		Repeat		Competency	
	Yes	No	Yes	No	Yes	No
19. Instills confidence in the patient by exhibiting self-confidence throughout the examination.	☐	☐	☐	☐	☐	☐
20. Places a lead marker in the appropriate area of the cassette/receptor (top/bottom/anteriorly/laterally), where it will be visualized on the finished radiograph, on the proper anatomical side (right/left), and in the appropriate position (face up/face down), depending on the patient's position.	☐	☐	☐	☐	☐	☐
21. Provides radiation protection (shield) for the patient (when appropriate), self, and others (closes doors).	☐	☐	☐	☐	☐	☐
22. Applies proper collimation and makes adjustments as necessary.	☐	☐	☐	☐	☐	☐
23. Properly measures the patient along the course of the central ray *for each projection.*	☐	☐	☐	☐	☐	☐
24. Sets the proper exposure techniques:	☐	☐	☐	☐	☐	☐

Conventional systems
• Sets the proper kVp, mA, and time, and makes adjustments as necessary.

or

	Procedure		Repeat		Competency	
	Yes	No	Yes	No	Yes	No

CR or DR systems
- Identifies the patient on the work-list (or manually types the patient information into the system).
- Selects appropriate body region, specific body part, and accurate view/projection.
- Double-checks preset parameters:
  —Adult vs. pediatric patients
  ◦ Small, medium, or large
  —Bucky/receptor (upright vs. table) *or* non-Bucky
  —AEC vs. fixed
  ◦ If AEC, checks ion chambers
  ◦ Density setting
  —kVp and mA; adjusts if necessary
  —Focal spot/filament size

	Procedure		Repeat		Competency	
	Yes	No	Yes	No	Yes	No
25. Exposes the cassette/receptor after telling the patient to hold still and after giving the patient proper breathing instructions (expiration) *for each projection.*	☐	☐	☐	☐	☐	☐
26. Provides each radiograph with the proper identification (flash) and/or processes each cassette (image) without difficulty (regardless of technology—film, CR, or DR).	☐	☐	☐	☐	☐	☐
27. Properly completes the examination by filling out all necessary paperwork, entering the examination in the computer, having the images checked by the appropriate staff members, answering any last-minute questions, and informing the patient that he or she is finished.	☐	☐	☐	☐	☐	☐
28. Exhibits the ability to adapt to new and difficult situations if and when necessary.	☐	☐	☐	☐	☐	☐
29. Accepts constructive criticism and uses it to his or her advantage.	☐	☐	☐	☐	☐	☐
30. Leaves the radiographic room neat and clean for the next examination.	☐	☐	☐	☐	☐	☐
31. Completes the examination within a reasonable time frame.	☐	☐	☐	☐	☐	☐

Comments:

_____

_____

RADIOGRAPHIC IMAGE QUALITY
The student is able to critique his or her radiographs as to whether they demonstrate:

	Procedure		Repeat		Competency	
	Yes	No	Yes	No	Yes	No
32. Proper technique/optimal density	☐	☐	☐	☐	☐	☐
33. Enhanced detail, without evidence of motion and without any visible artifacts	☐	☐	☐	☐	☐	☐
34. Proper positioning (all anatomy included, evidence of proper centering/alignment, etc.)	☐	☐	☐	☐	☐	☐
35. Proper marker placement	☐	☐	☐	☐	☐	☐
36. Evidence of proper collimation and radiation protection	☐	☐	☐	☐	☐	☐
37. Long vs. short scale of contrast	☐	☐	☐	☐	☐	☐

Comments:

_____

_____

(continued)

HIP ANATOMY
The student is able to identify:

	Procedure		Repeat		Competency	
	Yes	No	Yes	No	Yes	No
38. Acetabulum	☐	☐	☐	☐	☐	☐
39. Femoral head	☐	☐	☐	☐	☐	☐
40. Greater and lesser trochanters	☐	☐	☐	☐	☐	☐
41. Femoral neck	☐	☐	☐	☐	☐	☐
42. Ischial tuberosity	☐	☐	☐	☐	☐	☐
43. Obvious pathology	☐	☐	☐	☐	☐	☐

Comments:

_____

_____

| Procedure Evaluator Signature | Repeat Evaluator Signature | Competency Evaluator Signature |

| Date | Date | Date |

END TRAUMA HIP (CROSS-TABLE) EVALUATION

Student Name:_____

Procedure Grade	Repeat Grade	Competency Grade

PATIENT INFORMATION OR SIMULATED PROCEDURE *(circle if simulated)*

	Procedure	Repeat	Competency
Age			
Medical Record No.			
Ability to Cooperate			
Condition/Pathology			
Technical Factors Used			
Exposure Index			

FACILITY PREPARATION
The student:

	Procedure Yes	No	Repeat Yes	No	Competency Yes	No
1. Examines the radiographic room and cleans/straightens it before escorting the patient in.	☐	☐	☐	☐	☐	☐
2. Has all equipment and supplies (patient gown, shield, markers, lead blockers, etc.) readily available before escorting the patient in.	☐	☐	☐	☐	☐	☐
3. Is able to manipulate all radiographic equipment with ease, and centers the central ray to the cassette/receptor *for all projections*.	☐	☐	☐	☐	☐	☐
4. Adjusts the tube to the proper SID *for each projection*.	☐	☐	☐	☐	☐	☐
5. Selects cassettes/receptor of the appropriate sizes *for all projections*, according to patient size and examination.	☐	☐	☐	☐	☐	☐

Comments:

_____

_____

PATIENT PREPARATION
The student:

	Procedure Yes	No	Repeat Yes	No	Competency Yes	No
6. Identifies the correct patient and examination according to the requisition while establishing a good rapport with him or her.	☐	☐	☐	☐	☐	☐
7. Obtains and documents the patient's history before the examination.	▨	▨	▨	▨	☐	☐
8. Explains the examination in terms the patient fully understands and properly communicates with the patient throughout the examination.	☐	☐	☐	☐	☐	☐
9. Asks female patients of childbearing age the date of their last menstrual period and documents this; inquires about the possibility of pregnancy and has them sign pregnancy consent forms.	☐	☐	☐	☐	☐	☐
10. Removes all obscuring objects (shoes, zippers, jewelry, etc.) so as *not* to produce radiographic artifacts.	☐	☐	☐	☐	☐	☐

(continued)

	Procedure		Repeat		Competency	
	Yes	No	Yes	No	Yes	No
11. Respects the patient's modesty and provides ample comfort for him or her.	☐	☐	☐	☐	☐	☐

Comments:

_____

_____

PATIENT POSITIONING FOR TRAUMA OF THE LOWER EXTREMITY
AP or PA
The student:

	Procedure		Repeat		Competency	
	Yes	No	Yes	No	Yes	No
12. Places the patient in the truest AP or PA position possible.	☐	☐	☐	☐	☐	☐
13. Selects the appropriate receptor or places the cassette appropriately. For conventional cassettes, the flash must be high or low enough that it does not obscure any anatomy.	☐	☐	☐	☐	☐	☐
14. Centers the central ray to the midline of the affected area, making sure both the proximal and distal joints will be demonstrated on the finished radiograph (if required).	☐	☐	☐	☐	☐	☐
15. Centers the central ray perpendicularly or with the appropriate angle relative to the part being radiographed.	☐	☐	☐	☐	☐	☐

Lateral
The student:

	Procedure		Repeat		Competency	
	Yes	No	Yes	No	Yes	No
16. Places the patient in the truest lateral position possible or prepares the patient for a shoot-through radiograph.	☐	☐	☐	☐	☐	☐
17. Selects the appropriate receptor or places the cassette appropriately. For conventional cassettes, the flash must be high or low enough that it does not obscure any anatomy.	☐	☐	☐	☐	☐	☐
18. Centers the central ray to the midline of the affected area, making sure both the proximal and distal joints will be demonstrated on the finished radiograph (if required).	☐	☐	☐	☐	☐	☐
19. Centers the central ray perpendicularly or with the appropriate angle relative to the part being radiographed.	☐	☐	☐	☐	☐	☐

Comments:

_____

_____

IMPORTANT DETAILS
The student:

	Procedure		Repeat		Competency	
	Yes	No	Yes	No	Yes	No
20. Instills confidence in the patient by exhibiting self-confidence throughout the examination.	☐	☐	☐	☐	☐	☐
21. Places a lead marker in the appropriate area of the cassette/receptor (top/bottom/anteriorly/laterally), where it will be visualized on the finished radiograph, on the proper anatomical side (right/left), and in the appropriate position (face up/face down), depending on the patient's position.	☐	☐	☐	☐	☐	☐
22. Provides radiation protection (shield) for the patient, self, and others (closes doors).	☐	☐	☐	☐	☐	☐
23. Applies proper collimation and makes adjustments as necessary.	☐	☐	☐	☐	☐	☐
24. Properly measures the patient along the course of the central ray *for each projection.*	☐	☐	☐	☐	☐	☐
25. Sets the proper exposure techniques:	☐	☐	☐	☐	☐	☐

Conventional systems
• Sets the proper kVp, mA, and time, and makes adjustments as necessary.

	Procedure		Repeat		Competency	
	Yes	No	Yes	No	Yes	No

or

CR or DR systems
- Identifies the patient on the work-list (or manually types the patient information into the system).
- Selects appropriate body region, specific body part, and accurate view/projection.
- Double-checks preset parameters:
  —Adult vs. pediatric patients
    ◦ Small, medium, or large
  —Bucky/receptor (upright vs. table) *or* non-Bucky
  —AEC vs. fixed
    ◦ If AEC, checks ION chambers
    ◦ Density setting
  —kVp and mA; adjusts if necessary
  —Focal spot/filament size

	Procedure		Repeat		Competency	
	Yes	No	Yes	No	Yes	No
26. Exposes the cassette/receptor after telling the patient to hold still and supporting or immobilizing the area of interest if necessary *for each projection.*	☐	☐	☐	☐	☐	☐
27. Provides each radiograph with the proper identification (flash) and/or processes each cassette (image) without difficulty (regardless of technology—film, CR, or DR).	▣	▣	▣	▣	☐	☐
28. Properly completes the examination by filling out all necessary paperwork, entering the examination in the computer, having the images checked by the appropriate staff members, answering any last-minute questions, and informing the patient that he or she is finished.	▣	▣	▣	▣	☐	☐
29. Exhibits the ability to adapt to new and difficult situations if and when necessary.	▣	▣	▣	▣	☐	☐
30. Accepts constructive criticism and uses it to his or her advantage.	☐	☐	☐	☐	☐	☐
31. Leaves the radiographic room neat and clean for the next examination.	▣	▣	▣	▣	☐	☐
32. Completes the examination within a reasonable time frame.	☐	☐	☐	☐	☐	☐

Comments:

_____

_____

RADIOGRAPHIC IMAGE QUALITY
The student is able to critique his or her radiographs as to whether they demonstrate:

	Procedure		Repeat		Competency	
	Yes	No	Yes	No	Yes	No
33. Proper technique/optimal density	▣	▣	▣	▣	☐	☐
34. Enhanced detail, without evidence of motion and without any visible artifacts	▣	▣	▣	▣	☐	☐
35. Proper positioning (all anatomy included, evidence of proper centering/alignment, etc.)	▣	▣	▣	▣	☐	☐
36. Proper marker placement	▣	▣	▣	▣	☐	☐
37. Evidence of proper collimation and radiation protection	▣	▣	▣	▣	☐	☐
38. Long vs. short scale of contrast	▣	▣	▣	▣	☐	☐

Comments:

_____

_____

(continued)

TRAUMA LOWER EXTREMITY ANATOMY
The student is able to identify:

	Procedure		Repeat		Competency	
	Yes	No	Yes	No	Yes	No
39. _____	☐	☐	☐	☐	☐	☐
40. _____	☐	☐	☐	☐	☐	☐
41. _____	☐	☐	☐	☐	☐	☐
42. _____	☐	☐	☐	☐	☐	☐
43. _____	☐	☐	☐	☐	☐	☐
44. _____	☐	☐	☐	☐	☐	☐
45. _____	☐	☐	☐	☐	☐	☐
46. Obvious pathology	☐	☐	☐	☐	☐	☐

Comments:

_____

_____

_____ _____ _____
Procedure Evaluator Signature   Repeat Evaluator Signature   Competency Evaluator Signature

_____ _____ _____
Date   Date   Date

END TRAUMA LOWER EXTREMITY EVALUATION

Student Name:_____

Procedure Grade	Repeat Grade	Competency Grade

PATIENT INFORMATION OR SIMULATED PROCEDURE *(circle if simulated)*

	Procedure	Repeat	Competency
Age			
Medical Record No.			
Ability to Cooperate			
Condition/Pathology			
Technical Factors Used			
Exposure Index			

FACILITY PREPARATION
The student:

	Procedure Yes	Procedure No	Repeat Yes	Repeat No	Competency Yes	Competency No
1. Examines the radiographic room and cleans/straightens it before escorting the patient in.	☐	☐	☐	☐	☐	☐
2. Has all equipment and supplies (patient gown, shield, markers, tape, cassettes, etc.) readily available before escorting the patient in.	☐	☐	☐	☐	☐	☐
3. Is able to manipulate all radiographic equipment with ease, and centers the central ray to the cassette/receptor *for all projections.*	☐	☐	☐	☐	☐	☐
4. Adjusts the tube to the proper SID *for each projection.*	☐	☐	☐	☐	☐	☐
5. Selects the appropriate receptor or cassettes of the appropriate sizes *for all projections,* according to the patient's size and examination.	☐	☐	☐	☐	☐	☐

Comments:

_____

_____

PATIENT PREPARATION
The student:

	Procedure Yes	Procedure No	Repeat Yes	Repeat No	Competency Yes	Competency No
6. Identifies the correct patient and examination according to the requisition while establishing a good rapport with him or her.	☐	☐	☐	☐	☐	☐
7. Obtains and documents the patient's history before the examination.	▣	▣	▣	▣	☐	☐
8. Explains the examination in terms the patient fully understands and properly communicates with the patient throughout the examination.	☐	☐	☐	☐	☐	☐
9. If she intends to stay in the room during the procedure, asks the patient's mother/female guardian of childbearing age the date of her last menstrual period and documents this; inquires about the possibility of pregnancy and has her sign pregnancy consent forms.	☐	☐	☐	☐	☐	☐
10. Removes all obscuring objects (shoes, zippers, jewelry, etc.) so as *not* to produce radiographic artifacts.	☐	☐	☐	☐	☐	☐

(continued)

	Procedure		Repeat		Competency	
	Yes	No	Yes	No	Yes	No
11. Respects the patient's modesty and provides ample comfort for him or her.	☐	☐	☐	☐	☐	☐

Comments:

_____

_____

PATIENT POSITIONING FOR A PEDIATRIC LOWER EXTREMITY
AP or PA
The student:

	Procedure		Repeat		Competency	
	Yes	No	Yes	No	Yes	No
12. Places the patient in the supine or prone position on the radiographic table, without rotation.	☐	☐	☐	☐	☐	☐
13. Selects the appropriate receptor or places the cassette appropriately. For conventional cassettes, the flash must be away from any anatomy.	☐	☐	☐	☐	☐	☐
14. Centers the central ray to the midline (between the lateral surfaces) of the affected extremity.	☐	☐	☐	☐	☐	☐
15. Directs the central ray perpendicularly.	☐	☐	☐	☐	☐	☐

Lateral
The student:

	Procedure		Repeat		Competency	
	Yes	No	Yes	No	Yes	No
16. Places the patient in the true lateral position, without rotation.	☐	☐	☐	☐	☐	☐
17. Selects the appropriate receptor or places the cassette appropriately. For conventional cassettes, the flash must be away from any anatomy.	☐	☐	☐	☐	☐	☐
18. Centers the central ray midway between the anterior and posterior surfaces of the affected extremity.	☐	☐	☐	☐	☐	☐
19. Directs the central ray perpendicularly.	☐	☐	☐	☐	☐	☐

Comments:

_____

_____

IMPORTANT DETAILS
The student:

	Procedure		Repeat		Competency	
	Yes	No	Yes	No	Yes	No
20. Instills confidence in the patient and parent/guardian by exhibiting self-confidence throughout the examination.	☐	☐	☐	☐	☐	☐
21. Places lead markers in the appropriate area of the cassette/receptor (top/bottom/anteriorly/laterally), where they will be visualized, on the proper anatomical side (right/left), and in the appropriate position (face up/face down), depending on the patient's position.	☐	☐	☐	☐	☐	☐
22. Provides radiation protection (shield) for the patient, parent/guardian, self, and others (closes doors).	☐	☐	☐	☐	☐	☐
23. Applies proper collimation and makes adjustments as necessary.	☐	☐	☐	☐	☐	☐
24. Properly measures the patient along the course of the central ray.	☐	☐	☐	☐	☐	☐
25. Sets the proper exposure techniques:	☐	☐	☐	☐	☐	☐

Conventional systems
- Sets the proper kVp, mA, and time, and makes adjustments as necessary.

or

CR or DR systems
- Identifies the patient on the work-list (or manually types the patient information into the system).

- Selects appropriate body region, specific body part, and accurate view/projection.
- Double-checks preset parameters:
  - —Adult vs. pediatric patients
    - ○ Small, medium, or large
  - —Bucky/receptor (upright vs. table) *or* non-Bucky
  - —AEC vs. fixed
    - ○ If AEC, checks ion chambers
    - ○ Density setting
  - —kVp and mA; adjusts if necessary
  - —Focal spot/filament size

	Procedure Yes	Procedure No	Repeat Yes	Repeat No	Competency Yes	Competency No
26. Exposes the cassette/receptor after telling the patient to hold still and after giving him or her proper breathing instructions (if necessary) *for each projection.*	☐	☐	☐	☐	☐	☐
27. Provides each radiograph with the proper identification (flash) and/or processes each cassette (image) without difficulty (regardless of technology—film, CR, or DR).	☐	☐	☐	☐	☐	☐
28. Properly completes the examination by filling out all necessary paperwork, entering the examination in the computer, having images checked by the appropriate staff members, providing postprocedural instructions and answering last-minute questions, and informing the patient that he or she is finished.	☐	☐	☐	☐	☐	☐
29. Exhibits the ability to adapt to new and difficult situations if and when necessary.	☐	☐	☐	☐	☐	☐
30. Accepts constructive criticism and uses it to his or her advantage.	☐	☐	☐	☐	☐	☐
31. Leaves the radiographic room neat and clean for the next examination.	☐	☐	☐	☐	☐	☐
32. Completes the examination within a reasonable time frame.	☐	☐	☐	☐	☐	☐

Comments:

_____

_____

RADIOGRAPHIC IMAGE QUALITY

The student is able to critique his or her radiographs as to whether they demonstrate:

	Procedure Yes	Procedure No	Repeat Yes	Repeat No	Competency Yes	Competency No
33. Proper technique/optimal density	☐	☐	☐	☐	☐	☐
34. Enhanced detail, without evidence of motion and without any visible artifacts	☐	☐	☐	☐	☐	☐
35. Proper positioning (all anatomy included, evidence of proper centering/alignment, etc.)	☐	☐	☐	☐	☐	☐
36. Proper marker placement	☐	☐	☐	☐	☐	☐
37. Evidence of proper collimation and radiation protection	☐	☐	☐	☐	☐	☐
38. Long vs. short scale of contrast	☐	☐	☐	☐	☐	☐

Comments:

_____

_____

(continued)

PEDIATRIC LOWER EXTREMITY ANATOMY
The student is able to identify:

	Procedure		Repeat		Competency	
	Yes	No	Yes	No	Yes	No
39. _____		☐	☐	☐	☐	☐
40. _____	☐	☐	☐	☐	☐	☐
41. _____	☐	☐	☐	☐	☐	☐
42. _____	☐	☐	☐	☐	☐	☐
43. _____	☐	☐	☐	☐	☐	☐
44. _____	☐	☐	☐	☐	☐	☐
45. _____	☐	☐	☐	☐	☐	☐
46. Obvious pathology	☐	☐	☐	☐	☐	☐

Comments:

_____

_____

_____   _____   _____
Procedure Evaluator Signature   Repeat Evaluator Signature   Competency Evaluator Signature

_____   _____   _____
Date   Date   Date

END PEDIATRIC LOWER EXTREMITY (AGE 6 OR YOUNGER) EVALUATION

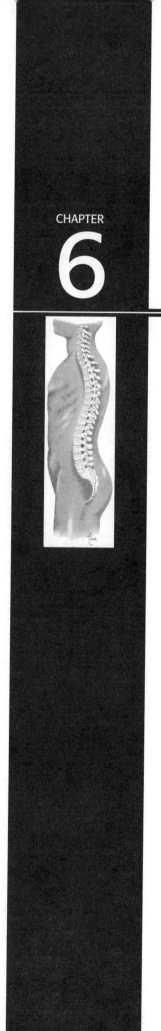

Spine, Pelvis, and Trunk

specific radiographic examinations.

Student Name:_____

Procedure Grade	Repeat Grade	Competency Grade

PATIENT INFORMATION OR SIMULATED PROCEDURE *(circle if simulated)*

	Procedure	Repeat	Competency
Age			
Medical Record No.			
Ability to Cooperate			
Condition/Pathology			
Technical Factors Used			
Exposure Index			

FACILITY PREPARATION
The student:

	Procedure Yes No	Repeat Yes No	Competency Yes No
1. Examines the radiographic room and cleans/straightens it before escorting the patient in.	☐ ☐	☐ ☐	☐ ☐
2. Has all equipment and supplies (patient gown, shield, markers, lead blockers, etc.) readily available before escorting the patient in.	☐ ☐	☐ ☐	☐ ☐
3. Is able to manipulate all radiographic equipment with ease, and centers the central ray to the cassette/receptor *for both projections.*	☐ ☐	☐ ☐	☐ ☐
4. Adjusts the tube to the proper SID *for each projection.*	☐ ☐	☐ ☐	☐ ☐
5. Selects cassettes/receptor of the appropriate sizes *for all projections,* according to the patient's size and examination.	☐ ☐	☐ ☐	☐ ☐

Comments:

_____

_____

PATIENT PREPARATION
The student:

	Procedure Yes No	Repeat Yes No	Competency Yes No
6. Identifies the correct patient and examination according to the requisition while establishing a good rapport with him or her.	☐ ☐	☐ ☐	☐ ☐
7. Obtains and documents the patient's history before the examination.	▨ ▨	▨ ▨	☐ ☐
8. Explains the examination in terms the patient fully understands and properly communicates with the patient throughout the examination.	☐ ☐	☐ ☐	☐ ☐
9. Asks female patients of childbearing age the date of their last menstrual period and documents this; inquires about the possibility of pregnancy and has them sign pregnancy consent forms.	☐ ☐	☐ ☐	☐ ☐
10. Removes all obscuring objects (snaps, zippers, jewelry, etc.) so as *not* to produce radiographic artifacts.	☐ ☐	☐ ☐	☐ ☐

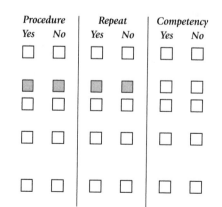

(continued)

	Procedure		Repeat		Competency	
	Yes	No	Yes	No	Yes	No
11. Respects the patient's modesty and provides ample comfort for him or her.	☐	☐	☐	☐	☐	☐

Comments:

_____

_____

PATIENT POSITIONING FOR A STERNUM
Right Anterior Oblique
The student:

	Procedure		Repeat		Competency	
	Yes	No	Yes	No	Yes	No
12. Places the patient in the RAO position, at an angle of 15–20°, against the upright Bucky/receptor.	☐	☐	☐	☐	☐	☐
13. Selects the appropriate receptor or places the upper border of the cassette lengthwise 2 inches above the patient's sternum. For conventional cassettes, the flash must be at the top and away from any anatomy.	☐	☐	☐	☐	☐	☐
14. Directs the central ray slightly to the left of the vertebral column.	☐	☐	☐	☐	☐	☐
15. Centers the central ray perpendicularly, midway between the manubrial notch and the xiphoid.	☐	☐	☐	☐	☐	☐

Lateral
The student:

	Procedure		Repeat		Competency	
	Yes	No	Yes	No	Yes	No
16. Places the patient in the left lateral position against the upright Bucky/receptor.	☐	☐	☐	☐	☐	☐
17. Selects the appropriate receptor or places the upper border of the cassette lengthwise 2 inches above the patient's sternum. For conventional cassettes, the flash must be at the top and away from any anatomy.	☐	☐	☐	☐	☐	☐
18. Rotates the arms and shoulders backward, out of the area of interest.	☐	☐	☐	☐	☐	☐
19. Directs the central ray to the lateral sternum.	☐	☐	☐	☐	☐	☐
20. Centers the central ray perpendicularly midway between the manubrial notch and the xiphoid.	☐	☐	☐	☐	☐	☐

Comments:

_____

_____

IMPORTANT DETAILS
The student:

	Procedure		Repeat		Competency	
	Yes	No	Yes	No	Yes	No
21. Instills confidence in the patient by exhibiting self-confidence throughout the examination.	☐	☐	☐	☐	☐	☐
22. Places a lead marker in the appropriate area of the cassette/receptor (top/bottom/anteriorly/laterally), where it will be visualized on the finished radiograph, on the proper anatomical side (right/left), and in the appropriate position (face up/face down), depending on the patient's position.	☐	☐	☐	☐	☐	☐
23. Provides radiation protection for himself or herself and others.	☐	☐	☐	☐	☐	☐
24. Applies proper collimation and makes adjustments as necessary.	☐	☐	☐	☐	☐	☐
25. Properly measures the patient along the course of the central ray *for each projection.*	☐	☐	☐	☐	☐	☐

	Procedure		Repeat		Competency	
	Yes	No	Yes	No	Yes	No
26. Sets the proper exposure techniques:	☐	☐	☐	☐	☐	☐

Conventional systems
- Sets the proper kVp, mA, and time and makes adjustments as necessary.

or

CR or DR systems
- Identifies the patient on the work-list (or manually types the patient information into the system).
- Selects appropriate body region, specific body part, and accurate view/projection.
- Double-checks preset parameters:
  —Adult vs. pediatric patients
   ○ Small, medium, or large
  —Bucky/receptor (upright vs. table) *or* non-Bucky
  —AEC vs. fixed
   ○ If AEC, checks ion chambers
   ○ Density setting
  —kVp and mA; adjusts if necessary
  —Focal spot/filament size

	Procedure		Repeat		Competency	
	Yes	No	Yes	No	Yes	No
27. Exposes the cassette/receptor after telling the patient to hold still and after giving him or her proper breathing instructions (RAO—shallow breathing; lateral—inspiration) *for each projection.*	☐	☐	☐	☐	☐	☐
28. Provides each radiograph with the proper identification (flash) and/or processes each cassette (image) without difficulty (regardless of technology—film, CR, or DR).	▢	▢	▢	▢	☐	☐
29. Properly completes the examination by filling out all necessary paperwork, entering the examination in the computer, having the images checked by the appropriate staff members, answering any last-minute questions, and informing the patient that he or she is finished.	▢	▢	▢	▢	☐	☐
30. Exhibits the ability to adapt to new and difficult situations if and when necessary.	▢	▢	▢	▢	☐	☐
31. Accepts constructive criticism and uses it to his or her advantage.	☐	☐	☐	☐	☐	☐
32. Leaves the radiographic room neat and clean for the next examination.	▢	▢	▢	▢	☐	☐
33. Completes the examination within a reasonable time frame.	☐	☐	☐	☐	☐	☐

Comments:

_____

_____

RADIOGRAPHIC IMAGE QUALITY
The student is able to critique his or her radiographs as to whether they demonstrate:

	Procedure		Repeat		Competency	
	Yes	No	Yes	No	Yes	No
34. Proper technique/optimal density	▢	▢	▢	▢	☐	☐
35. Enhanced detail, without evidence of motion and without any visible artifacts	▢	▢	▢	▢	☐	☐
36. Proper positioning (all anatomy included, evidence of proper centering/alignment, etc.)	▢	▢	▢	▢	☐	☐
37. Proper marker placement	▢	▢	▢	▢	☐	☐
38. Evidence of proper collimation and radiation protection	▢	▢	▢	▢	☐	☐
39. Long vs. short scale of contrast	▢	▢	▢	▢	☐	☐

(continued)

Comments:

_____

_____

STERNUM ANATOMY
The student is able to identify:

	Procedure		Repeat		Competency	
	Yes	No	Yes	No	Yes	No
40. Manubrial/jugular notch	☐	☐	☐	☐	☐	☐
41. Manubrium	☐	☐	☐	☐	☐	☐
42. Body/gladiolus	☐	☐	☐	☐	☐	☐
43. Xiphoid	☐	☐	☐	☐	☐	☐
44. Sternoclavicular (SC) joint articulation	☐	☐	☐	☐	☐	☐
45. Sternal angle	☐	☐	☐	☐	☐	☐
46. Obvious pathology	☐	☐	☐	☐	☐	☐

Comments:

_____

_____

_____   _____   _____
Procedure Evaluator Signature   Repeat Evaluator Signature   Competency Evaluator Signature

_____   _____   _____
Date   Date   Date

END STERNUM EVALUATION

Student Name:_____

Procedure Grade	Repeat Grade	Competency Grade

PATIENT INFORMATION OR SIMULATED PROCEDURE *(circle if simulated)*

	Procedure	Repeat	Competency
Age			
Medical Record No.			
Ability to Cooperate			
Condition/Pathology			
Technical Factors Used			
Exposure Index			

FACILITY PREPARATION
The student:

	Procedure Yes / No	Repeat Yes / No	Competency Yes / No
1. Examines the radiographic room and cleans/straightens it before escorting the patient in.	☐ ☐	☐ ☐	☐ ☐
2. Has all equipment and supplies (patient gown, shield, markers, lead blockers, etc.) readily available before escorting the patient in.	☐ ☐	☐ ☐	☐ ☐
3. Is able to manipulate all radiographic equipment with ease, and centers the central ray to the cassette/receptor *for all projections.*	☐ ☐	☐ ☐	☐ ☐
4. Adjusts the tube to the proper SID *for each projection.*	☐ ☐	☐ ☐	☐ ☐
5. Selects cassettes/receptor of the appropriate sizes *for both projections,* according to the patient's size and examination.	☐ ☐	☐ ☐	☐ ☐

Comments:

_____

_____

PATIENT PREPARATION
The student:

	Procedure Yes / No	Repeat Yes / No	Competency Yes / No
6. Identifies the correct patient and examination according to the requisition while establishing a good rapport with him or her.	☐ ☐	☐ ☐	☐ ☐
7. Obtains and documents the patient's history before the examination.	▧ ▧	▧ ▧	☐ ☐
8. Explains the examination in terms the patient fully understands and properly communicates with the patient throughout the examination.	☐ ☐	☐ ☐	☐ ☐
9. Asks female patients of childbearing age the date of their last menstrual period and documents this; inquires about the possibility of pregnancy and has them sign pregnancy consent forms.	☐ ☐	☐ ☐	☐ ☐
10. Removes all obscuring objects (snaps, zippers, jewelry, etc.) so as *not* to produce radiographic artifacts.	☐ ☐	☐ ☐	☐ ☐

(continued)

	Procedure		Repeat		Competency	
	Yes	No	Yes	No	Yes	No
11. Respects the patient's modesty and provides ample comfort for him or her.	☐	☐	☐	☐	☐	☐

Comments:

_____

_____

PATIENT POSITIONING FOR STERNOCLAVICULAR JOINTS
Posteroanterior
The student:

	Procedure		Repeat		Competency	
	Yes	No	Yes	No	Yes	No
12. Places the patient's chest against the upright Bucky/receptor.	☐	☐	☐	☐	☐	☐
13. Selects the appropriate receptor or places the cassette crosswise. For conventional cassettes, the flash must be away from any anatomy.	☐	☐	☐	☐	☐	☐
14. Centers the central ray to the midsagittal plane of the body.	☐	☐	☐	☐	☐	☐
15. Directs the central ray perpendicularly to the manubrial notch/T3.	☐	☐	☐	☐	☐	☐

Right Anterior Oblique
The student:

	Procedure		Repeat		Competency	
	Yes	No	Yes	No	Yes	No
16. Places the patient in the oblique position against the upright Bucky/receptor.	☐	☐	☐	☐	☐	☐
17. Rotates the patient enough to project the vertebral shadow behind the SC joint (approximately 10–15°).	☐	☐	☐	☐	☐	☐
18. Centers the central ray to the affected SC joint (level of T2–3).	☐	☐	☐	☐	☐	☐
19. Directs the central ray perpendicularly to the affected (side down) SC joint.	☐	☐	☐	☐	☐	☐

Left Anterior Oblique
The student:

	Procedure		Repeat		Competency	
	Yes	No	Yes	No	Yes	No
20. Places the patient in the oblique position against the upright Bucky/receptor.	☐	☐	☐	☐	☐	☐
21. Rotates the patient enough to project the vertebral shadow behind the SC joint (approximately 10–15°).	☐	☐	☐	☐	☐	☐
22. Centers the central ray to the affected SC joint (level of T2–3).	☐	☐	☐	☐	☐	☐
23. Directs the central ray perpendicularly to the affected (side down) SC joint.	☐	☐	☐	☐	☐	☐

Comments:

_____

_____

IMPORTANT DETAILS
The student:

	Procedure		Repeat		Competency	
	Yes	No	Yes	No	Yes	No
24. Instills confidence in the patient by exhibiting self-confidence throughout the examination.	☐	☐	☐	☐	☐	☐
25. Places a lead marker in the appropriate area of the cassette/receptor (top/bottom/anteriorly/laterally), where it will be visualized on the finished radiograph, on the proper anatomical side (right/left), and in the appropriate position (face up/face down), depending on the patient's position.	☐	☐	☐	☐	☐	☐

	Procedure		Repeat		Competency	
	Yes	No	Yes	No	Yes	No
26. Provides radiation protection (shield) for the patient, self, and others (closes doors).	☐	☐	☐	☐	☐	☐
27. Applies proper collimation and makes adjustments as necessary.	☐	☐	☐	☐	☐	☐
28. Properly measures the patient along the course of the central ray *for each projection.*	☐	☐	☐	☐	☐	☐
29. Sets the proper exposure techniques:	☐	☐	☐	☐	☐	☐

29. Sets the proper exposure techniques:

Conventional systems
- Sets the proper kVp, mA, and time and makes adjustments as necessary.

or

CR or DR systems
- Identifies the patient on the work-list (or manually types the patient information into the system).
- Selects appropriate body region, specific body part, and accurate view/projection.
- Double-checks preset parameters:
  —Adult vs. pediatric patients
    ○ Small, medium, or large
  —Bucky/receptor (upright vs. table) *or* non-Bucky
  —AEC vs. fixed
    ○ If AEC, checks ion chambers
    ○ Density setting
  —kVp and mA; adjusts if necessary
  —Focal spot/filament size

	Procedure		Repeat		Competency	
30. Exposes the cassette/receptor after telling the patient to hold still and after giving him or her proper breathing instructions (expiration) *for each projection.*	☐	☐	☐	☐	☐	☐
31. Provides each radiograph with the proper identification (flash) and/or processes each cassette (image) without difficulty (regardless of technology—film, CR, or DR).	▣	▣	▣	▣	☐	☐
32. Properly completes the examination by filling out all necessary paperwork, entering the examination in the computer, having the images checked by the appropriate staff members, answering any last-minute questions, and informing the patient that he or she is finished.	▣	▣	▣	▣	☐	☐
33. Exhibits the ability to adapt to new and difficult situations if and when necessary.	▣	▣	▣	▣	☐	☐
34. Accepts constructive criticism and uses it to his or her advantage.	☐	☐	☐	☐	☐	☐
35. Leaves the radiographic room neat and clean for the next examination.	▣	▣	▣	▣	☐	☐
36. Completes the examination within a reasonable time frame.	☐	☐	☐	☐	☐	☐

Comments:

_____

_____

RADIOGRAPHIC IMAGE QUALITY
The student is able to critique his or her radiographs as to whether they demonstrate:

	Procedure		Repeat		Competency	
	Yes	No	Yes	No	Yes	No
37. Proper technique/optimal density	▣	▣	▣	▣	☐	☐
38. Enhanced detail, without evidence of motion and without any visible artifacts	▣	▣	▣	▣	☐	☐
39. Proper positioning (all anatomy included, evidence of proper centering/ alignment, etc.)	▣	▣	▣	▣	☐	☐

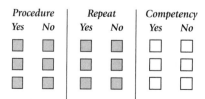

(continued)

	Procedure		Repeat		Competency	
	Yes	No	Yes	No	Yes	No
40. Proper marker placement	▢	▢	▢	▢	☐	☐
41. Evidence of proper collimation and radiation protection	▢	▢	▢	▢	☐	☐
42. Long vs. short scale of contrast	▢	▢	▢	▢	☐	☐

Comments:

_____

_____

STERNOCLAVICULAR ANATOMY
The student is able to identify:

	Procedure		Repeat		Competency	
	Yes	No	Yes	No	Yes	No
43. Medial end of clavicles	▢	▢	▢	▢	☐	☐
44. Manubrium	▢	▢	▢	▢	☐	☐
45. SC articulations	▢	▢	▢	▢	☐	☐
46. Obvious pathology	▢	▢	▢	▢	☐	☐

Comments:

_____

_____

Procedure Evaluator Signature	Repeat Evaluator Signature	Competency Evaluator Signature

Date	Date	Date

END STERNOCLAVICULAR JOINTS EVALUATION

Student Name:_____

Procedure Grade	Repeat Grade	Competency Grade

PATIENT INFORMATION OR SIMULATED PROCEDURE *(circle if simulated)*

	Procedure	Repeat	Competency
Age			
Medical Record No.			
Ability to Cooperate			
Condition/Pathology			
Technical Factors Used			
Exposure Index			

FACILITY PREPARATION
The student:

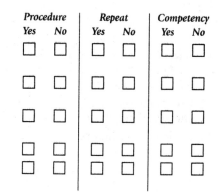

	Procedure		Repeat		Competency	
	Yes	No	Yes	No	Yes	No
1. Examines the radiographic room and cleans/straightens it before escorting the patient in.	☐	☐	☐	☐	☐	☐
2. Has all equipment and supplies (patient gown, shield, markers, lead blockers, etc.) readily available before escorting the patient in.	☐	☐	☐	☐	☐	☐
3. Is able to manipulate all radiographic equipment with ease, and centers the central ray to the cassette/receptor *for all projections.*	☐	☐	☐	☐	☐	☐
4. Adjusts the tube to the proper SID *for each projection.*	☐	☐	☐	☐	☐	☐
5. Selects cassettes/receptor of the appropriate sizes *for all projections,* according to the patient's size and examination.	☐	☐	☐	☐	☐	☐

Comments:

_____

_____

PATIENT PREPARATION
The student:

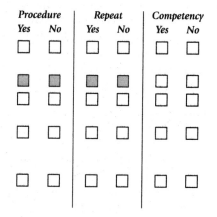

	Procedure		Repeat		Competency	
	Yes	No	Yes	No	Yes	No
6. Identifies the correct patient and examination according to the requisition while establishing a good rapport with him or her.	☐	☐	☐	☐	☐	☐
7. Obtains and documents the patient's history before the examination.	■	■	■	■	☐	☐
8. Explains the examination in terms the patient fully understands and properly communicates with the patient throughout the examination.	☐	☐	☐	☐	☐	☐
9. Asks female patients of childbearing age the date of their last menstrual period and documents this; inquires about the possibility of pregnancy and has them sign pregnancy consent forms.	☐	☐	☐	☐	☐	☐
10. Removes all obscuring objects (snaps, zippers, jewelry, etc.) so as *not* to produce radiographic artifacts.	☐	☐	☐	☐	☐	☐

(continued)

	Procedure		Repeat		Competency	
	Yes	No	Yes	No	Yes	No
11. Respects the patient's modesty and provides ample comfort for him or her.	☐	☐	☐	☐	☐	☐

Comments:

_____

_____

PATIENT POSITIONING POSITIONING FOR RIBS
Anterior Injury
Posteroanterior
The student:

	Procedure		Repeat		Competency	
	Yes	No	Yes	No	Yes	No
12. Places the patient's chest against the upright Bucky/receptor.	☐	☐	☐	☐	☐	☐
13. Selects the appropriate receptor or places the cassette lengthwise in the Bucky drawer. For conventional cassettes, the flash must be at the top and away from any anatomy.	☐	☐	☐	☐	☐	☐
14. Centers the central ray to the midsagittal plane of the body for bilateral examinations or midway between the midsagittal plane and the lateral rib margin for unilateral examinations.	☐	☐	☐	☐	☐	☐
15. Directs the central ray perpendicularly at the level of T6.	☐	☐	☐	☐	☐	☐

RAO or LAO
The student:

	Procedure		Repeat		Competency	
	Yes	No	Yes	No	Yes	No
16. Places the patient in the oblique position at an angle of 45° against the upright Bucky/receptor.	☐	☐	☐	☐	☐	☐
17. Selects the appropriate receptor or places the cassette lengthwise in the Bucky drawer. For conventional cassettes, the flash must be at the top and away from any anatomy.	☐	☐	☐	☐	☐	☐
18. Directs the central ray midway between the midsagittal plane and the lateral rib margin of the side of interest (side up).	☐	☐	☐	☐	☐	☐
19. Centers the central ray perpendicularly at the level of T6.	☐	☐	☐	☐	☐	☐

Cone-Down AP (for Ribs Below Diaphragm)
The student:

	Procedure		Repeat		Competency	
	Yes	No	Yes	No	Yes	No
20. Places the patient's back against the upright Bucky/receptor.	☐	☐	☐	☐	☐	☐
21. Selects the appropriate receptor or places the cassette lengthwise in the Bucky drawer. For conventional cassettes, the flash must be at the bottom and away from any anatomy.	☐	☐	☐	☐	☐	☐
22. Centers the central ray to the midsagittal plane of the body for bilateral examinations or midway between the midsagittal plane and the lateral rib margin for unilateral examinations.	☐	☐	☐	☐	☐	☐
23. Directs the central ray perpendicularly to the center of the cassette, with the bottom of the cassette/receptor at the top of the iliac crest.	☐	☐	☐	☐	☐	☐

Posterior Injury
Anteroposterior
The student:

	Procedure		Repeat		Competency	
	Yes	No	Yes	No	Yes	No
24. Places the patient's back against the upright Bucky/receptor.	☐	☐	☐	☐	☐	☐
25. Selects the appropriate receptor or places the cassette lengthwise in the Bucky drawer. For conventional cassettes, the flash must be at the top and away from any anatomy.	☐	☐	☐	☐	☐	☐

	Procedure Yes	No	Repeat Yes	No	Competency Yes	No
26. Centers the central ray to the midsagittal plane of the body for bilateral examinations or midway between the midsagittal plane and the lateral rib margin for unilateral examinations.	☐	☐	☐	☐	☐	☐
27. Directs the central ray perpendicularly at the level of T6.	☐	☐	☐	☐	☐	☐

RPO or LPO
The student:

	Procedure Yes	No	Repeat Yes	No	Competency Yes	No
28. Places the patient in the oblique position at an angle of 45° against the upright Bucky/receptor.	☐	☐	☐	☐	☐	☐
29. Selects the appropriate receptor or places the cassette lengthwise in the Bucky drawer. For conventional cassettes, the flash must be at the top and away from any anatomy.	☐	☐	☐	☐	☐	☐
30. Directs the central ray midway between the midsagittal plane and the lateral rib margin on the side of interest (side down).	☐	☐	☐	☐	☐	☐
31. Centers the central ray perpendicularly at the level of T6.	☐	☐	☐	☐	☐	☐

Cone-Down AP (for Ribs Below Diaphragm)
The student:

	Procedure Yes	No	Repeat Yes	No	Competency Yes	No
32. Places the patient's back against the upright Bucky/receptor.	☐	☐	☐	☐	☐	☐
33. Selects the appropriate receptor or places the cassette lengthwise in the Bucky drawer. For conventional cassettes, the flash must be at the bottom and away from any anatomy.	☐	☐	☐	☐	☐	☐
34. Centers the central ray to the midsagittal plane of the body for bilateral examinations or midway between the midsagittal plane and the lateral rib margin for unilateral examinations.	☐	☐	☐	☐	☐	☐
35. Directs the central ray perpendicularly to the center of the cassette, with the bottom of the cassette/receptor at the top of the iliac crest.	☐	☐	☐	☐	☐	☐

Comments:

_____

_____

IMPORTANT DETAILS
The student:

	Procedure Yes	No	Repeat Yes	No	Competency Yes	No
36. Instills confidence in the patient by exhibiting self-confidence throughout the examination.	☐	☐	☐	☐	☐	☐
37. Places a lead marker in the appropriate area of the cassette/receptor (top/bottom/anteriorly/laterally), where it will be visualized on the finished radiograph, on the proper anatomical side (right/left), and in the appropriate position (face up/face down), depending on the patient's position.	☐	☐	☐	☐	☐	☐
38. Provides radiation protection (shield) for the patient, self, and others (closes doors).	☐	☐	☐	☐	☐	☐
39. Applies proper collimation and makes adjustments as necessary.	☐	☐	☐	☐	☐	☐
40. Properly measures the patient along the course of the central ray *for each projection.*	☐	☐	☐	☐	☐	☐
41. Sets the proper exposure techniques:	☐	☐	☐	☐	☐	☐

(continued)

	Procedure		Repeat		Competency	
	Yes	No	Yes	No	Yes	No

Conventional systems
- Sets the proper kVp, mA, and time and makes adjustments as necessary.

or

CR or DR systems
- Identifies the patient on the work-list (or manually types the patient information into the system).
- Selects appropriate body region, specific body part, and accurate view/ projection.
- Double-checks preset parameters:
  —Adult vs. pediatric patients
    ◦ Small, medium, or large
  —Bucky/receptor (upright vs. table) *or* non-Bucky
  —AEC vs. fixed
    ◦ If AEC, checks ion chambers
    ◦ Density setting
  —kVp and mA; adjusts if necessary
  —Focal spot/filament size

	Procedure		Repeat		Competency	
42. Exposes the cassette/receptor after telling the patient to hold still and after giving him or her proper breathing instructions (above—inspiration; below—expiration) *for each projection.*	☐	☐	☐	☐	☐	☐
43. Provides each radiograph with the proper identification (flash) and/or processes each cassette (image) without difficulty (regardless of technology—film, CR, or DR).	▣	▣	▣	▣	☐	☐
44. Properly completes the examination by filling out all necessary paperwork, entering the examination in the computer, having the images checked by the appropriate staff members, answering any last-minute questions, and informing the patient that he or she is finished.	▣	▣	▣	▣	☐	☐
45. Exhibits the ability to adapt to new and difficult situations if and when necessary.	▣	▣	▣	▣	☐	☐
46. Accepts constructive criticism and uses it to his or her advantage.	☐	☐	☐	☐	☐	☐
47. Leaves the radiographic room neat and clean for the next examination.	▣	▣	▣	▣	☐	☐
48. Completes the examination within a reasonable time frame.	☐	☐	☐	☐	☐	☐

Comments:

_____

_____

RADIOGRAPHIC IMAGE QUALITY
The student is able to critique his or her radiographs as to whether they demonstrate:

	Procedure		Repeat		Competency	
	Yes	No	Yes	No	Yes	No
49. Proper technique/optimal density	▣	▣	▣	▣	☐	☐
50. Enhanced detail, without evidence of motion and without any visible artifacts	▣	▣	▣	▣	☐	☐
51. Proper positioning (all anatomy included, evidence of proper centering/ alignment, etc.)	▣	▣	▣	▣	☐	☐
52. Proper marker placement	▣	▣	▣	▣	☐	☐
53. Evidence of proper collimation and radiation protection	▣	▣	▣	▣	☐	☐
54. Long vs. short scale of contrast	▣	▣	▣	▣	☐	☐

Comments:

_____

_____

RIB ANATOMY
The student is able to identify:

	Procedure		Repeat		Competency	
	Yes	No	Yes	No	Yes	No
55. Costovertebral articulation	☐	☐	☐	☐	☐	☐
56. Costal cartilage (calcified)	☐	☐	☐	☐	☐	☐
57. Head of the rib	☐	☐	☐	☐	☐	☐
58. Rib neck	☐	☐	☐	☐	☐	☐
59. Rib tubercle	☐	☐	☐	☐	☐	☐
60. Angle	☐	☐	☐	☐	☐	☐
61. Shaft	☐	☐	☐	☐	☐	☐
62. True ribs	☐	☐	☐	☐	☐	☐
63. False ribs	☐	☐	☐	☐	☐	☐
64. Floating ribs	☐	☐	☐	☐	☐	☐
65. Obvious pathology	☐	☐	☐	☐	☐	☐

Comments:

_____

_____

_____   _____   _____
Procedure Evaluator Signature   Repeat Evaluator Signature   Competency Evaluator Signature

_____   _____   _____
Date   Date   Date

END RIBS EVALUATION

The objective of this evaluation is to determine the student's competency level when performing specific radiographic examinations.

Student Name:_____

Procedure Grade	Repeat Grade	Competency Grade

PATIENT INFORMATION OR SIMULATED PROCEDURE *(circle if simulated)*

	Procedure	Repeat	Competency
Age			
Medical Record No.			
Ability to Cooperate			
Condition/Pathology			
Technical Factors Used			
Exposure Index			

FACILITY PREPARATION
The student:

	Procedure		Repeat		Competency	
	Yes	No	Yes	No	Yes	No
1. Examines the radiographic room and cleans/straightens it before escorting the patient in.	☐	☐	☐	☐	☐	☐
2. Has all equipment and supplies (patient gown, shield, markers, lead blockers, etc.) readily available before escorting the patient in.	☐	☐	☐	☐	☐	☐
3. Is able to manipulate all radiographic equipment with ease, and centers the central ray to the cassette/receptor *for all projections.*	☐	☐	☐	☐	☐	☐
4. Adjusts the tube to the proper SID *for each projection.*	☐	☐	☐	☐	☐	☐
5. Selects cassettes/receptor of the appropriate sizes *for all projections,* according to the patient's size and examination.	☐	☐	☐	☐	☐	☐

Comments:

_____

_____

PATIENT PREPARATION
The student:

	Procedure		Repeat		Competency	
	Yes	No	Yes	No	Yes	No
6. Identifies the correct patient and examination according to the requisition while establishing a good rapport with him or her.	☐	☐	☐	☐	☐	☐
7. Obtains and documents the patient's history before the examination.	☑	☑	☑	☑	☐	☐
8. Explains the examination in terms the patient fully understands and properly communicates with the patient throughout the examination.	☐	☐	☐	☐	☐	☐
9. Asks female patients of childbearing age the date of their last menstrual period and documents this; inquires about the possibility of pregnancy and has them sign pregnancy consent forms.	☐	☐	☐	☐	☐	☐
10. Removes all obscuring objects (snaps, zippers, jewelry, etc.) so as *not* to produce radiographic artifacts.	☐	☐	☐	☐	☐	☐

(continued)

	Procedure		Repeat		Competency	
	Yes	No	Yes	No	Yes	No
11. Respects the patient's modesty and provides ample comfort for him or her.	☐	☐	☐	☐	☐	☐

Comments:

_____

_____

PATIENT POSITIONING FOR A CERVICAL SPINE
Anteroposterior
The student:

	Procedure		Repeat		Competency	
	Yes	No	Yes	No	Yes	No
12. Places the patient's back against the erect Bucky/receptor, or supine on the radiographic table, without rotation.	☐	☐	☐	☐	☐	☐
13. Selects the appropriate receptor or places the cassette lengthwise in the Bucky drawer. For conventional cassettes, the flash must be away from any anatomy.	☐	☐	☐	☐	☐	☐
14. Extends the head enough to place the occlusal plane and the mastoid tips in the same transverse plane, perpendicular to the cassette/receptor.	☐	☐	☐	☐	☐	☐
15. Centers the central ray to the midsagittal plane of the body.	☐	☐	☐	☐	☐	☐
16. Directs the central ray at an angle of 15° cephalad to the thyroid cartilage/C4.	☐	☐	☐	☐	☐	☐

RPO or LAO (for the Left Cervical Anatomy)
The student:

	Procedure		Repeat		Competency	
	Yes	No	Yes	No	Yes	No
17. Places the patient in the oblique (RPO for the anatomy farthest from cassette/receptor, and LAO for the anatomy closest to cassette/receptor) position, at an angle of 45°.	☐	☐	☐	☐	☐	☐
18. Selects the appropriate receptor or places the cassette lengthwise in the Bucky drawer. For conventional cassettes, the flash must be away from any anatomy.	☐	☐	☐	☐	☐	☐
19. Elevates the patient's chin/jaw slightly forward.	☐	☐	☐	☐	☐	☐
20. Centers the central ray to the center of the spine.	☐	☐	☐	☐	☐	☐
21. Directs the central ray at an angle of 15° cephalad for RPO and 15° caudal for LAO, centering to the thyroid cartilage/C4.	☐	☐	☐	☐	☐	☐

LPO or RAO (for the Right Cervical Anatomy)
The student:

	Procedure		Repeat		Competency	
	Yes	No	Yes	No	Yes	No
22. Places the patient in the oblique (LPO for the anatomy farthest from cassette/receptor, and RAO for the anatomy closest to cassette/receptor) position, at an angle of 45°.	☐	☐	☐	☐	☐	☐
23. Selects the appropriate receptor or places the cassette lengthwise in the Bucky drawer. For conventional cassettes, the flash must be away from any anatomy.	☐	☐	☐	☐	☐	☐
24. Elevates the patient's jaw/chin slightly forward.	☐	☐	☐	☐	☐	☐
25. Directs the central ray to the center of the spine.	☐	☐	☐	☐	☐	☐
26. Directs the central ray at an angle of 15° cephalad for LPO and 15° caudad for RAO, centering to the thyroid cartilage/C4.	☐	☐	☐	☐	☐	☐

Lateral
The student:

	Procedure		Repeat		Competency	
	Yes	No	Yes	No	Yes	No
27. Places the patient in the left lateral position against the upright Bucky/receptor, without rotation.	☐	☐	☐	☐	☐	☐

	Procedure		Repeat		Competency	
	Yes	No	Yes	No	Yes	No
28. Selects the appropriate receptor or places the cassette lengthwise with the top at the level of the external auditory meatus (EAM). For conventional cassettes, the flash must be away from any anatomy.	☐	☐	☐	☐	☐	☐
29. Elevates the patient's jaw/chin slightly forward.	☐	☐	☐	☐	☐	☐
30. Asks the patient to drop his or her shoulders and arms to the sides, reaching for the floor (and/or uses weights, if possible).	☐	☐	☐	☐	☐	☐
31. Directs the central ray to the center of the spine.	☐	☐	☐	☐	☐	☐
32. Centers the central ray perpendicularly, at the level of the thyroid cartilage/C4.	☐	☐	☐	☐	☐	☐

AP Open Mouth (Atlas and Axis [A&A])
The student:

	Procedure		Repeat		Competency	
	Yes	No	Yes	No	Yes	No
33. Places the patient's back against the erect Bucky/receptor, or supine on the radiographic table, without rotation.	☐	☐	☐	☐	☐	☐
34. Extends the head enough to place the occlusal plane and the mastoid tips in the same transverse plane, perpendicular to the cassette/receptor.	☐	☐	☐	☐	☐	☐
35. Instructs the patient to open his or her mouth as wide as possible, by dropping his or her jaw only, not tilting the entire head.	☐	☐	☐	☐	☐	☐
36. Centers the central ray to the midsagittal plane of the body.	☐	☐	☐	☐	☐	☐
37. Directs the central ray perpendicularly to the mouth opening.	☐	☐	☐	☐	☐	☐

Comments:

_____

_____

IMPORTANT DETAILS
The student:

	Procedure		Repeat		Competency	
	Yes	No	Yes	No	Yes	No
38. Instills confidence in the patient by exhibiting self-confidence throughout the examination.	☐	☐	☐	☐	☐	☐
39. Places a lead marker in the appropriate area of the cassette/receptor (top/bottom/anteriorly/laterally), where it will be visualized on the finished radiograph, on the proper anatomical side (right/left), and in the appropriate position (face up/face down), depending on the patient's position.	☐	☐	☐	☐	☐	☐
40. Provides radiation protection (shield) for the patient, self, and others (closes doors).	☐	☐	☐	☐	☐	☐
41. Applies proper collimation and makes adjustments as necessary, especially for the A&A, to decrease the dose to the thyroid and the lens of the eyes.	☐	☐	☐	☐	☐	☐
42. Properly measures the patient along the course of the central ray *for each projection.*	☐	☐	☐	☐	☐	☐
43. Sets the proper exposure techniques:	☐	☐	☐	☐	☐	☐

43. Sets the proper exposure techniques:

Conventional systems
- Sets the proper kVp, mA, and time and makes adjustments as necessary.

or

CR or DR systems
- Identifies the patient on the work-list (or manually types the patient information into the system).
- Selects appropriate body region, specific body part, and accurate view/projection.

(continued)

	Procedure		Repeat		Competency	
	Yes	No	Yes	No	Yes	No

- Double-checks preset parameters:
  —Adult vs. pediatric patients
  ◦ Small, medium, or large
  —Bucky/receptor (upright vs. table) *or* non-Bucky
  —AEC vs. fixed
  ◦ If AEC, checks ion chambers
  ◦ Density setting
  —kVp and mA; adjusts if necessary
  —Focal spot/filament size

44. Exposes the cassette/receptor after telling the patient to hold still and after giving him or her proper breathing instructions (expiration) *for each projection.*	☐	☐	☐	☐	☐	☐
45. Provides each radiograph with the proper identification (flash) and/or processes each cassette (image) without difficulty (regardless of technology—film, CR, or DR).	▨	▨	▨	▨	☐	☐
46. Properly completes the examination by filling out all necessary paperwork, entering the examination in the computer, having the images checked by the appropriate staff members, answering any last-minute questions, and informing the patient that he or she is finished.	▨	▨	▨	▨	☐	☐
47. Exhibits the ability to adapt to new and difficult situations if and when necessary.	▨	▨	▨	▨	☐	☐
48. Accepts constructive criticism and uses it to his or her advantage.	☐	☐	☐	☐	☐	☐
49. Leaves the radiographic room neat and clean for the next examination.	▨	▨	▨	▨	☐	☐
50. Completes the examination within a reasonable time frame.	☐	☐	☐	☐	☐	☐

Comments:

_____

_____

RADIOGRAPHIC IMAGE QUALITY
The student is able to critique his or her radiographs as to whether they demonstrate:

	Procedure		Repeat		Competency	
	Yes	No	Yes	No	Yes	No
51. Proper technique/optimal density	▨	▨	▨	▨	☐	☐
52. Enhanced detail, without evidence of motion and without any visible artifacts	▨	▨	▨	▨	☐	☐
53. Proper positioning (all anatomy included, evidence of proper centering/ alignment, etc.)	▨	▨	▨	▨	☐	☐
54. Proper marker placement	▨	▨	▨	▨	☐	☐
55. Evidence of proper collimation and radiation protection	▨	▨	▨	▨	☐	☐
56. Long vs. short scale of contrast	▨	▨	▨	▨	☐	☐

Comments:

_____

_____

CERVICAL SPINE ANATOMY
The student is able to identify:

	Procedure		Repeat		Competency	
	Yes	No	Yes	No	Yes	No
57. Odontoid process (dens)	☐	☐	☐	☐	☐	☐
58. Transverse process	☐	☐	☐	☐	☐	☐
59. Body	☐	☐	☐	☐	☐	☐
60. Spinous process	☐	☐	☐	☐	☐	☐
61. Superior and inferior articular processes	☐	☐	☐	☐	☐	☐
62. Zygapophyseal joints	☐	☐	☐	☐	☐	☐
63. Intervertebral disk space	☐	☐	☐	☐	☐	☐
64. Intervertebral foramen	☐	☐	☐	☐	☐	☐
65. Lamina vs. pedicle	☐	☐	☐	☐	☐	☐
66. Atlas	☐	☐	☐	☐	☐	☐
67. Axis	☐	☐	☐	☐	☐	☐
68. C1 through C7	☐	☐	☐	☐	☐	☐
69. Obvious pathology	☐	☐	☐	☐	☐	☐

Comments:

_____

_____

_____ _____ _____
Procedure Evaluator Signature   Repeat Evaluator Signature   Competency Evaluator Signature

_____ _____ _____
Date   Date   Date

END CERVICAL SPINE EVALUATION

Student Name:_____

Procedure Grade	Repeat Grade	Competency Grade

PATIENT INFORMATION OR SIMULATED PROCEDURE *(circle if simulated)*

	Procedure	Repeat	Competency
Age			
Medical Record No.			
Ability to Cooperate			
Condition/Pathology			
Technical Factors Used			
Exposure Index			

FACILITY PREPARATION
The student:

	Procedure Yes No	Repeat Yes No	Competency Yes No
1. Examines the radiographic room and cleans/straightens it before escorting the patient in.	☐ ☐	☐ ☐	☐ ☐
2. Has all equipment and supplies (patient gown, shield, markers, lead blockers, etc.) readily available before escorting the patient in.	☐ ☐	☐ ☐	☐ ☐
3. Is able to manipulate all radiographic equipment with ease, and centers the central ray to the cassette/receptor *for all projections.*	☐ ☐	☐ ☐	☐ ☐
4. Adjusts the tube to the proper SID *for each projection.*	☐ ☐	☐ ☐	☐ ☐
5. Selects cassettes/receptor of the appropriate sizes *for all projections,* according to the patient's size and examination.	☐ ☐	☐ ☐	☐ ☐

Comments:

_____

_____

PATIENT PREPARATION
The student:

	Procedure Yes No	Repeat Yes No	Competency Yes No
6. Identifies the correct patient and examination according to the requisition while establishing a good rapport with him or her.	☐ ☐	☐ ☐	☐ ☐
7. Obtains and documents the patient's history before the examination.	▨ ▨	▨ ▨	☐ ☐
8. Explains the examination in terms the patient fully understands and properly communicates with the patient throughout the examination.	☐ ☐	☐ ☐	☐ ☐
9. Asks female patients of childbearing age the date of their last menstrual period and documents this; inquires about the possibility of pregnancy and has them sign pregnancy consent forms.	☐ ☐	☐ ☐	☐ ☐
10. Removes all obscuring objects (snaps, zippers, jewelry, etc.) so as *not* to produce radiographic artifacts.	☐ ☐	☐ ☐	☐ ☐

(continued)

	Procedure		Repeat		Competency	
	Yes	No	Yes	No	Yes	No
11. Respects the patient's modesty and provides ample comfort for him or her.	☐	☐	☐	☐	☐	☐

Comments:

_____

_____

PATIENT POSITIONING FOR A TRAUMA CERVICAL SPINE
Anteroposterior
The student:

	Procedure		Repeat		Competency	
	Yes	No	Yes	No	Yes	No
12. Does not adjust the patient from the supine position on the radiographic table or stretcher.	☐	☐	☐	☐	☐	☐
13. Selects the appropriate receptor or places the cassette lengthwise in the Bucky drawer. For conventional cassettes, the flash must be away from any anatomy.	☐	☐	☐	☐	☐	☐
14. If possible, requests that the physician adjust the patient's head enough to place the occlusal plane and the mastoid tips in the same transverse plane, perpendicular to the cassette/receptor.	☐	☐	☐	☐	☐	☐
15. Centers the central ray to the midsagittal plane of the body.	☐	☐	☐	☐	☐	☐
16. Directs the central ray at an angle of 15° cephalad to the thyroid cartilage/C4.	☐	☐	☐	☐	☐	☐

Lateral
The student:

	Procedure		Repeat		Competency	
	Yes	No	Yes	No	Yes	No
17. Does not adjust the patient from the supine position on the radiographic table or stretcher.	☐	☐	☐	☐	☐	☐
18. Positions the radiographic tube for horizontal/cross-table radiographs.	☐	☐	☐	☐	☐	☐
19. Places the receptor/cassette with a grid holder as close to the patient's left side as possible, with the top of the cassette/receptor at the level of the EAM.	☐	☐	☐	☐	☐	☐
20. Asks the patient to drop his or her shoulders and arms to the sides, reaching for the feet, or has the attending physician pull the patient's arms down.	☐	☐	☐	☐	☐	☐
21. Directs the central ray to the center of the spine.	☐	☐	☐	☐	☐	☐
22. Centers the central ray perpendicularly to the thyroid cartilage/C4.	☐	☐	☐	☐	☐	☐

AP Open Mouth (A&A)
The student:

	Procedure		Repeat		Competency	
	Yes	No	Yes	No	Yes	No
23. After the AP and lateral are cleared by the attending radiologist, if possible extend the patient's head enough to place the occlusal plane and the mastoid tips in the same transverse plane, perpendicular to the cassette/receptor.	☐	☐	☐	☐	☐	☐
24. Instructs the patient to open his or her mouth as wide as possible.	☐	☐	☐	☐	☐	☐
25. Centers the central ray to the midsagittal plane of the body.	☐	☐	☐	☐	☐	☐
26. Directs the central ray perpendicularly to the mouth opening.	☐	☐	☐	☐	☐	☐

Comments:

_____

_____

IMPORTANT DETAILS
The student:

	Procedure		Repeat		Competency	
	Yes	No	Yes	No	Yes	No
27. Instills confidence in the patient by exhibiting self-confidence throughout the examination.	☐	☐	☐	☐	☐	☐
28. Places a lead marker in the appropriate area of the cassette/receptor (top/bottom/anteriorly/laterally), where it will be visualized on the finished radiograph, on the proper anatomical side (right/left), and in the appropriate position (face up/face down), depending on the patient's position.	☐	☐	☐	☐	☐	☐
29. Provides radiation protection (shield) for the patient, self, and others (closes doors).	☐	☐	☐	☐	☐	☐
30. Applies proper collimation and makes adjustments as necessary, especially for the A&A, to decrease the dose to the thyroid and the lens of the eyes.	☐	☐	☐	☐	☐	☐
31. Properly measures the patient along the course of the central ray *for each projection.*	☐	☐	☐	☐	☐	☐
32. Sets the proper exposure techniques:	☐	☐	☐	☐	☐	☐

Conventional systems
- Sets the proper kVp, mA, and time and makes adjustments as necessary.

or

CR or DR systems
- Identifies the patient on the work-list (or manually types the patient information into the system).
- Selects appropriate body region, specific body part, and accurate view/projection.
- Double-checks preset parameters:
  —Adult vs. pediatric patients
    ○ Small, medium, or large
  —Bucky/receptor (upright vs. table) *or* non-Bucky
  —AEC vs. fixed
    ○ If AEC, checks ion chambers
    ○ Density setting
  —kVp and mA; adjusts if necessary
  —Focal spot/filament size

	Procedure		Repeat		Competency	
33. Exposes the cassette/receptor after telling the patient to hold still and after giving him or her proper breathing instructions (expiration) *for each projection.*	☐	☐	☐	☐	☐	☐
34. Provides each radiograph with the proper identification (flash) and/or processes each cassette (image) without difficulty (regardless of technology—film, CR, or DR).	▨	▨	▨	▨	☐	☐
35. Properly completes the examination by filling out all necessary paperwork, entering the examination in the computer, having the images checked by the appropriate staff members, answering any last-minute questions, and informing the patient that he or she is finished.	▨	▨	▨	▨	☐	☐
36. Exhibits the ability to adapt to new and difficult situations if and when necessary.	▨	▨	▨	▨	☐	☐
37. Accepts constructive criticism and uses it to his or her advantage.	☐	☐	☐	☐	☐	☐
38. Leaves the radiographic room neat and clean for the next examination.	▨	▨	▨	▨	☐	☐
39. Completes the examination within a reasonable time frame.	☐	☐	☐	☐	☐	☐

Comments:

_____

_____

(continued)

RADIOGRAPHIC IMAGE QUALITY

The student is able to critique his or her radiographs as to whether they demonstrate:

	Procedure		Repeat		Competency	
	Yes	No	Yes	No	Yes	No
40. Proper technique/optimal density	☐	☐	☐	☐	☐	☐
41. Enhanced detail, without evidence of motion and without any visible artifacts	☐	☐	☐	☐	☐	☐
42. Proper positioning (all anatomy included, evidence of proper centering/ alignment, etc.)	☐	☐	☐	☐	☐	☐
43. Proper marker placement	☐	☐	☐	☐	☐	☐
44. Evidence of proper collimation and radiation protection	☐	☐	☐	☐	☐	☐
45. Long vs. short scale of contrast	☐	☐	☐	☐	☐	☐

Comments:

_____

_____

CERVICAL SPINE ANATOMY

The student is able to identify:

	Procedure		Repeat		Competency	
	Yes	No	Yes	No	Yes	No
46. Odontoid process	☐	☐	☐	☐	☐	☐
47. Transverse process	☐	☐	☐	☐	☐	☐
48. Body	☐	☐	☐	☐	☐	☐
49. Spinous process	☐	☐	☐	☐	☐	☐
50. Superior and inferior articular processes	☐	☐	☐	☐	☐	☐
51. Zygapophyseal joints	☐	☐	☐	☐	☐	☐
52. Intervertebral foramen	☐	☐	☐	☐	☐	☐
53. Intervertebral disk space	☐	☐	☐	☐	☐	☐
54. Atlas	☐	☐	☐	☐	☐	☐
55. Axis	☐	☐	☐	☐	☐	☐
56. C1 through C7	☐	☐	☐	☐	☐	☐
57. Obvious pathology	☐	☐	☐	☐	☐	☐

Comments:

_____

_____

_____ _____ _____
Procedure Evaluator Signature   Repeat Evaluator Signature   Competency Evaluator Signature

_____ _____ _____
Date   Date   Date

END TRAUMA WITH CROSS-TABLE LATERAL CERVICAL SPINE EVALUATION

Student Name:_____

	Procedure Grade	Repeat Grade	Competency Grade

PATIENT INFORMATION OR SIMULATED PROCEDURE *(circle if simulated)*

	Procedure	Repeat	Competency
Age			
Medical Record No.			
Ability to Cooperate			
Condition/Pathology			
Technical Factors Used			
Exposure Index			

FACILITY PREPARATION
The student:

	Procedure Yes	No	Repeat Yes	No	Competency Yes	No
1. Examines the radiographic room and cleans/straightens it before escorting the patient in.	☐	☐	☐	☐	☐	☐
2. Has all equipment and supplies (patient gown, shield, markers, lead blockers, etc.) readily available before escorting the patient in.	☐	☐	☐	☐	☐	☐
3. Is able to manipulate all radiographic equipment with ease, and centers the central ray to the cassette/receptor.	☐	☐	☐	☐	☐	☐
4. Adjusts the tube to the proper SID.	☐	☐	☐	☐	☐	☐
5. Selects a cassette/receptor of the appropriate size.	☐	☐	☐	☐	☐	☐

Comments:

_____

_____

PATIENT PREPARATION
The student:

	Procedure Yes	No	Repeat Yes	No	Competency Yes	No
6. Identifies the correct patient and examination according to the requisition while establishing a good rapport with him or her.	☐	☐	☐	☐	☐	☐
7. Obtains and documents the patient's history before the examination.	▨	▨	▨	▨	☐	☐
8. Explains the examination in terms the patient fully understands and properly communicates with the patient throughout the examination.	☐	☐	☐	☐	☐	☐
9. Asks female patients of childbearing age the date of their last menstrual period and documents this; inquires about the possibility of pregnancy and has them sign pregnancy consent forms.	☐	☐	☐	☐	☐	☐
10. Removes all obscuring objects (snaps, zippers, jewelry, etc.) so as *not* to produce radiographic artifacts.	☐	☐	☐	☐	☐	☐
11. Respects the patient's modesty and provides ample comfort for him or her.	☐	☐	☐	☐	☐	☐

Comments:

_____

_____

PATIENT POSITIONING FOR A SWIMMER'S LATERAL OF THE CERVICAL SPINE, USING THE TWINING METHOD
The student:

	Procedure		Repeat		Competency	
	Yes	No	Yes	No	Yes	No
12. Positions the radiographic tube for horizontal/shoot-through radiographs.	☐	☐	☐	☐	☐	☐
13. Places the receptor/cassette with a grid holder as close to the patient's left side as possible, with the top of the cassette/receptor at the level of the EAM (the cassette lengthwise in the Bucky drawer centered at C7–T1).	☐	☐	☐	☐	☐	☐
14. Asks the patient to drop the right shoulder and raise the left arm above the head.	☐	☐	☐	☐	☐	☐
15. Rotates the right shoulder anteriorly and the left posteriorly, just enough to prevent the shoulders from superimposing over the vertebrae.	☐	☐	☐	☐	☐	☐
16. Directs the central ray to the midaxillary plane, at the center of the spine.	☐	☐	☐	☐	☐	☐
17. Centers the central ray perpendicularly to T2, or at an angle of 5° caudad if the right shoulder cannot be depressed.	☐	☐	☐	☐	☐	☐

Comments:

_____

_____

IMPORTANT DETAILS
The student:

	Procedure		Repeat		Competency	
	Yes	No	Yes	No	Yes	No
18. Instills confidence in the patient by exhibiting self-confidence throughout the examination.	☐	☐	☐	☐	☐	☐
19. Places a lead marker in the appropriate area of the cassette/receptor (top/bottom/anteriorly/laterally), where it will be visualized on the finished radiograph, on the proper anatomical side (right/left), and in the appropriate position (face up/face down), depending on the patient's position.	☐	☐	☐	☐	☐	☐
20. Provides radiation protection (shield) for the patient, self, and others (closes doors).	☐	☐	☐	☐	☐	☐
21. Applies proper collimation and makes adjustments as necessary, especially for the A&A, to decrease the dose to the thyroid and the lens of the eyes.	☐	☐	☐	☐	☐	☐
22. Properly measures the patient along the course of the central ray *for each projection.*	☐	☐	☐	☐	☐	☐
23. Sets the proper exposure techniques:	☐	☐	☐	☐	☐	☐

Conventional systems
- Sets the proper kVp, mA, and time and makes adjustments as necessary.

or

CR or DR systems
- Identifies the patient on the work-list (or manually types the patient information into the system).
- Selects appropriate body region, specific body part, and accurate view/projection.
- Double-checks preset parameters:
  —Adult vs. pediatric patients
    ○ Small, medium, or large
  —Bucky/receptor (upright vs. table) *or* non-Bucky
  —AEC vs. fixed

	Procedure		Repeat		Competency	
	Yes	No	Yes	No	Yes	No
○ If AEC, checks ion chambers ○ Density setting —kVp and mA; adjusts if necessary —Focal spot/filament size						
24. Exposes the cassette/receptor after telling the patient to hold still and after giving him or her proper breathing instructions (expiration) *for each projection.*	☐	☐	☐	☐	☐	☐
25. Provides each radiograph with the proper identification (flash) and/or processes each cassette (image) without difficulty (regardless of technology—film, CR, or DR).	■	■	■	■	☐	☐
26. Properly completes the examination by filling out all necessary paperwork, entering the examination in the computer, having the images checked by the appropriate staff members, answering any last-minute questions, and informing the patient that he or she is finished.	■	■	■	■	☐	☐
27. Exhibits the ability to adapt to new and difficult situations if and when necessary.	■	■	■	■	☐	☐
28. Accepts constructive criticism and uses it to his or her advantage.	☐	☐	☐	☐	☐	☐
29. Leaves the radiographic room neat and clean for the next examination.	■	■	■	■	☐	☐
30. Completes the examination within a reasonable time frame.	☐	☐	☐	☐	☐	☐

Comments:

RADIOGRAPHIC IMAGE QUALITY
The student is able to critique his or her radiographs as to whether they demonstrate:

	Procedure		Repeat		Competency	
	Yes	No	Yes	No	Yes	No
31. Proper technique/optimal density	■	■	■	■	☐	☐
32. Enhanced detail, without evidence of motion and without any visible artifacts	■	■	■	■	☐	☐
33. Proper positioning (all anatomy included, evidence of proper centering/alignment, etc.)	■	■	■	■	☐	☐
34. Proper marker placement	■	■	■	■	☐	☐
35. Evidence of proper collimation and radiation protection	■	■	■	■	☐	☐
36. Long vs. short scale of contrast	■	■	■	■	☐	☐

Comments:

CERVICAL SPINE ANATOMY
The student is able to identify:

	Procedure		Repeat		Competency	
	Yes	No	Yes	No	Yes	No
37. Elevated humerus	■	■	■	■	☐	☐
38. Depressed humerus	■	■	■	■	☐	☐
39. C7	■	■	■	■	☐	☐
40. T1	■	■	■	■	☐	☐
41. Obvious pathology	■	■	■	■	☐	☐

(continued)

Comments:

_____

_____

_____

Procedure Evaluator Signature	Repeat Evaluator Signature	Competency Evaluator Signature
Date	Date	Date

Student Name:_____

Procedure Grade	Repeat Grade	Competency Grade

PATIENT INFORMATION OR SIMULATED PROCEDURE *(circle if simulated)*

	Procedure	Repeat	Competency
Age			
Medical Record No.			
Ability to Cooperate			
Condition/Pathology			
Technical Factors Used			
Exposure Index			

FACILITY PREPARATION
The student:

	Procedure Yes / No	Repeat Yes / No	Competency Yes / No
1. Examines the radiographic room and cleans/straightens it before escorting the patient in.	☐ ☐	☐ ☐	☐ ☐
2. Has all equipment and supplies (patient gown, shield, markers, lead blockers, etc.) readily available before escorting the patient in.	☐ ☐	☐ ☐	☐ ☐
3. Is able to manipulate all radiographic equipment with ease, and centers the central ray to the cassette/receptor *for both projections.*	☐ ☐	☐ ☐	☐ ☐
4. Adjusts the tube to the proper SID *for each projection.*	☐ ☐	☐ ☐	☐ ☐
5. Selects cassettes/receptor of the appropriate sizes *for both projections,* according to the patient's size and examination.	☐ ☐	☐ ☐	☐ ☐

Comments:

_____

_____

PATIENT PREPARATION
The student:

	Procedure Yes / No	Repeat Yes / No	Competency Yes / No
6. Identifies the correct patient and examination according to the requisition while establishing a good rapport with him or her.	☐ ☐	☐ ☐	☐ ☐
7. Obtains and documents the patient's history before the examination.	▣ ▣	▣ ▣	☐ ☐
8. Explains the examination in terms the patient fully understands and properly communicates with the patient throughout the examination.	☐ ☐	☐ ☐	☐ ☐
9. Asks female patients of childbearing age the date of their last menstrual period and documents this; inquires about the possibility of pregnancy and has them sign pregnancy consent forms.	☐ ☐	☐ ☐	☐ ☐
10. Removes all obscuring objects (snaps, zippers, jewelry, etc.) so as *not* to produce radiographic artifacts.	☐ ☐	☐ ☐	☐ ☐

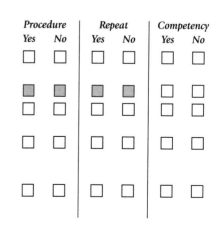

(continued)

	Procedure		Repeat		Competency	
	Yes	No	Yes	No	Yes	No
11. Respects the patient's modesty and provides ample comfort for him or her.	☐	☐	☐	☐	☐	☐

Comments:

_____

_____

PATIENT POSITIONING FOR FLEXION AND EXTENSION LATERALS OF A CERVICAL SPINE

Flexion
The student:

	Procedure		Repeat		Competency	
	Yes	No	Yes	No	Yes	No
12. Places the patient in the left lateral position against the upright Bucky/receptor, without rotation.	☐	☐	☐	☐	☐	☐
13. Places the top of the cassette/receptor at the level of the EAM (the cassette lengthwise in the Bucky drawer).	☐	☐	☐	☐	☐	☐
14. Instructs the patient to flex his or her neck by bringing his or her chin as close to the chest as possible.	☐	☐	☐	☐	☐	☐
15. Asks the patient to drop his or her shoulders and arms to the sides, reaching for the floor.	☐	☐	☐	☐	☐	☐
16. Directs the central ray to the center of the spine.	☐	☐	☐	☐	☐	☐
17. Centers the central ray perpendicularly at the level of the thyroid cartilage/C4.	☐	☐	☐	☐	☐	☐

Extension
The student:

	Procedure		Repeat		Competency	
	Yes	No	Yes	No	Yes	No
18. Places the patient in the left lateral position against the upright Bucky/receptor, without rotation.	☐	☐	☐	☐	☐	☐
19. Places the top of the cassette/receptor at the level of the EAM (the cassette lengthwise in the Bucky drawer).	☐	☐	☐	☐	☐	☐
20. Instructs the patient to extend his or her neck by elevating his or her chin as much as possible.	☐	☐	☐	☐	☐	☐
21. Asks the patient to drop his or her shoulders and arms to the sides, reaching for the floor.	☐	☐	☐	☐	☐	☐
22. Directs the central ray to the center of the spine.	☐	☐	☐	☐	☐	☐
23. Centers the central ray perpendicularly at the level of the thyroid cartilage/C4.	☐	☐	☐	☐	☐	☐

Comments:

_____

_____

IMPORTANT DETAILS
The student:

	Procedure		Repeat		Competency	
	Yes	No	Yes	No	Yes	No
24. Instills confidence in the patient by exhibiting self-confidence throughout the examination.	☐	☐	☐	☐	☐	☐
25. Places a lead marker in the appropriate area of the cassette/receptor (top/bottom/anteriorly/laterally), where it will be visualized on the finished radiograph, on the proper anatomical side (right/left), and in the appropriate position (face up/face down), depending on the patient's position.	☐	☐	☐	☐	☐	☐
26. Provides radiation protection (shield) for the patient, self, and others (closes doors).	☐	☐	☐	☐	☐	☐

	Procedure		Repeat		Competency	
	Yes	No	Yes	No	Yes	No
27. Applies proper collimation and makes adjustments as necessary, especially for the A&A, to decrease the dose to the thyroid and the lens of the eyes.	☐	☐	☐	☐	☐	☐
28. Properly measures the patient along the course of the central ray *for each projection.*	☐	☐	☐	☐	☐	☐
29. Sets the proper exposure techniques:	☐	☐	☐	☐	☐	☐

29. Sets the proper exposure techniques:

Conventional systems
- Sets the proper kVp, mA, and time and makes adjustments as necessary.

or

CR or DR systems
- Identifies the patient on the work-list (or manually types the patient information into the system).
- Selects appropriate body region, specific body part, and accurate view/ projection.
- Double-checks preset parameters:
  —Adult vs. pediatric patients
    ◦ Small, medium, or large
  —Bucky/receptor (upright vs. table) *or* non-Bucky
  —AEC vs. fixed
    ◦ If AEC, checks ion chambers
    ◦ Density setting
  —kVp and mA; adjusts if necessary
  —Focal spot/filament size

	Procedure		Repeat		Competency	
30. Exposes the cassette/receptor after telling the patient to hold still and after giving him or her proper breathing instructions (expiration) *for each projection.*	☐	☐	☐	☐	☐	☐
31. Provides each radiograph with the proper identification (flash) and/or processes each cassette (image) without difficulty (regardless of technology—film, CR, or DR).	▦	▦	▦	▦	☐	☐
32. Properly completes the examination by filling out all necessary paperwork, entering the examination in the computer, having the images checked by the appropriate staff members, answering any last-minute questions, and informing the patient that he or she is finished.	▦	▦	▦	▦	☐	☐
33. Exhibits the ability to adapt to new and difficult situations if and when necessary.	▦	▦	▦	▦	☐	☐
34. Accepts constructive criticism and uses it to his or her advantage.	☐	☐	☐	☐	☐	☐
35. Leaves the radiographic room neat and clean for the next examination.	▦	▦	▦	▦	☐	☐
36. Completes the examination within a reasonable time frame.	☐	☐	☐	☐	☐	☐

Comments:

_____

_____

RADIOGRAPHIC IMAGE QUALITY
The student is able to critique his or her radiographs as to whether they demonstrate:

	Procedure		Repeat		Competency	
	Yes	No	Yes	No	Yes	No
37. Proper technique/optimal density	▦	▦	▦	▦	☐	☐
38. Enhanced detail, without evidence of motion and without any visible artifacts	▦	▦	▦	▦	☐	☐
39. Proper positioning (all anatomy included, evidence of proper centering/ alignment, etc.)	▦	▦	▦	▦	☐	☐

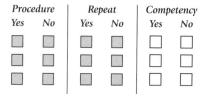

(continued)

	Procedure		Repeat		Competency	
	Yes	No	Yes	No	Yes	No
40. Proper marker placement	☐	☐	☐	☐	☐	☐
41. Evidence of proper collimation and radiation protection	☐	☐	☐	☐	☐	☐
42. Long vs. short scale of contrast	☐	☐	☐	☐	☐	☐

Comments:

_____

_____

CERVICAL SPINE ANATOMY
The student is able to identify:

	Procedure		Repeat		Competency	
	Yes	No	Yes	No	Yes	No
43. Atlas vs. axis	☐	☐	☐	☐	☐	☐
44. Intervertebral disk space	☐	☐	☐	☐	☐	☐
45. Intervertebral foramen	☐	☐	☐	☐	☐	☐
46. Body	☐	☐	☐	☐	☐	☐
47. Spinous process	☐	☐	☐	☐	☐	☐
48. Superior and inferior articular processes	☐	☐	☐	☐	☐	☐
49. Zygapophyseal joints	☐	☐	☐	☐	☐	☐
50. Obvious pathology	☐	☐	☐	☐	☐	☐

Comments:

_____

_____

_____   _____   _____
Procedure Evaluator Signature   Repeat Evaluator Signature   Competency Evaluator Signature

_____   _____   _____
Date   Date   Date

END FLEXION AND EXTENSION CERVICAL SPINE EVALUATION

Student Name:_____

Procedure Grade	Repeat Grade	Competency Grade

PATIENT INFORMATION OR SIMULATED PROCEDURE *(circle if simulated)*

	Procedure	Repeat	Competency
Age			
Medical Record No.			
Ability to Cooperate			
Condition/Pathology			
Technical Factors Used			
Exposure Index			

FACILITY PREPARATION
The student:

	Procedure Yes / No	Repeat Yes / No	Competency Yes / No
1. Examines the radiographic room and cleans/straightens it before escorting the patient in.	☐ ☐	☐ ☐	☐ ☐
2. Has all equipment and supplies (patient gown, shield, markers, lead blockers, etc.) readily available before escorting the patient in.	☐ ☐	☐ ☐	☐ ☐
3. Is able to manipulate all radiographic equipment with ease, and centers the central ray to the cassette/receptor *for all projections.*	☐ ☐	☐ ☐	☐ ☐
4. Adjusts the tube to the proper SID *for each projection.*	☐ ☐	☐ ☐	☐ ☐
5. Selects cassettes/receptor of the appropriate sizes *for all projections,* according to the patient's size and examination.	☐ ☐	☐ ☐	☐ ☐

Comments:

_____

_____

PATIENT PREPARATION
The student:

	Procedure Yes / No	Repeat Yes / No	Competency Yes / No
6. Identifies the correct patient and examination according to the requisition while establishing a good rapport with him or her.	☐ ☐	☐ ☐	☐ ☐
7. Obtains and documents the patient's history before the examination.	▣ ▣	▣ ▣	☐ ☐
8. Explains the examination in terms the patient fully understands and properly communicates with the patient throughout the examination.	☐ ☐	☐ ☐	☐ ☐
9. Asks female patients of childbearing age the date of their last menstrual period and documents this; inquires about the possibility of pregnancy and has them sign pregnancy consent forms.	☐ ☐	☐ ☐	☐ ☐
10. Removes all obscuring objects (snaps, zippers, jewelry, etc.) so as *not* to produce radiographic artifacts.	☐ ☐	☐ ☐	☐ ☐

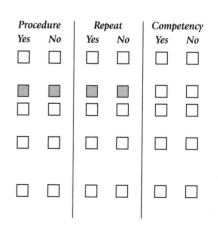

(continued)

	Procedure		Repeat		Competency	
	Yes	No	Yes	No	Yes	No
11. Respects the patient's modesty and provides ample comfort for him or her while positioning him or her to begin the examination.	☐	☐	☐	☐	☐	☐

Comments:

_____

_____

PATIENT POSITIONING FOR A LARYNX (SOFT TISSUE NECK)
Anteroposterior
The student:

	Procedure		Repeat		Competency	
	Yes	No	Yes	No	Yes	No
12. Places the patient's back against the upright Bucky/receptor (or supine on the radiographic table), without rotation.	☐	☐	☐	☐	☐	☐
13. Selects the appropriate receptor or places the cassette lengthwise in the Bucky drawer. For conventional cassettes, the flash must be away from any anatomy.	☐	☐	☐	☐	☐	☐
14. Extends the head enough to prevent the mandible from obscuring the laryngeal area.	☐	☐	☐	☐	☐	☐
15. Centers the central ray to the midsagittal plane of the body.	☐	☐	☐	☐	☐	☐
16. Directs the central ray perpendicularly at the level of the laryngeal prominence.	☐	☐	☐	☐	☐	☐

Lateral
The student:

	Procedure		Repeat		Competency	
	Yes	No	Yes	No	Yes	No
17. Places the patient in the left lateral position against the upright Bucky/receptor, without rotation.	☐	☐	☐	☐	☐	☐
18. Selects the appropriate receptor or places the cassette lengthwise in the Bucky drawer. For conventional cassettes, the flash must be away from any anatomy.	☐	☐	☐	☐	☐	☐
19. Extends the patient's jaw slightly forward.	☐	☐	☐	☐	☐	☐
20. Requests the patient to drop his or her shoulders and arms to the sides, reaching for the floor.	☐	☐	☐	☐	☐	☐
21. Directs the central ray to the center of the spine.	☐	☐	☐	☐	☐	☐
22. Centers the central ray perpendicularly to the level of the laryngeal prominence.	☐	☐	☐	☐	☐	☐

Comments:

_____

_____

IMPORTANT DETAILS
The student:

	Procedure		Repeat		Competency	
	Yes	No	Yes	No	Yes	No
23. Instills confidence in the patient by exhibiting self-confidence throughout the examination.	☐	☐	☐	☐	☐	☐
24. Places lead markers in the appropriate area of the cassette/receptor (top/bottom/anteriorly/laterally), where they will be visualized, on the proper anatomical side (right/left), and in the appropriate position (face up/face down), depending on the patient's position.	☐	☐	☐	☐	☐	☐
25. Provides radiation protection (shield) for the patient, self, and others (closes doors).	☐	☐	☐	☐	☐	☐
26. Applies proper collimation and makes adjustments as necessary.	☐	☐	☐	☐	☐	☐

	Procedure		Repeat		Competency	
	Yes	No	Yes	No	Yes	No
27. Properly measures the patient along the course of the central ray.	☐	☐	☐	☐	☐	☐
28. Sets the proper exposure techniques:	☐	☐	☐	☐	☐	☐

Conventional systems
- Sets the proper kVp, mA, and time and makes adjustments as necessary.

or

CR or DR systems
- Identifies the patient on the work-list (or manually types the patient information into the system).
- Selects appropriate body region, specific body part, and accurate view/ projection.
- Double-checks preset parameters:
  —Adult vs. pediatric patients
  ○ Small, medium, or large
  —Bucky/receptor (upright vs. table) *or* non-Bucky
  —AEC vs. fixed
  ○ If AEC, checks ion chambers
  ○ Density setting
  —kVp and mA; adjusts if necessary
  —Focal spot/filament size

	Procedure		Repeat		Competency	
29. Exposes the cassette/receptor after telling the patient to hold still and after giving him or her proper breathing instructions (during inspiration) *for each projection*.	☐	☐	☐	☐	☐	☐
30. Provides each radiograph with the proper identification (flash) and/or processes each cassette (image) without difficulty (regardless of technology—film, CR, or DR).	☑	☑	☑	☑	☐	☐
31. Properly completes the examination by filling out all necessary paperwork, entering the examination in the computer, having images checked by the appropriate staff members, providing postprocedural instructions and answering last-minute questions, and informing the patient that he or she is finished.	☑	☑	☑	☑	☐	☐
32. Exhibits the ability to adapt to new and difficult situations if and when necessary.	☑	☑	☑	☑	☐	☐
33. Accepts constructive criticism and uses it to his or her advantage.	☐	☐	☐	☐	☐	☐
34. Leaves the radiographic room neat and clean for the next examination.	☑	☑	☑	☑	☐	☐
35. Completes the examination within a reasonable time frame.	☐	☐	☐	☐	☐	☐

Comments:

_____

_____

RADIOGRAPHIC IMAGE QUALITY
The student is able to critique his or her radiographs as to whether they demonstrate:

	Procedure		Repeat		Competency	
	Yes	No	Yes	No	Yes	No
36. Proper technique/optimal density	☑	☑	☑	☑	☐	☐
37. Enhanced detail, without evidence of motion and without any visible artifacts	☑	☑	☑	☑	☐	☐
38. Proper positioning (all anatomy included, evidence of proper centering/ alignment, etc.)	☑	☑	☑	☑	☐	☐
39. Proper marker placement	☑	☑	☑	☑	☐	☐
40. Evidence of proper collimation and radiation protection	☑	☑	☑	☑	☐	☐
41. Long vs. short scale of contrast	☑	☑	☑	☑	☐	☐

(continued)

Comments:

_____

_____

_____

LARYNX (SOFT TISSUE) ANATOMY
The student is able to identify:

	Procedure		Repeat		Competency	
	Yes	No	Yes	No	Yes	No
42. Air-filled pharynx	☐	☐	☐	☐	☐	☐
43. Hyoid bone	☐	☐	☐	☐	☐	☐
44. Larynx	☐	☐	☐	☐	☐	☐
45. Trachea	☐	☐	☐	☐	☐	☐
46. Cervical spine	☐	☐	☐	☐	☐	☐
47. Obvious pathology/foreign body	☐	☐	☐	☐	☐	☐

Comments:

_____

_____

_____   _____   _____
Procedure Evaluator Signature   Repeat Evaluator Signature   Competency Evaluator Signature

_____   _____   _____
Date   Date   Date

END LARYNX/UPPER AIRWAY (SOFT TISSUE NECK) EVALUATION

Student Name:_____

Procedure Grade	Repeat Grade	Competency Grade

PATIENT INFORMATION OR SIMULATED PROCEDURE *(circle if simulated)*

	Procedure	Repeat	Competency
Age			
Medical Record No.			
Ability to Cooperate			
Condition/Pathology			
Technical Factors Used			
Exposure Index			

FACILITY PREPARATION
The student:

	Procedure Yes No	Repeat Yes No	Competency Yes No
1. Examines the radiographic room and cleans/straightens it before escorting the patient in.	☐ ☐	☐ ☐	☐ ☐
2. Has all equipment and supplies (patient gown, shield, markers, lead blockers, etc.) readily available before escorting the patient in.	☐ ☐	☐ ☐	☐ ☐
3. Remembers to use the anode heel effect, is able to manipulate all radiographic equipment with ease, and centers the central ray to the cassette/receptor *for both projections.*	☐ ☐	☐ ☐	☐ ☐
4. Adjusts the tube to the proper SID *for each projection.*	☐ ☐	☐ ☐	☐ ☐
5. Selects cassettes/receptor of the appropriate sizes *for both projections,* according to the patient's size and examination.	☐ ☐	☐ ☐	☐ ☐

Comments:

_____

_____

PATIENT PREPARATION
The student:

	Procedure Yes No	Repeat Yes No	Competency Yes No
6. Identifies the correct patient and examination according to the requisition while establishing a good rapport with him or her.	☐ ☐	☐ ☐	☐ ☐
7. Obtains and documents the patient's history before the examination.	▨ ▨	▨ ▨	☐ ☐
8. Explains the examination in terms the patient fully understands and properly communicates with the patient throughout the examination.	☐ ☐	☐ ☐	☐ ☐
9. Asks female patients of childbearing age the date of their last menstrual period and documents this; inquires about the possibility of pregnancy and has them sign pregnancy consent forms.	☐ ☐	☐ ☐	☐ ☐
10. Removes all obscuring objects (snaps, zippers, jewelry, etc.) so as *not* to produce radiographic artifacts.	☐ ☐	☐ ☐	☐ ☐

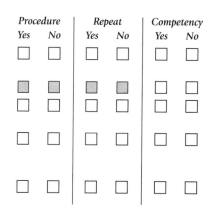

(continued)

	Procedure		Repeat		Competency	
	Yes	No	Yes	No	Yes	No
11. Respects the patient's modesty and provides ample comfort for him or her.	☐	☐	☐	☐	☐	☐

Comments:

_____

_____

PATIENT POSITIONING FOR A THORACIC SPINE
Anteroposterior
The student:

	Procedure		Repeat		Competency	
	Yes	No	Yes	No	Yes	No
12. Places the patient in the supine position on the radiographic table without rotation.	☐	☐	☐	☐	☐	☐
13. Selects the appropriate receptor or places the upper edge of the cassette lengthwise approximately 1–2 inches above the patient's shoulders. For conventional cassettes, the flash must be at the top and away from any anatomy.	☐	☐	☐	☐	☐	☐
14. If possible, uses the anode heel effect and instructs the patient to flex his or her hips and knees slightly.	☐	☐	☐	☐	☐	☐
15. Centers the central ray to the midsagittal plane of the body.	☐	☐	☐	☐	☐	☐
16. Directs the central ray perpendicularly at the level of T6, or 3–4 inches below the manubrial notch.	☐	☐	☐	☐	☐	☐

Lateral
The student:

	Procedure		Repeat		Competency	
	Yes	No	Yes	No	Yes	No
17. Places the patient in the left lateral position on the table, without rotation.	☐	☐	☐	☐	☐	☐
18. Selects the appropriate receptor or places the cassette lengthwise in the Bucky drawer.	☐	☐	☐	☐	☐	☐
19. Instructs the patient to flex his or her hips and knees up to a comfortable position.	☐	☐	☐	☐	☐	☐
20. Supports the patient's waist so that the spine is parallel to the table, places a support between the patient's knees, and supports the patient's head to avoid rotation.	☐	☐	☐	☐	☐	☐
21. Adjusts the patient's arms so that they are at right angles to the body.	☐	☐	☐	☐	☐	☐
22. Directs the central ray to the center of the spine.	☐	☐	☐	☐	☐	☐
23. Centers the central ray perpendicularly to T6, or if the spine is not supported, angles the central ray cephalad until it is perpendicular to the spine, usually 10–15°.	☐	☐	☐	☐	☐	☐
24. Places a lead blocker behind the patient.	☐	☐	☐	☐	☐	☐

Comments:

_____

_____

IMPORTANT DETAILS
The student:

	Procedure		Repeat		Competency	
	Yes	No	Yes	No	Yes	No
25. Instills confidence in the patient by exhibiting self-confidence throughout the examination.	☐	☐	☐	☐	☐	☐
26. Places a lead marker in the appropriate area of the cassette/receptor (top/bottom/anteriorly/laterally), where it will be visualized on the finished radiograph, on the proper anatomical side (right/left), and in the appropriate position (face up/face down), depending on the patient's position.	☐	☐	☐	☐	☐	☐

	Procedure Yes	Procedure No	Repeat Yes	Repeat No	Competency Yes	Competency No
27. Provides radiation protection (shield) for the patient, self, and others (closes doors).	☐	☐	☐	☐	☐	☐
28. Applies proper collimation and makes adjustments as necessary.	☐	☐	☐	☐	☐	☐
29. Properly measures the patient along the course of the central ray *for each projection.*	☐	☐	☐	☐	☐	☐
30. Sets the proper exposure techniques:	☐	☐	☐	☐	☐	☐

30. Sets the proper exposure techniques:

Conventional systems
- Sets the proper kVp, mA, and time and makes adjustments as necessary.

or

CR or DR systems
- Identifies the patient on the work-list (or manually types the patient information into the system).
- Selects appropriate body region, specific body part, and accurate view/ projection.
- Double-checks preset parameters:
  —Adult vs. pediatric patients
    ○ Small, medium, or large
  —Bucky/receptor (upright vs. table) *or* non-Bucky
  —AEC vs. fixed
    ○ If AEC, checks ion chambers
    ○ Density setting
  —kVp and mA; adjusts if necessary
  —Focal spot/filament size

	Procedure Yes	Procedure No	Repeat Yes	Repeat No	Competency Yes	Competency No
31. Exposes the cassette/receptor after telling the patient to hold still and after giving him or her proper breathing instructions (AP—inspiration; lateral—shallow breathing) *for each projection.*	☐	☐	☐	☐	☐	☐
32. Provides each radiograph with the proper identification (flash) and/or processes each cassette (image) without difficulty (regardless of technology—film, CR, or DR).	▣	▣	▣	▣	☐	☐
33. Properly completes the examination by filling out all necessary paperwork, entering the examination in the computer, having the images checked by the appropriate staff members, answering any last-minute questions, and informing the patient that he or she is finished.	▣	▣	▣	▣	☐	☐
34. Exhibits the ability to adapt to new and difficult situations if and when necessary.	▣	▣	▣	▣	☐	☐
35. Accepts constructive criticism and uses it to his or her advantage.	☐	☐	☐	☐	☐	☐
36. Leaves the radiographic room neat and clean for the next examination.	▣	▣	▣	▣	☐	☐
37. Completes the examination within a reasonable time frame.	☐	☐	☐	☐	☐	☐

Comments:

RADIOGRAPHIC IMAGE QUALITY
The student is able to critique his or her radiographs as to whether they demonstrate:

	Procedure Yes	Procedure No	Repeat Yes	Repeat No	Competency Yes	Competency No
38. Proper technique/optimal density	▣	▣	▣	▣	☐	☐
39. Enhanced detail, without evidence of motion and without any visible artifacts	▣	▣	▣	▣	☐	☐
40. Proper positioning (all anatomy included, evidence of proper centering/ alignment, etc.)	▣	▣	▣	▣	☐	☐

(continued)

	Procedure		Repeat		Competency	
	Yes	No	Yes	No	Yes	No
41. Proper marker placement	☐	☐	☐	☐	☐	☐
42. Evidence of proper collimation and radiation protection	☐	☐	☐	☐	☐	☐
43. Long vs. short scale of contrast	☐	☐	☐	☐	☐	☐

Comments:

_____

_____

THORACIC SPINE ANATOMY
The student is able to identify:

	Procedure		Repeat		Competency	
	Yes	No	Yes	No	Yes	No
44. Lamina	☐	☐	☐	☐	☐	☐
45. Pedicle	☐	☐	☐	☐	☐	☐
46. Body	☐	☐	☐	☐	☐	☐
47. Spinous process	☐	☐	☐	☐	☐	☐
48. Superior and inferior articular processes	☐	☐	☐	☐	☐	☐
49. Zygapophyseal joints	☐	☐	☐	☐	☐	☐
50. Transverse process	☐	☐	☐	☐	☐	☐
51. Intervertebral disk space	☐	☐	☐	☐	☐	☐
52. Intervertebral foramen	☐	☐	☐	☐	☐	☐
53. T12 and the 12th rib	☐	☐	☐	☐	☐	☐
54. Obvious pathology	☐	☐	☐	☐	☐	☐

Comments:

_____

_____

Procedure Evaluator Signature	Repeat Evaluator Signature	Competency Evaluator Signature
Date	Date	Date

END THORACIC SPINE EVALUATION

Student Name:_____

Procedure Grade	Repeat Grade	Competency Grade

PATIENT INFORMATION OR SIMULATED PROCEDURE *(circle if simulated)*

	Procedure	Repeat	Competency
Age			
Medical Record No.			
Ability to Cooperate			
Condition/Pathology			
Technical Factors Used			
Exposure Index			

FACILITY PREPARATION
The student:

	Procedure Yes	No	Repeat Yes	No	Competency Yes	No
1. Examines the radiographic room and cleans/straightens it before escorting the patient in.	☐	☐	☐	☐	☐	☐
2. Has all equipment and supplies (patient gown, shield, markers, lead blockers, etc.) readily available before escorting the patient in.	☐	☐	☐	☐	☐	☐
3. Is able to manipulate all radiographic equipment with ease, and centers the central ray to the cassette/receptor *for all projections.*	☐	☐	☐	☐	☐	☐
4. Adjusts the tube to the proper SID *for each projection.*	☐	☐	☐	☐	☐	☐
5. Selects cassettes/receptor of the appropriate sizes *for all projections,* according to the patient's size and examination.	☐	☐	☐	☐	☐	☐

Comments:

_____

_____

PATIENT PREPARATION
The student:

	Procedure Yes	No	Repeat Yes	No	Competency Yes	No
6. Identifies the correct patient and examination according to the requisition while establishing a good rapport with him or her.	☐	☐	☐	☐	☐	☐
7. Obtains and documents the patient's history before the examination.	▨	▨	▨	▨	☐	☐
8. Explains the examination in terms the patient fully understands and properly communicates with the patient throughout the examination.	☐	☐	☐	☐	☐	☐
9. Asks female patients of childbearing age the date of their last menstrual period and documents this; inquires about the possibility of pregnancy and has them sign pregnancy consent forms.	☐	☐	☐	☐	☐	☐
10. Removes all obscuring objects (snaps, zippers, belts, etc.) so as *not* to produce radiographic artifacts.	☐	☐	☐	☐	☐	☐

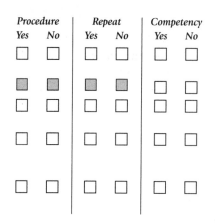

(continued)

	Procedure		Repeat		Competency	
	Yes	No	Yes	No	Yes	No
11. Respects the patient's modesty and provides ample comfort for him or her.	☐	☐	☐	☐	☐	☐

Comments:

_____

_____

PATIENT POSITIONING FOR A LUMBAR SPINE
Anteroposterior
The student:

	Procedure		Repeat		Competency	
	Yes	No	Yes	No	Yes	No
12. Places the patient in the supine position on the radiographic table, without rotation.	☐	☐	☐	☐	☐	☐
13. Selects the appropriate receptor or places the cassette lengthwise in the Bucky drawer. For conventional cassettes, the flash must be at the bottom away from any anatomy.	☐	☐	☐	☐	☐	☐
14. Instructs the patient to flex his or her hips and knees slightly, just enough to place the feet flat on the table.	☐	☐	☐	☐	☐	☐
15. Centers the central ray to the midsagittal plane of the body.	☐	☐	☐	☐	☐	☐
16. Directs the central ray perpendicularly at the level of the iliac crest.	☐	☐	☐	☐	☐	☐

Right Posterior Oblique
The student:

	Procedure		Repeat		Competency	
	Yes	No	Yes	No	Yes	No
17. Places the patient in the oblique position, at an angle of 45°.	☐	☐	☐	☐	☐	☐
18. Selects the appropriate receptor or places the cassette lengthwise in the Bucky drawer. For conventional cassettes, the flash must be away from any anatomy.	☐	☐	☐	☐	☐	☐
19. Ensures that the patient's shoulders and hips lie in the same plane, adjusting if necessary.	☐	☐	☐	☐	☐	☐
20. Directs the central ray to the center of the spine, 2 inches medially from the raised anterosuperior iliac spine (ASIS).	☐	☐	☐	☐	☐	☐
21. Directs the central ray perpendicularly at a level 2 inches above the iliac crest (L3).	☐	☐	☐	☐	☐	☐

Left Posterior Oblique
The student:

	Procedure		Repeat		Competency	
	Yes	No	Yes	No	Yes	No
22. Places the patient in the oblique position, at an angle of 45°.	☐	☐	☐	☐	☐	☐
23. Selects the appropriate receptor or places the cassette lengthwise in the Bucky drawer. For conventional cassettes, the flash must be away from any anatomy.	☐	☐	☐	☐	☐	☐
24. Ensures that the patient's shoulders and hips lie in the same plane, adjusting if necessary.	☐	☐	☐	☐	☐	☐
25. Directs the central ray to the center of the spine, 2 inches medially from the raised ASIS.	☐	☐	☐	☐	☐	☐
26. Directs the central ray perpendicularly at a level 2 inches above the iliac crest (L3).	☐	☐	☐	☐	☐	☐

Lateral
The student:

	Procedure		Repeat		Competency	
	Yes	No	Yes	No	Yes	No
27. Places the patient in the left lateral position on the radiographic table, without rotation.	☐	☐	☐	☐	☐	☐

	Procedure		Repeat		Competency	
	Yes	No	Yes	No	Yes	No
28. Selects the appropriate receptor or places the cassette lengthwise in the Bucky drawer. For conventional cassettes, the flash must be away from any anatomy.	☐	☐	☐	☐	☐	☐
29. Instructs the patient to flex his or her hips and knees up toward his or her chest.	☐	☐	☐	☐	☐	☐
30. Supports the patient's waist so that the spine is parallel, and places a support between the patient's knees to avoid rotation.	☐	☐	☐	☐	☐	☐
31. Adjusts the patient's arms so that they are at right angles to the body.	☐	☐	☐	☐	☐	☐
32. Directs the central ray to the center of the spine, 3 inches anteriorly from the spinous process.	☐	☐	☐	☐	☐	☐
33. Centers the central ray perpendicularly at the level of the iliac crest, or if the spine is not supported/parallel, angles the central ray caudad until it is perpendicular to the spine, usually 5° for males and 8° for females.	☐	☐	☐	☐	☐	☐
34. Places a lead blocker behind the patient.	☐	☐	☐	☐	☐	☐

Lumbosacral Junction/Interspace (L-S Spot)
The student:

	Procedure		Repeat		Competency	
	Yes	No	Yes	No	Yes	No
35. Places the patient in the (opposite) lateral position, without rotation.	☐	☐	☐	☐	☐	☐
36. Selects the appropriate receptor or places the cassette lengthwise in the Bucky drawer. For conventional cassettes, the flash must be away from any anatomy.	☐	☐	☐	☐	☐	☐
37. Instructs the patient to flex his or her hips and knees up toward his or her chest.	☐	☐	☐	☐	☐	☐
38. Supports the patient's waist so that the spine is parallel, and places a support between the patient's knees to avoid rotation.	☐	☐	☐	☐	☐	☐
39. Adjusts the patient's arms so that they are at right angles to the body.	☐	☐	☐	☐	☐	☐
40. Centers the central ray 1.5 inches inferiorly from the crest and 2 inches posteriorly from the ASIS.	☐	☐	☐	☐	☐	☐
41. Centers the central ray perpendicularly to the L-S articulation, or if the spine is not supported/parallel, angles the central ray caudad until it is perpendicular to the spine, usually 5° for males and 8° for females.	☐	☐	☐	☐	☐	☐
42. Places a lead blocker behind the patient.	☐	☐	☐	☐	☐	☐

Comments:

_____

_____

IMPORTANT DETAILS
The student:

	Procedure		Repeat		Competency	
	Yes	No	Yes	No	Yes	No
43. Instills confidence in the patient by exhibiting self-confidence throughout the examination.	☐	☐	☐	☐	☐	☐
44. Places a lead marker in the appropriate area of the cassette/receptor (top/bottom/anteriorly/laterally), where it will be visualized on the finished radiograph, on the proper anatomical side (right/left), and in the appropriate position (face up/face down), depending on the patient's position.	☐	☐	☐	☐	☐	☐
45. Provides radiation protection (shield) for the patient (when appropriate), self, and others (closes doors).	☐	☐	☐	☐	☐	☐
46. Applies proper collimation and makes adjustments as necessary.	☐	☐	☐	☐	☐	☐

(continued)

	Procedure		Repeat		Competency	
	Yes	No	Yes	No	Yes	No
47. Properly measures the patient along the course of the central ray *for each projection.*	☐	☐	☐	☐	☐	☐
48. Sets the proper exposure techniques:	☐	☐	☐	☐	☐	☐

Conventional systems
- Sets the proper kVp, mA, and time and makes adjustments as necessary.

or

CR or DR systems
- Identifies the patient on the work-list (or manually types the patient information into the system).
- Selects appropriate body region, specific body part, and accurate view/ projection.
- Double-checks preset parameters:
  —Adult vs. pediatric patients
  ○ Small, medium, or large
  —Bucky/receptor (upright vs. table) *or* non-Bucky
  —AEC vs. fixed
  ○ If AEC, checks ion chambers
  ○ Density setting
  —kVp and mA; adjusts if necessary
  —Focal spot/filament size

	Procedure		Repeat		Competency	
49. Exposes the cassette/receptor after telling the patient to hold still and after giving him or her proper breathing instructions (expiration) *for each projection.*	☐	☐	☐	☐	☐	☐
50. Provides each radiograph with the proper identification (flash) and/or processes each cassette (image) without difficulty (regardless of technology—film, CR, or DR).	☑	☑	☑	☑	☐	☐
51. Properly completes the examination by filling out all necessary paperwork, entering the examination in the computer, having the images checked by the appropriate staff members, answering any last-minute questions, and informing the patient that he or she is finished.	☑	☑	☑	☑	☐	☐
52. Exhibits the ability to adapt to new and difficult situations if and when necessary.	☑	☑	☑	☑	☐	☐
53. Accepts constructive criticism and uses it to his or her advantage.	☐	☐	☐	☐	☐	☐
54. Leaves the radiographic room neat and clean for the next examination.	☑	☑	☑	☑	☐	☐
55. Completes the examination within a reasonable time frame.	☐	☐	☐	☐	☐	☐

Comments:

_____

_____

RADIOGRAPHIC IMAGE QUALITY

The student is able to critique his or her radiographs as to whether they demonstrate:

	Procedure		Repeat		Competency	
	Yes	No	Yes	No	Yes	No
56. Proper technique/optimal density	☑	☑	☑	☑	☐	☐
57. Enhanced detail, without evidence of motion and without any visible artifacts	☑	☑	☑	☑	☐	☐
58. Proper positioning (all anatomy included, evidence of proper centering/ alignment, etc.)	☑	☑	☑	☑	☐	☐
59. Proper marker placement	☑	☑	☑	☑	☐	☐
60. Evidence of proper collimation and radiation protection	☑	☑	☑	☑	☐	☐
61. Long vs. short scale of contrast	☑	☑	☑	☑	☐	☐

Comments:

_____

_____

LUMBAR SPINE ANATOMY
The student is able to identify:

	Procedure		Repeat		Competency	
	Yes	No	Yes	No	Yes	No
62. Lamina (body)	☐	☐	☐	☐	☐	☐
63. Pedicle (eye)	☐	☐	☐	☐	☐	☐
64. Body	☐	☐	☐	☐	☐	☐
65. Spinous process	☐	☐	☐	☐	☐	☐
66. Superior (ear) and inferior (foot) articular processes	☐	☐	☐	☐	☐	☐
67. Zygapophyseal joints	☐	☐	☐	☐	☐	☐
68. Transverse process (nose)	☐	☐	☐	☐	☐	☐
69. Intervertebral disk space	☐	☐	☐	☐	☐	☐
70. Intervertebral foramen	☐	☐	☐	☐	☐	☐
71. Sacrum	☐	☐	☐	☐	☐	☐
72. Lumbosacral articulation	☐	☐	☐	☐	☐	☐
73. Pars interarticulares (neck)	☐	☐	☐	☐	☐	☐
74. Obvious pathology	☐	☐	☐	☐	☐	☐

Comments:

_____

_____

Procedure Evaluator Signature   Repeat Evaluator Signature   Competency Evaluator Signature

Date   Date   Date

END LUMBAR SPINE EVALUATION

Student Name:_____

Procedure Grade	Repeat Grade	Competency Grade

PATIENT INFORMATION OR SIMULATED PROCEDURE *(circle if simulated)*

	Procedure	Repeat	Competency
Age			
Medical Record No.			
Ability to Cooperate			
Condition/Pathology			
Technical Factors Used			
Exposure Index			

FACILITY PREPARATION
The student:

	Procedure Yes / No	Repeat Yes / No	Competency Yes / No
1. Examines the radiographic room and cleans/straightens it before escorting the patient in.	☐ ☐	☐ ☐	☐ ☐
2. Has all equipment and supplies (patient gown, shield, markers, lead blockers, etc.) readily available before escorting the patient in.	☐ ☐	☐ ☐	☐ ☐
3. Is able to manipulate all radiographic equipment with ease, and centers the central ray to the cassette/receptor *for both projections.*	☐ ☐	☐ ☐	☐ ☐
4. Adjusts the tube to the proper SID *for each projection.*	☐ ☐	☐ ☐	☐ ☐
5. Selects cassettes/receptor of the appropriate sizes *for both projections,* according to the patient's size and examination.	☐ ☐	☐ ☐	☐ ☐

Comments:

_____

_____

PATIENT PREPARATION
The student:

	Procedure Yes / No	Repeat Yes / No	Competency Yes / No
6. Identifies the correct patient and examination according to the requisition while establishing a good rapport with him or her.	☐ ☐	☐ ☐	☐ ☐
7. Obtains and documents the patient's history before the examination.	▥ ▥	▥ ▥	☐ ☐
8. Explains the examination in terms the patient fully understands and properly communicates with the patient throughout the examination.	☐ ☐	☐ ☐	☐ ☐
9. Asks female patients of childbearing age the date of their last menstrual period and documents this; inquires about the possibility of pregnancy and has them sign pregnancy consent forms.	☐ ☐	☐ ☐	☐ ☐
10. Removes all obscuring objects (snaps, zippers, belts, etc.) so as *not* to produce radiographic artifacts.	☐ ☐	☐ ☐	☐ ☐

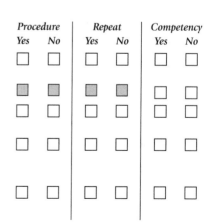

(continued)

	Procedure		Repeat		Competency	
	Yes	No	Yes	No	Yes	No
11. Respects the patient's modesty and provides ample comfort for him or her.	☐	☐	☐	☐	☐	☐

Comments:

_____

_____

PATIENT POSITIONING FOR FLEXION AND EXTENSION LATERALS OF A LUMBAR SPINE

Flexion

The student:

	Procedure		Repeat		Competency	
	Yes	No	Yes	No	Yes	No
12. Places the patient in the left lateral position on the radiographic table, without rotation.	☐	☐	☐	☐	☐	☐
13. Selects the appropriate receptor or places the cassette lengthwise in the Bucky drawer. For conventional cassettes, the flash must be away from any anatomy.	☐	☐	☐	☐	☐	☐
14. Instructs the patient to draw his or her hips and knees up toward his or her shoulders as much as possible.	☐	☐	☐	☐	☐	☐
15. Supports the patient's waist so that the spine is parallel, and places a support between the patient's knees to avoid rotation.	☐	☐	☐	☐	☐	☐
16. Adjusts the patient's arms so that they are at right angles to the body.	☐	☐	☐	☐	☐	☐
17. Directs the central ray 2 inches posteriorly from the midaxillary line.	☐	☐	☐	☐	☐	☐
18. Centers the central ray perpendicularly at the level of the iliac crest (L3).	☐	☐	☐	☐	☐	☐
19. Places a lead blocker behind the patient.	☐	☐	☐	☐	☐	☐

Extension

The student:

	Procedure		Repeat		Competency	
	Yes	No	Yes	No	Yes	No
20. Places the patient in the left lateral position on the radiographic table, without rotation.	☐	☐	☐	☐	☐	☐
21. Selects the appropriate receptor or places the cassette lengthwise in the Bucky drawer. For conventional cassettes, the flash must be away from any anatomy.	☐	☐	☐	☐	☐	☐
22. Instructs the patient to extend his or her hips and knees backward as much as possible.	☐	☐	☐	☐	☐	☐
23. Supports the patient's waist so that the spine is parallel, and places a support between the patient's knees to avoid rotation.	☐	☐	☐	☐	☐	☐
24. Adjusts the patient's arms so that they are at right angles to the body.	☐	☐	☐	☐	☐	☐
25. Directs the central ray 2 inches posteriorly from the midaxillary line.	☐	☐	☐	☐	☐	☐
26. Centers the central ray perpendicularly at the level of the iliac crest (L3).	☐	☐	☐	☐	☐	☐
27. Places a lead blocker behind the patient.	☐	☐	☐	☐	☐	☐

Comments:

_____

_____

IMPORTANT DETAILS

The student:

	Procedure		Repeat		Competency	
	Yes	No	Yes	No	Yes	No
28. Instills confidence in the patient by exhibiting self-confidence throughout the examination.	☐	☐	☐	☐	☐	☐

	Procedure		Repeat		Competency	
	Yes	No	Yes	No	Yes	No
29. Places a lead marker in the appropriate area of the cassette/receptor (top/bottom/anteriorly/laterally), where it will be visualized on the finished radiograph, on the proper anatomical side (right/left), and in the appropriate position (face up/face down), depending on the patient's position.	☐	☐	☐	☐	☐	☐
30. Provides radiation protection (shield) for the patient (when appropriate), self, and others (closes doors).	☐	☐	☐	☐	☐	☐
31. Applies proper collimation and makes adjustments as necessary.	☐	☐	☐	☐	☐	☐
32. Properly measures the patient along the course of the central ray *for each projection.*	☐	☐	☐	☐	☐	☐
33. Sets the proper exposure techniques:	☐	☐	☐	☐	☐	☐

33. Sets the proper exposure techniques:

Conventional systems
- Sets the proper kVp, mA, and time and makes adjustments as necessary.

or

CR or DR systems
- Identifies the patient on the work-list (or manually types the patient information into the system).
- Selects appropriate body region, specific body part, and accurate view/ projection.
- Double-checks preset parameters:
  —Adult vs. pediatric patients
  ○ Small, medium, or large
  —Bucky/receptor (upright vs. table) *or* non-Bucky
  —AEC vs. fixed
  ○ If AEC, checks ion chambers
  ○ Density setting
  —kVp and mA; adjusts if necessary
  —Focal spot/filament size

	Procedure		Repeat		Competency	
	Yes	No	Yes	No	Yes	No
34. Exposes the cassette/receptor after telling the patient to hold still and after giving him or her proper breathing instructions (expiration) *for each projection.*	☐	☐	☐	☐	☐	☐
35. Provides each radiograph with the proper identification (flash) and/or processes each cassette (image) without difficulty (regardless of technology—film, CR, or DR).	▨	▨	▨	▨	☐	☐
36. Properly completes the examination by filling out all necessary paperwork, entering the examination in the computer, having the images checked by the appropriate staff members, answering any last-minute questions, and informing the patient that he or she is finished.	▨	▨	▨	▨	☐	☐
37. Exhibits the ability to adapt to new and difficult situations if and when necessary.	▨	▨	▨	▨	☐	☐
38. Accepts constructive criticism and uses it to his or her advantage.	☐	☐	☐	☐	☐	☐
39. Leaves the radiographic room neat and clean for the next examination.	▨	▨	▨	▨	☐	☐
40. Completes the examination within a reasonable time frame.	☐	☐	☐	☐	☐	☐

Comments:

_____

_____

(continued)

RADIOGRAPHIC IMAGE QUALITY

The student is able to critique his or her radiographs as to whether they demonstrate:

	Procedure Yes	Procedure No	Repeat Yes	Repeat No	Competency Yes	Competency No
41. Proper technique/optimal density	☐	☐	☐	☐	☐	☐
42. Enhanced detail, without evidence of motion and without any visible artifacts	☐	☐	☐	☐	☐	☐
43. Proper positioning (all anatomy included, evidence of proper centering/alignment, etc.)	☐	☐	☐	☐	☐	☐
44. Proper marker placement	☐	☐	☐	☐	☐	☐
45. Evidence of proper collimation and radiation protection	☐	☐	☐	☐	☐	☐
46. Long vs. short scale of contrast	☐	☐	☐	☐	☐	☐

Comments:

_____

_____

LUMBAR SPINE ANATOMY

The student is able to identify:

	Procedure Yes	Procedure No	Repeat Yes	Repeat No	Competency Yes	Competency No
47. Body	☐	☐	☐	☐	☐	☐
48. Spinous process	☐	☐	☐	☐	☐	☐
49. Superior and inferior articular processes	☐	☐	☐	☐	☐	☐
50. Intervertebral disk space	☐	☐	☐	☐	☐	☐
51. Intervertebral foramen	☐	☐	☐	☐	☐	☐
52. Sacrum	☐	☐	☐	☐	☐	☐
53. Lumbosacral articulation	☐	☐	☐	☐	☐	☐
54. Obvious pathology	☐	☐	☐	☐	☐	☐

Comments:

_____

_____

_____	_____	_____
Procedure Evaluator Signature	Repeat Evaluator Signature	Competency Evaluator Signature
_____	_____	_____
Date	Date	Date

END FLEXION AND EXTENSION LUMBAR SPINE EVALUATION

Student Name: _____

	Procedure Grade	Repeat Grade	Competency Grade

PATIENT INFORMATION OR SIMULATED PROCEDURE *(circle if simulated)*

	Procedure	Repeat	Competency
Age			
Medical Record No.			
Ability to Cooperate			
Condition/Pathology			
Technical Factors Used			
Exposure Index			

FACILITY PREPARATION
The student:

	Procedure		Repeat		Competency	
	Yes	No	Yes	No	Yes	No
1. Examines the radiographic room and cleans/straightens it before escorting the patient in.	☐	☐	☐	☐	☐	☐
2. Has all equipment and supplies (patient gown, shield, markers, lead blockers, etc.) readily available before escorting the patient in.	☐	☐	☐	☐	☐	☐
3. Is able to manipulate all radiographic equipment with ease, and centers the central ray to the cassette/receptor *for all projections*.	☐	☐	☐	☐	☐	☐
4. Adjusts the tube to the proper SID *for each projection*.	☐	☐	☐	☐	☐	☐
5. Selects cassettes/receptor of the appropriate sizes *for all projections*, according to the patient's size and examination.	☐	☐	☐	☐	☐	☐

Comments:

_____

_____

PATIENT PREPARATION
The student:

	Procedure		Repeat		Competency	
	Yes	No	Yes	No	Yes	No
6. Identifies the correct patient and examination according to the requisition while establishing a good rapport with him or her.	☐	☐	☐	☐	☐	☐
7. Obtains and documents the patient's history before the examination.	■	■	■	■	☐	☐
8. Explains the examination in terms the patient fully understands and properly communicates with the patient throughout the examination.	☐	☐	☐	☐	☐	☐
9. Asks female patients of childbearing age the date of their last menstrual period and documents this; inquires about the possibility of pregnancy and has them sign pregnancy consent forms.	☐	☐	☐	☐	☐	☐
10. Removes all obscuring objects (snaps, zippers, belts, etc.) so as *not* to produce radiographic artifacts.	☐	☐	☐	☐	☐	☐

(continued)

	Procedure		Repeat		Competency	
	Yes	No	Yes	No	Yes	No
11. Respects the patient's modesty and provides ample comfort for him or her.	☐	☐	☐	☐	☐	☐

Comments:

_____

_____

PATIENT POSITIONING FOR A SCOLIOSIS SERIES
AP or PA in the Normal Erect Position
The student:

	Procedure		Repeat		Competency	
	Yes	No	Yes	No	Yes	No
12. Places the patient in the supine/prone position against the erect Bucky/receptor, without rotation.	☐	☐	☐	☐	☐	☐
13. Places the cassette/receptor so that the bottom edge includes approximately 2 inches of the iliac crest (the cassette lengthwise in the Bucky drawer).	☐	☐	☐	☐	☐	☐
14. Instructs the patient to distribute his or her weight evenly on both feet.	☐	☐	☐	☐	☐	☐
15. Centers the central ray to the midsagittal plane of the body.	☐	☐	☐	☐	☐	☐
16. Directs the central ray perpendicularly to the center of the cassette/receptor.	☐	☐	☐	☐	☐	☐

AP or PA in the Supported Erect Position
The student:

	Procedure		Repeat		Competency	
	Yes	No	Yes	No	Yes	No
17. Places the patient in the supine/prone position against the erect Bucky/receptor, without rotation.	☐	☐	☐	☐	☐	☐
18. Places the cassette/receptor so that the bottom edge includes approximately 2 inches of the iliac crest (the cassette lengthwise in the Bucky drawer).	☐	☐	☐	☐	☐	☐
19. Assists the patient in elevating the foot of the convex side of the curve (the foot of the bulging or protruding side of the curve—if the patient's curve protrudes out left, the left foot is elevated on a support) approximately 3–4 inches by using appropriate support under the patient's foot.	☐	☐	☐	☐	☐	☐
20. Centers the central ray to the midsagittal plane of the body.	☐	☐	☐	☐	☐	☐
21. Directs the central ray perpendicularly to the center of the cassette/receptor.	☐	☐	☐	☐	☐	☐

Lateral
The student:

	Procedure		Repeat		Competency	
	Yes	No	Yes	No	Yes	No
22. Places the patient in the lateral position against the erect Bucky/receptor, without rotation.	☐	☐	☐	☐	☐	☐
23. Places the cassette/receptor so that the bottom edge includes approximately 2 inches of the iliac crest (the cassette lengthwise in the Bucky drawer).	☐	☐	☐	☐	☐	☐
24. Instructs the patient to distribute his or her weight evenly on both feet.	☐	☐	☐	☐	☐	☐
25. Centers the central ray to the midcoronal plane of the body.	☐	☐	☐	☐	☐	☐
26. Directs the central ray perpendicularly to the center of the cassette/receptor.	☐	☐	☐	☐	☐	☐

Comments:

_____

_____

_____

IMPORTANT DETAILS
The student:

	Procedure		Repeat		Competency	
	Yes	No	Yes	No	Yes	No
27. Instills confidence in the patient by exhibiting self-confidence throughout the examination.	☐	☐	☐	☐	☐	☐
28. Places a lead marker in the appropriate area of the cassette/receptor (top/bottom/anteriorly/laterally), where it will be visualized on the finished radiograph, on the proper anatomical side (right/left), and in the appropriate position (face up/face down), depending on the patient's position.	☐	☐	☐	☐	☐	☐
29. Provides radiation protection (shield) for the patient *(extremely important for adolescents)*, self, and others (closes doors).	☐	☐	☐	☐	☐	☐
30. Applies proper collimation and makes adjustments as necessary.	☐	☐	☐	☐	☐	☐
31. Properly measures the patient along the course of the central ray *for each projection.*	☐	☐	☐	☐	☐	☐
32. Sets the proper exposure techniques:	☐	☐	☐	☐	☐	☐

Conventional systems
- Sets the proper kVp, mA, and time and makes adjustments as necessary.

or

CR or DR systems
- Identifies the patient on the work-list (or manually types the patient information into the system).
- Selects appropriate body region, specific body part, and accurate view/projection.
- Double-checks preset parameters:
  —Adult vs. pediatric patients
    ○ Small, medium, or large
  —Bucky/receptor (upright vs. table) *or* non-Bucky
  —AEC vs. fixed
    ○ If AEC, checks ion chambers
    ○ Density setting
  —kVp and mA; adjusts if necessary
  —Focal spot/filament size

	Procedure		Repeat		Competency	
33. Exposes the cassette/receptor after telling the patient to hold still and after giving him or her proper breathing instructions (expiration) *for each projection.*	☐	☐	☐	☐	☐	☐
34. Provides each radiograph with the proper identification (flash) and/or processes each cassette (image) without difficulty (regardless of technology—film, CR, or DR).	▨	▨	▨	▨	☐	☐
35. Properly completes the examination by filling out all necessary paperwork, entering the examination in the computer, having the images checked by the appropriate staff members, answering any last-minute questions, and informing the patient that he or she is finished.	▨	▨	▨	▨	☐	☐
36. Exhibits the ability to adapt to new and difficult situations if and when necessary.	▨	▨	▨	▨	☐	☐
37. Accepts constructive criticism and uses it to his or her advantage.	☐	☐	☐	☐	☐	☐
38. Leaves the radiographic room neat and clean for the next examination.	▨	▨	▨	▨	☐	☐
39. Completes the examination within a reasonable time frame.	☐	☐	☐	☐	☐	☐

(continued)

Comments:

_____

_____

RADIOGRAPHIC IMAGE QUALITY
The student is able to critique his or her radiographs as to whether they demonstrate:

	Procedure		Repeat		Competency	
	Yes	No	Yes	No	Yes	No
40. Proper technique/optimal density	☐	☐	☐	☐	☐	☐
41. Enhanced detail, without evidence of motion and without any visible artifacts	☐	☐	☐	☐	☐	☐
42. Proper positioning (all anatomy included, evidence of proper centering/alignment, etc.)	☐	☐	☐	☐	☐	☐
43. Proper marker placement	☐	☐	☐	☐	☐	☐
44. Evidence of proper collimation and radiation protection	☐	☐	☐	☐	☐	☐
45. Long vs. short scale of contrast	☐	☐	☐	☐	☐	☐

Comments:

_____

_____

LUMBAR/THORACIC ANATOMY
The student is able to identify:

	Procedure		Repeat		Competency	
	Yes	No	Yes	No	Yes	No
46. Thoracic vs. lumbar vertebrae	☐	☐	☐	☐	☐	☐
47. Iliac crest	☐	☐	☐	☐	☐	☐
48. Transverse process	☐	☐	☐	☐	☐	☐
49. Intervertebral disk space	☐	☐	☐	☐	☐	☐
50. Intervertebral foramen	☐	☐	☐	☐	☐	☐
51. Spinous process	☐	☐	☐	☐	☐	☐
52. Body	☐	☐	☐	☐	☐	☐
53. Obvious pathology	☐	☐	☐	☐	☐	☐

Comments:

_____

_____

Procedure Evaluator Signature	Repeat Evaluator Signature	Competency Evaluator Signature
Date	Date	Date

END SCOLIOSIS SERIES EVALUATION

Student Name:_____

	Procedure Grade	Repeat Grade	Competency Grade

PATIENT INFORMATION OR SIMULATED PROCEDURE *(circle if simulated)*

	Procedure	Repeat	Competency
Age			
Medical Record No.			
Ability to Cooperate			
Condition/Pathology			
Technical Factors Used			
Exposure Index			

FACILITY PREPARATION
The student:

	Procedure Yes	No	Repeat Yes	No	Competency Yes	No
1. Examines the radiographic room and cleans/straightens it before escorting the patient in.	☐	☐	☐	☐	☐	☐
2. Has all equipment and supplies (patient gown, shield, markers, lead blockers, etc.) readily available before escorting the patient in.	☐	☐	☐	☐	☐	☐
3. Is able to manipulate all radiographic equipment with ease, and centers the central ray to the cassette/receptor.	☐	☐	☐	☐	☐	☐
4. Adjusts the tube to the proper SID.	☐	☐	☐	☐	☐	☐
5. Selects a cassette/receptor of the appropriate size.	☐	☐	☐	☐	☐	☐

Comments:

_____

_____

PATIENT PREPARATION
The student:

	Procedure Yes	No	Repeat Yes	No	Competency Yes	No
6. Identifies the correct patient and examination according to the requisition while establishing a good rapport with him or her.	☐	☐	☐	☐	☐	☐
7. Obtains and documents the patient's history before the examination.	☐	☐	☐	☐	☐	☐
8. Explains the examination in terms the patient fully understands and properly communicates with the patient throughout the examination.	☐	☐	☐	☐	☐	☐
9. Asks female patients of childbearing age the date of their last menstrual period and documents this; inquires about the possibility of pregnancy and has them sign pregnancy consent forms.	☐	☐	☐	☐	☐	☐
10. Removes all obscuring objects (snaps, zippers, belts, etc.) so as *not* to produce radiographic artifacts.	☐	☐	☐	☐	☐	☐

(continued)

	Procedure		Repeat		Competency	
	Yes	No	Yes	No	Yes	No
11. Respects the patient's modesty and provides ample comfort for him or her.	☐	☐	☐	☐	☐	☐

Comments:

_____

_____

PATIENT POSITIONING FOR A PELVIS
The student:

	Procedure		Repeat		Competency	
	Yes	No	Yes	No	Yes	No
12. Places the patient in the supine position on the radiographic table, without rotation.	☐	☐	☐	☐	☐	☐
13. Places the cassette/receptor with the top of the cassette/receptor 1–2 inches above the iliac crest (the cassette crosswise in the Bucky drawer).	☐	☐	☐	☐	☐	☐
14. Rotates the legs internally, approximately 15°.	☐	☐	☐	☐	☐	☐
15. Centers the central ray to the midsagittal plane of the body.	☐	☐	☐	☐	☐	☐
16. Centers the central ray perpendicularly to the pelvis, midway between the crest and the symphysis pubis.	☐	☐	☐	☐	☐	☐

Comments:

_____

_____

IMPORTANT DETAILS
The student:

	Procedure		Repeat		Competency	
	Yes	No	Yes	No	Yes	No
17. Instills confidence in the patient by exhibiting self-confidence throughout the examination.	☐	☐	☐	☐	☐	☐
18. Places a lead marker in the appropriate area of the cassette/receptor (top/bottom/anteriorly/laterally), where it will be visualized on the finished radiograph, on the proper anatomical side (right/left), and in the appropriate position (face up/face down), depending on the patient's position.	☐	☐	☐	☐	☐	☐
19. Provides radiation protection for himself or herself and others (closes doors).	☐	☐	☐	☐	☐	☐
20. Applies proper collimation and makes adjustments as necessary.	☐	☐	☐	☐	☐	☐
21. Properly measures the patient along the course of the central ray.	☐	☐	☐	☐	☐	☐
22. Sets the proper exposure techniques:	☐	☐	☐	☐	☐	☐

Conventional systems
- Sets the proper kVp, mA, and time and makes adjustments as necessary.

or

CR or DR systems
- Identifies the patient on the work-list (or manually types the patient information into the system).
- Selects appropriate body region, specific body part, and accurate view/ projection.
- Double-checks preset parameters:
  —Adult vs. pediatric patients
    ○ Small, medium, or large
  —Bucky/receptor (upright vs. table) *or* non-Bucky
  —AEC vs. fixed
    ○ If AEC, checks ion chambers
    ○ Density setting

	Procedure		Repeat		Competency	
	Yes	No	Yes	No	Yes	No

—kVp and mA; adjusts if necessary
—Focal spot/filament size

	Yes	No	Yes	No	Yes	No
23. Exposes the cassette/receptor after telling the patient to hold still and after giving him or her proper breathing instructions (expiration) *for each projection.*	☐	☐	☐	☐	☐	☐
24. Provides each radiograph with the proper identification (flash) and/or processes each cassette (image) without difficulty (regardless of technology—film, CR, or DR).	☐	☐	☐	☐	☐	☐
25. Properly completes the examination by filling out all necessary paperwork, entering the examination in the computer, having the images checked by the appropriate staff members, answering any last-minute questions, and informing the patient that he or she is finished.	☐	☐	☐	☐	☐	☐
26. Exhibits the ability to adapt to new and difficult situations if and when necessary.	☐	☐	☐	☐	☐	☐
27. Accepts constructive criticism and uses it to his or her advantage.	☐	☐	☐	☐	☐	☐
28. Leaves the radiographic room neat and clean for the next examination.	☐	☐	☐	☐	☐	☐
29. Completes the examination within a reasonable time frame.	☐	☐	☐	☐	☐	☐

Comments:

_____

_____

RADIOGRAPHIC IMAGE QUALITY

The student is able to critique his or her radiographs as to whether they demonstrate:

	Procedure		Repeat		Competency	
	Yes	No	Yes	No	Yes	No
30. Proper technique/optimal density	☐	☐	☐	☐	☐	☐
31. Enhanced detail, without evidence of motion and without any visible artifacts	☐	☐	☐	☐	☐	☐
32. Proper positioning (all anatomy included, evidence of proper centering/alignment, etc.)	☐	☐	☐	☐	☐	☐
33. Proper marker placement	☐	☐	☐	☐	☐	☐
34. Evidence of proper collimation and radiation protection	☐	☐	☐	☐	☐	☐
35. Long vs. short scale of contrast	☐	☐	☐	☐	☐	☐

Comments:

_____

_____

PELVIS ANATOMY

The student is able to identify:

	Procedure		Repeat		Competency	
	Yes	No	Yes	No	Yes	No
36. Acetabulum	☐	☐	☐	☐	☐	☐
37. Femoral head	☐	☐	☐	☐	☐	☐
38. Greater and lesser trochanters	☐	☐	☐	☐	☐	☐
39. Femoral neck	☐	☐	☐	☐	☐	☐
40. Ischial tuberosity	☐	☐	☐	☐	☐	☐
41. Ischial spine	☐	☐	☐	☐	☐	☐
42. Pubic symphysis	☐	☐	☐	☐	☐	☐
43. Obturator foramen	☐	☐	☐	☐	☐	☐
44. Sacroiliac (SI) articulation	☐	☐	☐	☐	☐	☐

(continued)

	Procedure		Repeat		Competency	
	Yes	*No*	*Yes*	*No*	*Yes*	*No*
45. Ilium	▨	▨	▨	▨	☐	☐
46. Obvious pathology	▨	▨	▨	▨	☐	☐

Comments:

_____

_____

Procedure Evaluator Signature	Repeat Evaluator Signature	Competency Evaluator Signature

Date	Date	Date

END PELVIS EVALUATION

The objective of this evaluation is to determine the student's competency level when performing specific radiographic examinations.

Student Name:_____

Procedure Grade	Repeat Grade	Competency Grade

PATIENT INFORMATION OR SIMULATED PROCEDURE *(circle if simulated)*

	Procedure	Repeat	Competency
Age			
Medical Record No.			
Ability to Cooperate			
Condition/Pathology			
Technical Factors Used			
Exposure Index			

FACILITY PREPARATION
The student:

	Procedure Yes	No	Repeat Yes	No	Competency Yes	No
1. Examines the radiographic room and cleans/straightens it before escorting the patient in.	☐	☐	☐	☐	☐	☐
2. Has all equipment and supplies (patient gown, shield, markers, lead blockers, etc.) readily available before escorting the patient in.	☐	☐	☐	☐	☐	☐
3. Is able to manipulate all radiographic equipment with ease, and centers the central ray to the cassette/receptor *for all projections*.	☐	☐	☐	☐	☐	☐
4. Adjusts the tube to the proper SID *for each projection*.	☐	☐	☐	☐	☐	☐
5. Selects cassettes/receptor of the appropriate sizes *for all projections*, according to the patient's size and examination.	☐	☐	☐	☐	☐	☐

Comments:

_____

_____

PATIENT PREPARATION
The student:

	Procedure Yes	No	Repeat Yes	No	Competency Yes	No
6. Identifies the correct patient and examination according to the requisition while establishing a good rapport with him or her.	☐	☐	☐	☐	☐	☐
7. Obtains and documents the patient's history before the examination.	▦	▦	▦	▦	☐	☐
8. Explains the examination in terms the patient fully understands and properly communicates with the patient throughout the examination.	☐	☐	☐	☐	☐	☐
9. Asks female patients of childbearing age the date of their last menstrual period and documents this; inquires about the possibility of pregnancy and has them sign pregnancy consent forms.	☐	☐	☐	☐	☐	☐
10. Removes all obscuring objects (snaps, zippers, belts, etc.) so as *not* to produce radiographic artifacts.	☐	☐	☐	☐	☐	☐

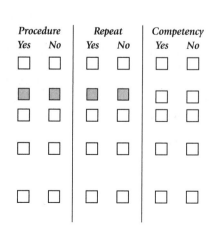

(continued)

	Procedure		Repeat		Competency	
	Yes	No	Yes	No	Yes	No
11. Respects the patient's modesty and provides ample comfort for him or her.	☐	☐	☐	☐	☐	☐

Comments:

_____

_____

PATIENT POSITIONING FOR SACROILIAC JOINTS
Anteroposterior
The student:

	Procedure		Repeat		Competency	
	Yes	No	Yes	No	Yes	No
12. Places the patient in the supine position on the radiographic table without rotation.	☐	☐	☐	☐	☐	☐
13. Places the cassette/receptor with the top of the cassette/receptor 1–2 inches above the iliac crest (the cassette crosswise in the Bucky drawer).	☐	☐	☐	☐	☐	☐
14. Rotates the legs internally, approximately 15°.	☐	☐	☐	☐	☐	☐
15. Centers the central ray to the midsagittal plane of the body.	☐	☐	☐	☐	☐	☐
16. Directs the central ray at an angle of 30–35° cephalad, entering 3 inches above the symphysis pubis.	☐	☐	☐	☐	☐	☐

Right Posterior Oblique
The student:

	Procedure		Repeat		Competency	
	Yes	No	Yes	No	Yes	No
17. Places the patient in the oblique position, at an angle of 25°.	☐	☐	☐	☐	☐	☐
18. Selects the appropriate receptor or places the cassette lengthwise in the Bucky drawer. For conventional cassettes, the flash must be away from any anatomy.	☐	☐	☐	☐	☐	☐
19. Ensures that the patient's shoulders and hips lie in the same plane, adjusting if necessary.	☐	☐	☐	☐	☐	☐
20. Centers the central ray 1 inch medially from the ASIS of the elevated/left side.	☐	☐	☐	☐	☐	☐
21. Directs the central ray perpendicularly to the ASIS.	☐	☐	☐	☐	☐	☐

Left Posterior Oblique
The student:

	Procedure		Repeat		Competency	
	Yes	No	Yes	No	Yes	No
22. Places the patient in the oblique position, at an angle of 25°.	☐	☐	☐	☐	☐	☐
23. Selects the appropriate receptor or places the cassette lengthwise in the Bucky drawer. For conventional cassettes, the flash must be away from any anatomy.	☐	☐	☐	☐	☐	☐
24. Ensures that the patient's shoulders and hips lie in the same plane, adjusting if necessary.	☐	☐	☐	☐	☐	☐
25. Centers the central ray 1 inch medially from the ASIS of the elevated/right side.	☐	☐	☐	☐	☐	☐
26. Directs the central ray perpendicularly to the ASIS.	☐	☐	☐	☐	☐	☐

Comments:

_____

_____

IMPORTANT DETAILS
The student:

	Procedure Yes	Procedure No	Repeat Yes	Repeat No	Competency Yes	Competency No
27. Instills confidence in the patient by exhibiting self-confidence throughout the examination.	☐	☐	☐	☐	☐	☐
28. Places a lead marker in the appropriate area of the cassette/receptor (top/bottom/anteriorly/laterally), where it will be visualized on the finished radiograph, on the proper anatomical side (right/left), and in the appropriate position (face up/face down), depending on the patient's position.	☐	☐	☐	☐	☐	☐
29. Provides radiation protection for himself or herself and others (closes doors).	☐	☐	☐	☐	☐	☐
30. Applies proper collimation and makes adjustments as necessary.	☐	☐	☐	☐	☐	☐
31. Properly measures the patient along the course of the central ray *for each projection.*	☐	☐	☐	☐	☐	☐
32. Sets the proper exposure techniques:	☐	☐	☐	☐	☐	☐

Conventional systems
- Sets the proper kVp, mA, and time and makes adjustments as necessary.

or

CR or DR systems
- Identifies the patient on the work-list (or manually types the patient information into the system).
- Selects appropriate body region, specific body part, and accurate view/projection.
- Double-checks preset parameters:
  - —Adult vs. pediatric patients
    - ○ Small, medium, or large
  - —Bucky/receptor (upright vs. table) *or* non-Bucky
  - —AEC vs. fixed
    - ○ If AEC, checks ion chambers
    - ○ Density setting
  - —kVp and mA; adjusts if necessary
  - —Focal spot/filament size

	Procedure Yes	Procedure No	Repeat Yes	Repeat No	Competency Yes	Competency No
33. Exposes the cassette/receptor after telling the patient to hold still and after giving him or her proper breathing instructions (expiration) *for each projection.*	☐	☐	☐	☐	☐	☐
34. Provides each radiograph with the proper identification (flash) and/or processes each cassette (image) without difficulty (regardless of technology—film, CR, or DR).	▨	▨	▨	▨	☐	☐
35. Properly completes the examination by filling out all necessary paperwork, entering the examination in the computer, having the images checked by the appropriate staff members, answering any last-minute questions, and informing the patient that he or she is finished.	▨	▨	▨	▨	☐	☐
36. Exhibits the ability to adapt to new and difficult situations if and when necessary.	▨	▨	▨	▨	☐	☐
37. Accepts constructive criticism and uses it to his or her advantage.	☐	☐	☐	☐	☐	☐
38. Leaves the radiographic room neat and clean for the next examination.	▨	▨	▨	▨	☐	☐
39. Completes the examination within a reasonable time frame.	☐	☐	☐	☐	☐	☐

Comments:

_____

_____

(continued)

RADIOGRAPHIC IMAGE QUALITY
The student is able to critique his or her radiographs as to whether they demonstrate:

	Procedure		Repeat		Competency	
	Yes	No	Yes	No	Yes	No
40. Proper technique/optimal density	■	■	■	■	☐	☐
41. Enhanced detail, without evidence of motion and without any visible artifacts	■	■	■	■	☐	☐
42. Proper positioning (all anatomy included, evidence of proper centering/alignment, etc.)	■	■	■	■	☐	☐
43. Proper marker placement	■	■	■	■	☐	☐
44. Evidence of proper collimation and radiation protection	■	■	■	■	☐	☐
45. Long vs. short scale of contrast	■	■	■	■	☐	☐

Comments:

_____

_____

PELVIS ANATOMY
The student is able to identify:

	Procedure		Repeat		Competency	
	Yes	No	Yes	No	Yes	No
46. Ilium	■	■	■	■	☐	☐
47. Sacrum	■	■	■	■	☐	☐
48. SI articulation	■	■	■	■	☐	☐
49. Lumbar vertebrae	■	■	■	■	☐	☐
50. Obvious pathology	■	■	■	■	☐	☐

Comments:

_____

_____

Procedure Evaluator Signature	Repeat Evaluator Signature	Competency Evaluator Signature
Date	Date	Date

END SACROILIAC JOINTS EVALUATION

specific radiographic examinations.

Student Name:_____

Procedure Grade	Repeat Grade	Competency Grade

PATIENT INFORMATION OR SIMULATED PROCEDURE *(circle if simulated)*

	Procedure	Repeat	Competency
Age			
Medical Record No.			
Ability to Cooperate			
Condition/Pathology			
Technical Factors Used			
Exposure Index			

FACILITY PREPARATION
The student:

	Procedure Yes No	Repeat Yes No	Competency Yes No
1. Examines the radiographic room and cleans/straightens it before escorting the patient in.	☐ ☐	☐ ☐	☐ ☐
2. Has all equipment and supplies (patient gown, shield, markers, lead blockers, etc.) readily available before escorting the patient in.	☐ ☐	☐ ☐	☐ ☐
3. Is able to manipulate all radiographic equipment with ease, and centers the central ray to the cassette/receptor *for both projections.*	☐ ☐	☐ ☐	☐ ☐
4. Adjusts the tube to the proper SID *for each projection.*	☐ ☐	☐ ☐	☐ ☐
5. Selects cassettes/receptor of the appropriate sizes *for both projections,* according to the patient's size and examination.	☐ ☐	☐ ☐	☐ ☐

Comments:

_____

_____

PATIENT PREPARATION
The student:

	Procedure Yes No	Repeat Yes No	Competency Yes No
6. Identifies the correct patient and examination according to the requisition while establishing a good rapport with him or her.	☐ ☐	☐ ☐	☐ ☐
7. Obtains and documents the patient's history before the examination.	▨ ▨	▨ ▨	☐ ☐
8. Explains the examination in terms the patient fully understands and properly communicates with the patient throughout the examination.	☐ ☐	☐ ☐	☐ ☐
9. Asks female patients of childbearing age the date of their last menstrual period and documents this; inquires about the possibility of pregnancy and has them sign pregnancy consent forms.	☐ ☐	☐ ☐	☐ ☐
10. Removes all obscuring objects (snaps, zippers, belts, etc.) so as *not* to produce radiographic artifacts.	☐ ☐	☐ ☐	☐ ☐

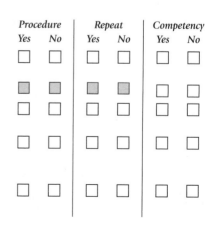

(continued)

	Procedure		Repeat		Competency	
	Yes	No	Yes	No	Yes	No
11. Respects the patient's modesty and provides ample comfort for him or her.	☐	☐	☐	☐	☐	☐

Comments:

_____

_____

PATIENT POSITIONING FOR A SACRUM
Anteroposterior
The student:

	Procedure		Repeat		Competency	
	Yes	No	Yes	No	Yes	No
12. Places the patient in the supine position on the radiographic table, without rotation.	☐	☐	☐	☐	☐	☐
13. Places the cassette/receptor with the top of the cassette/receptor 1–2 inches above the iliac crest (the cassette lengthwise in the Bucky drawer).	☐	☐	☐	☐	☐	☐
14. Places a support under the patient's knees.	☐	☐	☐	☐	☐	☐
15. Centers the central ray to the midsagittal plane of the body.	☐	☐	☐	☐	☐	☐
16. Directs the central ray at an angle of 15° cephalad, entering midway between the ASIS and the symphysis pubis.	☐	☐	☐	☐	☐	☐

Lateral
The student:

	Procedure		Repeat		Competency	
	Yes	No	Yes	No	Yes	No
17. Places the patient in the left lateral position without rotation.	☐	☐	☐	☐	☐	☐
18. Selects the appropriate receptor or places the cassette lengthwise in the Bucky drawer. For conventional cassettes, the flash must be away from any anatomy.	☐	☐	☐	☐	☐	☐
19. Instructs the patient to flex his or her hips and knees up toward his or her chest.	☐	☐	☐	☐	☐	☐
20. Supports the patient's waist so that the spine is parallel, and places a support between the patient's knees to avoid rotation.	☐	☐	☐	☐	☐	☐
21. Adjusts the patient's arms so that they are at right angles to the body.	☐	☐	☐	☐	☐	☐
22. Centers the central ray 2 inches anteriorly from the posterior surface, approximately 3 inches posteriorly from the midaxillary plane.	☐	☐	☐	☐	☐	☐
23. Centers the central ray perpendicularly to the ASIS.						
24. Places a lead blocker behind the patient.	☐	☐	☐	☐	☐	☐

Comments:

_____

_____

IMPORTANT DETAILS
The student:

	Procedure		Repeat		Competency	
	Yes	No	Yes	No	Yes	No
25. Instills confidence in the patient by exhibiting self-confidence throughout the examination.	☐	☐	☐	☐	☐	☐
26. Places a lead marker in the appropriate area of the cassette/receptor (top/bottom/anteriorly/laterally), where it will be visualized on the finished radiograph, on the proper anatomical side (right/left), and in the appropriate position (face up/face down), depending on the patient's position.	☐	☐	☐	☐	☐	☐
27. Provides radiation protection for himself or herself and others (closes doors).	☐	☐	☐	☐	☐	☐

	Procedure		Repeat		Competency	
	Yes	No	Yes	No	Yes	No
28. Applies proper collimation and makes adjustments as necessary.	☐	☐	☐	☐	☐	☐
29. Properly measures the patient along the course of the central ray *for each projection.*	☐	☐	☐	☐	☐	☐
30. Sets the proper exposure techniques:	☐	☐	☐	☐	☐	☐

Conventional systems
- Sets the proper kVp, mA, and time and makes adjustments as necessary.

or

CR or DR systems
- Identifies the patient on the work-list (or manually types the patient information into the system).
- Selects appropriate body region, specific body part, and accurate view/ projection.
- Double-checks preset parameters:
  —Adult vs. pediatric patients
   ◦ Small, medium, or large
  —Bucky/receptor (upright vs. table) *or* non-Bucky
  —AEC vs. fixed
   ◦ If AEC, checks ion chambers
   ◦ Density setting
  —kVp and mA; adjusts if necessary
  —Focal spot/filament size

	Procedure		Repeat		Competency	
31. Exposes the cassette/receptor after telling the patient to hold still and after giving him or her proper breathing instructions (expiration) *for each projection.*	☐	☐	☐	☐	☐	☐
32. Provides each radiograph with the proper identification (flash) and/or processes each cassette (image) without difficulty (regardless of technology—film, CR, or DR).	▣	▣	▣	▣	☐	☐
33. Properly completes the examination by filling out all necessary paper-work, entering the examination in the computer, having the images checked by the appropriate staff members, answering any last-minute questions, and informing the patient that he or she is finished.	▣	▣	▣	▣	☐	☐
34. Exhibits the ability to adapt to new and difficult situations if and when necessary.	▣	▣	▣	▣	☐	☐
35. Accepts constructive criticism and uses it to his or her advantage.	☐	☐	☐	☐	☐	☐
36. Leaves the radiographic room neat and clean for the next examination.	▣	▣	▣	▣	☐	☐
37. Completes the examination within a reasonable time frame.	☐	☐	☐	☐	☐	☐

Comments:

_____

_____

RADIOGRAPHIC IMAGE QUALITY

The student is able to critique his or her radiographs as to whether they demonstrate:

	Procedure		Repeat		Competency	
	Yes	No	Yes	No	Yes	No
38. Proper technique/optimal density	▣	▣	▣	▣	☐	☐
39. Enhanced detail, without evidence of motion and without any visible artifacts	▣	▣	▣	▣	☐	☐
40. Proper positioning (all anatomy included, evidence of proper centering/ alignment, etc.)	▣	▣	▣	▣	☐	☐
41. Proper marker placement	▣	▣	▣	▣	☐	☐
42. Evidence of proper collimation and radiation protection	▣	▣	▣	▣	☐	☐
43. Long vs. short scale of contrast	▣	▣	▣	▣	☐	☐

(continued)

Comments:

_____

_____

SACRUM ANATOMY
The student is able to identify:

	Procedure		Repeat		Competency	
	Yes	No	Yes	No	Yes	No
44. Sacral ala	☐	☐	☐	☐	☐	☐
45. Sacral apex	☐	☐	☐	☐	☐	☐
46. Sacral foramen	☐	☐	☐	☐	☐	☐
47. SI articulation	☐	☐	☐	☐	☐	☐
48. L5–S1 articulation	☐	☐	☐	☐	☐	☐
49. Coccyx	☐	☐	☐	☐	☐	☐
50. Sacral–coccygeal articulation	☐	☐	☐	☐	☐	☐
51. Obvious pathology	☐	☐	☐	☐	☐	☐

Comments:

_____

_____

_____   _____   _____
Procedure Evaluator Signature   Repeat Evaluator Signature   Competency Evaluator Signature

_____   _____   _____
Date   Date   Date

END SACRUM EVALUATION

Student Name:_____

Procedure Grade	Repeat Grade	Competency Grade

PATIENT INFORMATION OR SIMULATED PROCEDURE *(circle if simulated)*

	Procedure	Repeat	Competency
Age			
Medical Record No.			
Ability to Cooperate			
Condition/Pathology			
Technical Factors Used			
Exposure Index			

FACILITY PREPARATION
The student:

	Procedure Yes	Procedure No	Repeat Yes	Repeat No	Competency Yes	Competency No
1. Examines the radiographic room and cleans/straightens it before escorting the patient in.	☐	☐	☐	☐	☐	☐
2. Has all equipment and supplies (patient gown, shield, markers, lead blockers, etc.) readily available before escorting the patient in.	☐	☐	☐	☐	☐	☐
3. Is able to manipulate all radiographic equipment with ease, and centers the central ray to the cassette/receptor *for both projections.*	☐	☐	☐	☐	☐	☐
4. Adjusts the tube to the proper SID *for each projection.*	☐	☐	☐	☐	☐	☐
5. Selects cassettes/receptor of the appropriate sizes *for both projections,* according to the patient's size and examination.	☐	☐	☐	☐	☐	☐

Comments:

_____

_____

PATIENT PREPARATION
The student:

	Procedure Yes	Procedure No	Repeat Yes	Repeat No	Competency Yes	Competency No
6. Identifies the correct patient and examination according to the requisition while establishing a good rapport with him or her.	☐	☐	☐	☐	☐	☐
7. Obtains and documents the patient's history before the examination.	☐	☐	☐	☐	☐	☐
8. Explains the examination in terms the patient fully understands and properly communicates with the patient throughout the examination.	☐	☐	☐	☐	☐	☐
9. Asks female patients of childbearing age the date of their last menstrual period and documents this; inquires about the possibility of pregnancy and has them sign pregnancy consent forms.	☐	☐	☐	☐	☐	☐
10. Removes all obscuring objects (snaps, zippers, belts, etc.) so as *not* to produce radiographic artifacts.	☐	☐	☐	☐	☐	☐

(continued)

	Procedure		Repeat		Competency	
	Yes	No	Yes	No	Yes	No
11. Respects the patient's modesty and provides ample comfort for him or her.	☐	☐	☐	☐	☐	☐

Comments:

_____

_____

PATIENT POSITIONING FOR A COCCYX
Anteroposterior
The student:

	Procedure		Repeat		Competency	
	Yes	No	Yes	No	Yes	No
12. Places the patient in the supine position on the radiographic table, without rotation.	☐	☐	☐	☐	☐	☐
13. Places the cassette/receptor with the top of the cassette/receptor near the iliac crest (the cassette lengthwise in the Bucky drawer).	☐	☐	☐	☐	☐	☐
14. Places a support under the patient's knees.	☐	☐	☐	☐	☐	☐
15. Centers the central ray to the midsagittal plane of the body.	☐	☐	☐	☐	☐	☐
16. Directs the central ray at an angle of 10° caudad, entering 2 inches above the symphysis pubis.	☐	☐	☐	☐	☐	☐

Lateral
The student:

	Procedure		Repeat		Competency	
	Yes	No	Yes	No	Yes	No
17. Places the patient in the left lateral position, without rotation.	☐	☐	☐	☐	☐	☐
18. Selects the appropriate receptor or places the cassette lengthwise in the Bucky drawer. For conventional cassettes, the flash must be away from any anatomy.	☐	☐	☐	☐	☐	☐
19. Instructs the patient to flex his or her hips and knees up toward his or her chest.	☐	☐	☐	☐	☐	☐
20. Supports the patient's waist so that the spine is parallel, and places a support between the patient's knees to avoid rotation.	☐	☐	☐	☐	☐	☐
21. Adjusts the patient's arms so that they are at right angles to the body.	☐	☐	☐	☐	☐	☐
22. Centers the central ray 2 inches anteriorly from the posterior surface, approximately 5 inches posteriorly from the midaxillary plane.	☐	☐	☐	☐	☐	☐
23. Centers the central ray perpendicularly 1/2 inch superiorly from the tip of the coccyx.	☐	☐	☐	☐	☐	☐
24. Places a lead blocker behind the patient.	☐	☐	☐	☐	☐	☐

Comments:

_____

_____

IMPORTANT DETAILS
The student:

	Procedure		Repeat		Competency	
	Yes	No	Yes	No	Yes	No
25. Instills confidence in the patient by exhibiting self-confidence throughout the examination.	☐	☐	☐	☐	☐	☐
26. Places a lead marker in the appropriate area of the cassette/receptor (top/bottom/anteriorly/laterally), where it will be visualized on the finished radiograph, on the proper anatomical side (right/left), and in the appropriate position (face up/face down), depending on the patient's position.	☐	☐	☐	☐	☐	☐
27. Provides radiation protection for himself or herself and others (closes doors).	☐	☐	☐	☐	☐	☐

	Procedure		Repeat		Competency	
	Yes	No	Yes	No	Yes	No
28. Applies proper collimation and makes adjustments as necessary.	☐	☐	☐	☐	☐	☐
29. Properly measures the patient along the course of the central ray *for each projection.*	☐	☐	☐	☐	☐	☐
30. Sets the proper exposure techniques:	☐	☐	☐	☐	☐	☐

30. Sets the proper exposure techniques:

Conventional systems
- Sets the proper kVp, mA, and time and makes adjustments as necessary.

or

CR or DR systems
- Identifies the patient on the work-list (or manually types the patient information into the system).
- Selects appropriate body region, specific body part, and accurate view/projection.
- Double-checks preset parameters:
  - —Adult vs. pediatric patients
    - ○ Small, medium, or large
  - —Bucky/receptor (upright vs. table) *or* non-Bucky
  - —AEC vs. fixed
    - ○ If AEC, checks ion chambers
    - ○ Density setting
  - —kVp and mA; adjusts if necessary
  - —Focal spot/filament size

	Procedure		Repeat		Competency	
	Yes	No	Yes	No	Yes	No
31. Exposes the cassette/receptor after telling the patient to hold still and after giving him or her proper breathing instructions (expiration) *for each projection.*	☐	☐	☐	☐	☐	☐
32. Provides each radiograph with the proper identification (flash) and/or processes each cassette (image) without difficulty (regardless of technology—film, CR, or DR).	▥	▥	▥	▥	☐	☐
33. Properly completes the examination by filling out all necessary paperwork, entering the examination in the computer, having the images checked by the appropriate staff members, answering any last-minute questions, and informing the patient that he or she is finished.	▥	▥	▥	▥	☐	☐
34. Exhibits the ability to adapt to new and difficult situations if and when necessary.	▥	▥	▥	▥	☐	☐
35. Accepts constructive criticism and uses it to his or her advantage.	☐	☐	☐	☐	☐	☐
36. Leaves the radiographic room neat and clean for the next examination.	▥	▥	▥	▥	☐	☐
37. Completes the examination within a reasonable time frame.	☐	☐	☐	☐	☐	☐

Comments:

_____

_____

RADIOGRAPHIC IMAGE QUALITY
The student is able to critique his or her radiographs as to whether they demonstrate:

	Procedure		Repeat		Competency	
	Yes	No	Yes	No	Yes	No
38. Proper technique/optimal density	▥	▥	▥	▥	☐	☐
39. Enhanced detail, without evidence of motion and without any visible artifacts	▥	▥	▥	▥	☐	☐
40. Proper positioning (all anatomy included, evidence of proper centering/alignment, etc.)	▥	▥	▥	▥	☐	☐
41. Proper marker placement	▥	▥	▥	▥	☐	☐
42. Evidence of proper collimation and radiation protection	▥	▥	▥	▥	☐	☐
43. Long vs. short scale of contrast	▥	▥	▥	▥	☐	☐

(continued)

Comments:

_____

_____

COCCYX ANATOMY
The student is able to identify:

	Procedure		Repeat		Competency	
	Yes	No	Yes	No	Yes	No
44. Sacrum	☐	☐	☐	☐	☐	☐
45. SI articulation	☐	☐	☐	☐	☐	☐
46. L5–S1 articulation	☐	☐	☐	☐	☐	☐
47. Coccyx	☐	☐	☐	☐	☐	☐
48. Sacral–coccygeal articulation	☐	☐	☐	☐	☐	☐
49. Obvious pathology	☐	☐	☐	☐	☐	☐

Comments:

_____

_____

_____ _____ _____
Procedure Evaluator Signature   Repeat Evaluator Signature   Competency Evaluator Signature

_____ _____ _____
Date   Date   Date

END COCCYX EVALUATION

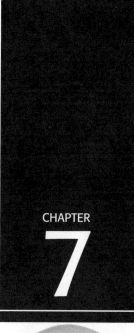

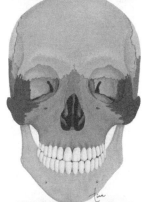

Head

Note: All head work may be performed on the radiographic table or the upright Bucky, with the exception of work on paranasal sinuses, which should be performed in the upright position, unless the patient's condition dictates otherwise.

specific radiographic examinations.

Student Name:_____

Procedure Grade	Repeat Grade	Competency Grade

PATIENT INFORMATION OR SIMULATED PROCEDURE *(circle if simulated)*

	Procedure	Repeat	Competency
Age			
Medical Record No.			
Ability to Cooperate			
Condition/Pathology			
Technical Factors Used			
Exposure Index			

FACILITY PREPARATION
The student:

	Procedure Yes / No	Repeat Yes / No	Competency Yes / No
1. Examines the radiographic room and cleans/straightens it before escorting the patient in.	☐ ☐	☐ ☐	☐ ☐
2. Has all equipment and supplies (shield, markers, supplies to clean the upright Bucky/receptor and table, etc.) readily available before escorting the patient in.	☐ ☐	☐ ☐	☐ ☐
3. Is able to manipulate all radiographic equipment with ease, and centers the central ray to the cassette/receptor *for all projections.*	☐ ☐	☐ ☐	☐ ☐
4. Adjusts the tube to the proper SID *for each projection.*	☐ ☐	☐ ☐	☐ ☐
5. Selects cassettes/receptor of the appropriate sizes *for all projections,* according to the patient's size and examination.	☐ ☐	☐ ☐	☐ ☐

Comments:

_____

_____

PATIENT PREPARATION
The student:

	Procedure Yes / No	Repeat Yes / No	Competency Yes / No
6. Identifies the correct patient and examination according to the requisition while establishing a good rapport with him or her.	☐ ☐	☐ ☐	☐ ☐
7. Obtains and documents the patient's history before the examination.	▨ ▨	▨ ▨	☐ ☐
8. Explains the examination in terms the patient fully understands and properly communicates with the patient throughout the examination.	☐ ☐	☐ ☐	☐ ☐
9. Asks female patients of childbearing age the date of their last menstrual period and documents this; inquires about the possibility of pregnancy and has them sign pregnancy consent forms.	☐ ☐	☐ ☐	☐ ☐
10. Removes all obscuring objects (hair pins, jewelry, dentures, etc.) so as *not* to produce radiographic artifacts.	☐ ☐	☐ ☐	☐ ☐

(continued)

	Procedure		Repeat		Competency	
	Yes	No	Yes	No	Yes	No
11. Respects the patient's modesty and provides ample comfort for him or her, and *cleans the Bucky/receptor in front of the patient.*	☐	☐	☐	☐	☐	☐

Comments:

_____

_____

PATIENT POSITIONING FOR A SKULL
PA or PA Axial (Caldwell)
The student:

	Procedure		Repeat		Competency	
	Yes	No	Yes	No	Yes	No
12. Places the patient in the prone position against the Bucky/receptor.	☐	☐	☐	☐	☐	☐
13. Selects the appropriate receptor or places the cassette so that the upper border of the cassette/receptor is 2 inches above the vertex. For conventional cassettes, the flash must be away from any anatomy.	☐	☐	☐	☐	☐	☐
14. Places the patient's nose and forehead in contact with the Bucky/receptor.	☐	☐	☐	☐	☐	☐
15. Ensures that the orbitomeatal line is perpendicular to the cassette/receptor.	☐	☐	☐	☐	☐	☐
16. Ensures that the midsagittal line is perpendicular to the cassette/receptor.	☐	☐	☐	☐	☐	☐
17. Ensures that the head is not tilted or rotated.	☐	☐	☐	☐	☐	☐
18. Centers the central ray to the midsagittal plane.	☐	☐	☐	☐	☐	☐
19. Directs the central ray at an angle of 15° caudad to the nasion.	☐	☐	☐	☐	☐	☐

Right Lateral
The student:

	Procedure		Repeat		Competency	
	Yes	No	Yes	No	Yes	No
20. Places the patient in the semiprone position.	☐	☐	☐	☐	☐	☐
21. Selects the appropriate receptor or places the cassette so that the upper border of the cassette/receptor is 1–2 inches above the vertex. For conventional cassettes, the flash must be away from any anatomy.	☐	☐	☐	☐	☐	☐
22. Places the patient's right side against the Bucky/receptor.	☐	☐	☐	☐	☐	☐
23. Ensures that the infraorbitomeatal line is parallel to the transverse axis of the cassette/receptor.	☐	☐	☐	☐	☐	☐
24. Ensures that the head is not tilted and that the interpupillary line is perpendicular and the midsagittal line is parallel to the cassette/receptor.	☐	☐	☐	☐	☐	☐
25. Centers the central ray 2 inches superiorly and anteriorly to the external auditory meatus (EAM), and if the sella turcica is the primary interest, centers the central ray 3/4 inch superiorly and anteriorly to the EAM.	☐	☐	☐	☐	☐	☐
26. Directs the central ray perpendicularly.	☐	☐	☐	☐	☐	☐

Left Lateral
The student:

	Procedure		Repeat		Competency	
	Yes	No	Yes	No	Yes	No
27. Places the patient in the semiprone position.	☐	☐	☐	☐	☐	☐
28. Selects the appropriate receptor or places the cassette so that the upper border of the cassette/receptor is 1–2 inches above the vertex. For conventional cassettes, the flash must be away from any anatomy.	☐	☐	☐	☐	☐	☐
29. Places the patient's left side against the Bucky/receptor.	☐	☐	☐	☐	☐	☐
30. Ensures that the infraorbitomeatal line is parallel to the transverse axis of the cassette/receptor.	☐	☐	☐	☐	☐	☐
31. Ensures that the head is not tilted and that the interpupillary line is perpendicular and the midsagittal line is parallel to the cassette/receptor.	☐	☐	☐	☐	☐	☐
32. Centers the central ray 2 inches to the EAM, and if the sella turcica is the primary interest, centers the central ray 3/4 inch superiorly and anteriorly to the EAM.	☐	☐	☐	☐	☐	☐

	Procedure		Repeat		Competency	
	Yes	No	Yes	No	Yes	No
33. Directs the central ray perpendicularly.	☐	☐	☐	☐	☐	☐

AP Axial (Towne)
The student:

	Procedure		Repeat		Competency	
	Yes	No	Yes	No	Yes	No
34. Places the patient in the supine position.	☐	☐	☐	☐	☐	☐
35. Selects the appropriate receptor or places the cassette so that the upper border of the cassette/receptor is at the vertex. For conventional cassettes, the flash must be away from any anatomy.	☐	☐	☐	☐	☐	☐
36. Instructs the patient to tuck his or her chin and ensures that the orbitomeatal line is perpendicular to the cassette/receptor.	☐	☐	☐	☐	☐	☐
37. Ensures that the midsagittal plane is perpendicular to the cassette/receptor.	☐	☐	☐	☐	☐	☐
38. Ensures that the head is not tilted or rotated.	☐	☐	☐	☐	☐	☐
39. Centers the central ray to the midsagittal plane.	☐	☐	☐	☐	☐	☐
40. Directs the central ray at an angle of 30° caudad so that it passes through the EAM and exits at the foramen magnum, and if the infraorbitomeatal line (IOML) is perpendicular to the cassette/receptor, angles the CR 37°.	☐	☐	☐	☐	☐	☐

Submentovertical (Base/Schuller Method)
The student:

	Procedure		Repeat		Competency	
	Yes	No	Yes	No	Yes	No
41. Places the patient in the supine position, approximately 6–12 inches away from the Bucky/receptor, and sets the technique before positioning the patient.	☐	☐	☐	☐	☐	☐
42. Selects the appropriate receptor. For conventional cassettes, the flash must be away from any anatomy.	☐	☐	☐	☐	☐	☐
43. Ensures that the midsagittal line is perpendicular to the cassette/receptor.	☐	☐	☐	☐	☐	☐
44. Instructs the patient to extend his or her head back to rest it on the vertex and ensures that the infraorbitomeatal line is parallel to the cassette/receptor.	☐	☐	☐	☐	☐	☐
45. Ensures that the head is not tilted or rotated.	☐	☐	☐	☐	☐	☐
46. Centers the central ray to the midsagittal plane.	☐	☐	☐	☐	☐	☐
47. Directs the central ray perpendicularly to the IOML, centered midway between the angles of the mandible, 3/4 inch anteriorly from the EAM, passing through the sella turcica.	☐	☐	☐	☐	☐	☐

Comments:

_____

_____

IMPORTANT DETAILS
The student:

	Procedure		Repeat		Competency	
	Yes	No	Yes	No	Yes	No
48. Instills confidence in the patient by exhibiting self-confidence throughout the examination.	☐	☐	☐	☐	☐	☐
49 Places a lead marker in the appropriate area of the cassette/receptor (top/bottom/anteriorly/laterally), where it will be visualized on the finished radiograph, on the proper anatomical side (right/left), and in the appropriate position (face up/face down), depending on the patient's position.	☐	☐	☐	☐	☐	☐

(continued)

	Procedure		Repeat		Competency	
	Yes	No	Yes	No	Yes	No
50. Provides radiation protection (shield) for the patient, self, and others (closes doors).	☐	☐	☐	☐	☐	☐
51 Applies proper collimation and makes adjustments as necessary.	☐	☐	☐	☐	☐	☐
52. Properly measures the patient along the course of the central ray *for each projection.*	☐	☐	☐	☐	☐	☐
53. Sets the proper exposure techniques:	☐	☐	☐	☐	☐	☐

Conventional systems
* Sets the proper kVp, mA, and time and makes adjustments as necessary.

or

CR or DR systems
* Identifies the patient on the work-list (or manually types the patient information into the system).
* Selects appropriate body region, specific body part, and accurate view/projection.
* Double-checks preset parameters:
  —Adult vs. pediatric patients
    ○ Small, medium, or large
  —Bucky/receptor (upright vs. table) *or* non-Bucky
  —AEC vs. fixed
    ○ If AEC, checks ion chambers
    ○ Density setting
  —kVp and mA; adjusts if necessary
  —Focal spot/filament size

	Procedure		Repeat		Competency	
54. Exposes the cassette/receptor after telling the patient to hold still and after giving him or her proper breathing instructions (suspended) *for each projection.*	☐	☐	☐	☐	☐	☐
55. Provides each radiograph with the proper identification (flash) and/or processes each cassette (image) without difficulty (regardless of technology—film, CR, or DR).	▨	▨	▨	▨	☐	☐
56. Properly completes the examination by filling out all necessary paperwork, entering the examination in the computer, having the images checked by the appropriate staff members, answering any last-minute questions, and informing the patient that he or she is finished.	▨	▨	▨	▨	☐	☐
57. Exhibits the ability to adapt to new and difficult situations if and when necessary.	▨	▨	▨	▨	☐	☐
58. Accepts constructive criticism and uses it to his or her advantage.	☐	☐	☐	☐	☐	☐
59. Leaves the radiographic room neat and clean for the next examination.	▨	▨	▨	▨	☐	☐
60. Completes the examination within a reasonable time frame.	☐	☐	☐	☐	☐	☐

Comments:

_____

_____

RADIOGRAPHIC IMAGE QUALITY
The student is able to critique his or her radiographs as to whether they demonstrate:

	Procedure		Repeat		Competency	
	Yes	No	Yes	No	Yes	No
61. Proper technique/optimal density	▨	▨	▨	▨	☐	☐
62. Enhanced detail, without evidence of motion and without any visible artifacts	▨	▨	▨	▨	☐	☐
63. Proper positioning (all anatomy included, evidence of proper centering/alignment, etc.)	▨	▨	▨	▨	☐	☐

	Procedure		Repeat		Competency	
	Yes	No	Yes	No	Yes	No
64. Proper marker placement	☐	☐	☐	☐	☐	☐
65. Evidence of proper collimation and radiation protection	☐	☐	☐	☐	☐	☐
66. Long vs. short scale of contrast	☐	☐	☐	☐	☐	☐

Comments:

_____

_____

SKULL ANATOMY
The student is able to identify:

	Procedure		Repeat		Competency	
	Yes	No	Yes	No	Yes	No
67. Coronal suture	☐	☐	☐	☐	☐	☐
68. Squamous suture	☐	☐	☐	☐	☐	☐
68. Lambdoidal suture	☐	☐	☐	☐	☐	☐
69. Sagittal suture	☐	☐	☐	☐	☐	☐
70. Anterior and posterior clinoid processes	☐	☐	☐	☐	☐	☐
71. Sella turcica	☐	☐	☐	☐	☐	☐
72. Temporomandibular joint (TMJ)	☐	☐	☐	☐	☐	☐
73. Mandibular body	☐	☐	☐	☐	☐	☐
74. Frontal sinus	☐	☐	☐	☐	☐	☐
75. Ethmoid sinus	☐	☐	☐	☐	☐	☐
76. Sphenoid sinus	☐	☐	☐	☐	☐	☐
77. Maxillary sinus	☐	☐	☐	☐	☐	☐
78. Parietal bone	☐	☐	☐	☐	☐	☐
79. Temporal bone	☐	☐	☐	☐	☐	☐
80. Frontal bone	☐	☐	☐	☐	☐	☐
81. Occipital bone	☐	☐	☐	☐	☐	☐
82. Foramen magnum	☐	☐	☐	☐	☐	☐
83. Odontoid	☐	☐	☐	☐	☐	☐
84. Superior and inferior orbital margins	☐	☐	☐	☐	☐	☐
85. Nasal bones	☐	☐	☐	☐	☐	☐
86. Nasal septum	☐	☐	☐	☐	☐	☐
87. Petrous ridge	☐	☐	☐	☐	☐	☐
88. Zygomatic arches	☐	☐	☐	☐	☐	☐
89. Mastoid air cells	☐	☐	☐	☐	☐	☐
90. Obvious pathology	☐	☐	☐	☐	☐	☐

Comments:

_____

_____

_____ _____ _____
Procedure Evaluator Signature   Repeat Evaluator Signature   Competency Evaluator Signature

_____ _____ _____
Date   Date   Date

END SKULL EVALUATION

Student Name:_____

Procedure Grade	Repeat Grade	Competency Grade

PATIENT INFORMATION OR SIMULATED PROCEDURE *(circle if simulated)*

	Procedure	Repeat	Competency
Age			
Medical Record No.			
Ability to Cooperate			
Condition/Pathology			
Technical Factors Used			
Exposure Index			

FACILITY PREPARATION
The student:

	Procedure Yes / No	Repeat Yes / No	Competency Yes / No
1. Examines the radiographic room and cleans/straightens it before escorting the patient in.	☐ ☐	☐ ☐	☐ ☐
2. Has all equipment and supplies (shield, markers, supplies to clean the upright Bucky/receptor and table, etc.) readily available before escorting the patient in.	☐ ☐	☐ ☐	☐ ☐
3. Is able to manipulate all radiographic equipment with ease, and centers the central ray to the cassette/receptor *for all projections.*	☐ ☐	☐ ☐	☐ ☐
4. Adjusts the tube to the proper SID *for each projection.*	☐ ☐	☐ ☐	☐ ☐
5. Selects cassettes/receptor of the appropriate sizes *for all projections,* according to the patient's size and examination.	☐ ☐	☐ ☐	☐ ☐

Comments:

_____

_____

PATIENT PREPARATION
The student:

	Procedure Yes / No	Repeat Yes / No	Competency Yes / No
6. Identifies the correct patient and examination according to the requisition while establishing a good rapport with him or her.	☐ ☐	☐ ☐	☐ ☐
7. Obtains and documents the patient's history before the examination.	☐ ☐	☐ ☐	☐ ☐
8. Explains the examination in terms the patient fully understands and properly communicates with the patient throughout the examination.	☐ ☐	☐ ☐	☐ ☐
9. Asks female patients of childbearing age the date of their last menstrual period and documents this; inquires about the possibility of pregnancy and has them sign pregnancy consent forms.	☐ ☐	☐ ☐	☐ ☐
10. Removes all obscuring objects (hair pins, jewelry, dentures, etc.) so as *not* to produce radiographic artifacts.	☐ ☐	☐ ☐	☐ ☐

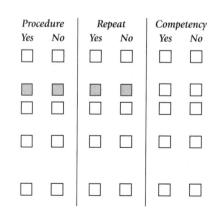

(continued)

	Procedure		Repeat		Competency	
	Yes	No	Yes	No	Yes	No
11. Respects the patient's modesty and provides ample comfort for him or her, and *cleans the Bucky/receptor in front of the patient.*	☐	☐	☐	☐	☐	☐

Comments:

_____

_____

PATIENT POSITIONING FOR FACIAL BONES
Parietoacanthial (Waters)
The student:

	Procedure		Repeat		Competency	
	Yes	No	Yes	No	Yes	No
12. Places the patient in the prone position against the Bucky/receptor.	☐	☐	☐	☐	☐	☐
13. Selects the appropriate receptor. For conventional cassettes, the flash must be away from any anatomy.	☐	☐	☐	☐	☐	☐
14. Instructs the patient to extend his or her neck and rest his or her head with the tip of the chin on the cassette/receptor.	☐	☐	☐	☐	☐	☐
15. Ensures that the mentomeatal line is perpendicular to the cassette/receptor, and the orbitomeatal line forms a 37° angle to the cassette/receptor.	☐	☐	☐	☐	☐	☐
16. Ensures that the midsagittal line is perpendicular to the cassette/receptor.	☐	☐	☐	☐	☐	☐
17. Ensures that the head is not tilted or rotated.	☐	☐	☐	☐	☐	☐
18. Centers the central ray to the midsagittal plane.	☐	☐	☐	☐	☐	☐
19. Directs the central ray perpendicularly to the acanthion.	☐	☐	☐	☐	☐	☐

Affected Lateral
The student:

	Procedure		Repeat		Competency	
	Yes	No	Yes	No	Yes	No
20. Places the patient in the semiprone position.	☐	☐	☐	☐	☐	☐
21. Selects the appropriate receptor . For conventional cassettes, the flash must be away from any anatomy.	☐	☐	☐	☐	☐	☐
22. Places the patient's affected side against the Bucky/receptor.	☐	☐	☐	☐	☐	☐
23. Ensures that the infraorbitomeatal line is parallel to the transverse axis of the cassette/receptor.	☐	☐	☐	☐	☐	☐
24. Ensures that the head is not tilted and that the interpupillary line is perpendicular and the midsagittal line is parallel to the cassette/receptor.	☐	☐	☐	☐	☐	☐
25. Centers the central ray to the zygoma (entering at the upper malar bone).	☐	☐	☐	☐	☐	☐
26. Directs the central ray perpendicularly.	☐	☐	☐	☐	☐	☐

PA (Caldwell)
The student:

	Procedure		Repeat		Competency	
	Yes	No	Yes	No	Yes	No
27. Places the patient in the prone position against the Bucky/receptor.	☐	☐	☐	☐	☐	☐
28. Selects the appropriate receptor or places the cassette so that the upper border of the cassette/receptor is 2 inches above the vertex. For conventional cassettes, the flash must be away from any anatomy.	☐	☐	☐	☐	☐	☐
29. Places the patient's nose and forehead in contact with the Bucky/receptor.	☐	☐	☐	☐	☐	☐
30. Ensures that the orbitomeatal line is perpendicular to the cassette/receptor.	☐	☐	☐	☐	☐	☐
31. Ensures that the midsagittal line is perpendicular to the cassette/receptor.	☐	☐	☐	☐	☐	☐
32. Ensures that the head is not tilted or rotated.	☐	☐	☐	☐	☐	☐
33. Centers the central ray to the midsagittal plane.	☐	☐	☐	☐	☐	☐
34. Directs the central ray at an angle of 15° caudad to the nasion.	☐	☐	☐	☐	☐	☐

Submentovertical (Base) for the Zygomatic Arches
The student:

	Procedure		Repeat		Competency	
	Yes	No	Yes	No	Yes	No
35. Places the patient in the supine position, approximately 6–12 inches away from the Bucky/receptor, and sets a decreased technique from the normal submentovertex (SMV) technique before positioning the patient.	☐	☐	☐	☐	☐	☐
36. Selects the appropriate receptor. For conventional cassettes, the flash must be away from any anatomy.	☐	☐	☐	☐	☐	☐
37. Ensures that the midsagittal line is perpendicular to the cassette/receptor.	☐	☐	☐	☐	☐	☐
38. Instructs the patient to extend his or her head back to rest it on the vertex and ensures that the infraorbitomeatal line is parallel to the cassette/receptor.	☐	☐	☐	☐	☐	☐
39. Ensures that the head is not tilted or rotated.	☐	☐	☐	☐	☐	☐
40. Centers the central ray to the midsagittal plane.	☐	☐	☐	☐	☐	☐
41. Directs the central ray perpendicularly to the IOML, centered midway between the zygomatic arches, passing a coronal plane lying approximately 1 inch posteriorly to the outer canthi.	☐	☐	☐	☐	☐	☐

Comments:

_____

_____

IMPORTANT DETAILS
The student:

	Procedure		Repeat		Competency	
	Yes	No	Yes	No	Yes	No
42. Instills confidence in the patient by exhibiting self-confidence throughout the examination.	☐	☐	☐	☐	☐	☐
43. Places a lead marker in the appropriate area of the cassette/receptor (top/bottom/anteriorly/laterally), where it will be visualized on the finished radiograph, on the proper anatomical side (right/left), and in the appropriate position (face up/face down), depending on the patient's position.	☐	☐	☐	☐	☐	☐
44. Provides radiation protection (shield) for the patient, self, and others (closes doors).	☐	☐	☐	☐	☐	☐
45. Applies proper collimation and makes adjustments as necessary.	☐	☐	☐	☐	☐	☐
45. Properly measures the patient along the course of the central ray *for each projection.*	☐	☐	☐	☐	☐	☐
47. Sets the proper exposure techniques:	☐	☐	☐	☐	☐	☐

Conventional systems
- Sets the proper kVp, mA, and time and makes adjustments as necessary.

or

CR or DR systems
- Identifies the patient on the work-list (or manually types the patient information into the system).
- Selects appropriate body region, specific body part, and accurate view/projection.
- Double-checks preset parameters:
  —Adult vs. pediatric patients
  ○ Small, medium, or large
  —Bucky/receptor (upright vs. table) *or* non-Bucky
  —AEC vs. fixed
  ○ If AEC, checks ion chambers
  ○ Density setting
  —kVp and mA; adjusts if necessary
  —Focal spot/filament size

(continued)

	Procedure		Repeat		Competency	
	Yes	No	Yes	No	Yes	No

48. Exposes the cassette/receptor after telling the patient to hold still and after giving him or her proper breathing instructions (suspended) *for each projection.*

49. Provides each radiograph with the proper identification (flash) and/or processes each cassette (image) without difficulty (regardless of technology—film, CR, or DR).

50. Properly completes the examination by filling out all necessary paperwork, entering the examination in the computer, having the images checked by the appropriate staff members, answering any last-minute questions, and informing the patient that he or she is finished.

51. Exhibits the ability to adapt to new and difficult situations if and when necessary.

52. Accepts constructive criticism and uses it to his or her advantage.

53. Leaves the radiographic room neat and clean for the next examination.

54. Completes the examination within a reasonable time frame.

Comments:

_____

RADIOGRAPHIC IMAGE QUALITY
The student is able to critique his or her radiographs as to whether they demonstrate:

	Procedure		Repeat		Competency	
	Yes	No	Yes	No	Yes	No

55. Proper technique/optimal density

56. Enhanced detail, without evidence of motion and without any visible artifacts

57. Proper positioning (all anatomy included, evidence of proper centering/ alignment, etc.)

58. Proper marker placement

59. Evidence of proper collimation and radiation protection

60. Long vs. short scale of contrast

Comments:

_____

FACIAL BONE ANATOMY
The student is able to identify:

	Procedure		Repeat		Competency	
	Yes	No	Yes	No	Yes	No

61. Anterior and posterior clinoid processes

62. Sella turcica

63. Dorsum sellae

64. TMJ

65. Mandibular body

66. Mandibular rami

67. Mandibular angle

68. Mandibular symphysis

69. Frontal sinus

70. Ethmoid sinus

	Procedure		Repeat		Competency	
	Yes	No	Yes	No	Yes	No
71. Sphenoid sinus	☐	☐	☐	☐	☐	☐
72. Maxillary sinus	☐	☐	☐	☐	☐	☐
73. Frontal bone	☐	☐	☐	☐	☐	☐
74. Odontoid	☐	☐	☐	☐	☐	☐
75. Superior and inferior orbital margins	☐	☐	☐	☐	☐	☐
76. Nasal bones	☐	☐	☐	☐	☐	☐
77. Nasal septum	☐	☐	☐	☐	☐	☐
78. Petrous ridge/pyramid	☐	☐	☐	☐	☐	☐
79. Zygomatic arches	☐	☐	☐	☐	☐	☐
80. Obvious pathology	☐	☐	☐	☐	☐	☐

Comments:

_____

_____

Procedure Evaluator Signature   Repeat Evaluator Signature   Competency Evaluator Signature

Date   Date   Date

END FACIAL BONES EVALUATION

Student Name:_____

Procedure Grade	Repeat Grade	Competency Grade

PATIENT INFORMATION OR SIMULATED PROCEDURE *(circle if simulated)*

	Procedure	Repeat	Competency
Age			
Medical Record No.			
Ability to Cooperate			
Condition/Pathology			
Technical Factors Used			
Exposure Index			

FACILITY PREPARATION
The student:

	Procedure Yes	No	Repeat Yes	No	Competency Yes	No
1. Examines the radiographic room and cleans/straightens it before escorting the patient in.	☐	☐	☐	☐	☐	☐
2. Has all equipment and supplies (shield, markers, supplies to clean the upright Bucky/receptor and table, etc.) readily available before escorting the patient in.	☐	☐	☐	☐	☐	☐
3. Is able to manipulate all radiographic equipment with ease, and centers the central ray to the cassette/receptor *for all projections.*	☐	☐	☐	☐	☐	☐
4. Adjusts the tube to the proper SID *for each projection.*	☐	☐	☐	☐	☐	☐
5. Selects cassettes/receptor of the appropriate sizes *for all projections,* according to the patient's size and examination.	☐	☐	☐	☐	☐	☐

Comments:

_____

_____

PATIENT PREPARATION
The student:

	Procedure Yes	No	Repeat Yes	No	Competency Yes	No
6. Identifies the correct patient and examination according to the requisition while establishing a good rapport with him or her.	☐	☐	☐	☐	☐	☐
7. Obtains and documents the patient's history before the examination.	▨	▨	▨	▨	☐	☐
8. Explains the examination in terms the patient fully understands and properly communicates with the patient throughout the examination.	☐	☐	☐	☐	☐	☐
9. Asks female patients of childbearing age the date of their last menstrual period and documents this; inquires about the possibility of pregnancy and has them sign pregnancy consent forms.	☐	☐	☐	☐	☐	☐
10. Removes all obscuring objects (hair pins, jewelry, dentures, etc.) so as *not* to produce radiographic artifacts.	☐	☐	☐	☐	☐	☐

(continued)

	Procedure		Repeat		Competency	
	Yes	No	Yes	No	Yes	No
11. Respects the patient's modesty and provides ample comfort for him or her, and *cleans the Bucky/receptor in front of the patient.*	☐	☐	☐	☐	☐	☐

Comments:

_____

_____

PATIENT POSITIONING FOR ORBITS
Parietoacanthial (Waters)
The student:

	Procedure		Repeat		Competency	
	Yes	No	Yes	No	Yes	No
12. Places the patient in the prone position against the Bucky/receptor.	☐	☐	☐	☐	☐	☐
13. Selects the appropriate receptor. For conventional cassettes, the flash must be away from any anatomy.	☐	☐	☐	☐	☐	☐
14. Instructs the patient to extend his or her neck and rest his or her head with the tip of the chin on the cassette/receptor.	☐	☐	☐	☐	☐	☐
15. Ensures that the mentomeatal line is perpendicular to the cassette/receptor, and the orbitomeatal line forms a 37° angle to the cassette/receptor.	☐	☐	☐	☐	☐	☐
16. Ensures that the midsagittal line is perpendicular to the cassette/receptor.	☐	☐	☐	☐	☐	☐
17. Ensures that the head is not tilted or rotated.	☐	☐	☐	☐	☐	☐
18. Centers the central ray to the midsagittal plane.	☐	☐	☐	☐	☐	☐
19. Directs the central ray perpendicularly to the acanthion.	☐	☐	☐	☐	☐	☐

Affected Lateral
The student:

	Procedure		Repeat		Competency	
	Yes	No	Yes	No	Yes	No
20. Places the patient in the semiprone position.						
21. Selects the appropriate receptor. For conventional cassettes, the flash must be away from any anatomy.	☐	☐	☐	☐	☐	☐
22. Places the patient's affected side against the Bucky/receptor.	☐	☐	☐	☐	☐	☐
23. Ensures that the infraorbitomeatal line is parallel to the transverse axis of the cassette/receptor.	☐	☐	☐	☐	☐	☐
24. Ensures that the head is not tilted and that the interpupillary line is perpendicular and the midsagittal line is parallel to the cassette/receptor.	☐	☐	☐	☐	☐	☐
25. Centers the central ray to the zygoma, entering at the upper malar bone.	☐	☐	☐	☐	☐	☐
26. Directs the central ray perpendicularly.	☐	☐	☐	☐	☐	☐

PA (Caldwell)
The student:

	Procedure		Repeat		Competency	
	Yes	No	Yes	No	Yes	No
27. Places the patient in the prone position against the Bucky/receptor	☐	☐	☐	☐	☐	☐
28. Selects the appropriate receptor or places the cassette so that the upper border of the cassette/receptor is 2 inches above the vertex. For conventional cassettes, the flash must be away from any anatomy.	☐	☐	☐	☐	☐	☐
29. Places the patient's nose and forehead in contact with the Bucky/receptor.	☐	☐	☐	☐	☐	☐
30. Ensures that the orbitomeatal line is perpendicular to the cassette/receptor.	☐	☐	☐	☐	☐	☐
31. Ensures that the midsagittal line is perpendicular to the cassette/receptor.	☐	☐	☐	☐	☐	☐
32. Ensures that the head is not tilted or rotated.	☐	☐	☐	☐	☐	☐
33. Centers the central ray to the midsagittal plane.	☐	☐	☐	☐	☐	☐
34. Directs the central ray at an angle of 15° caudad to the nasion.	☐	☐	☐	☐	☐	☐

Submentovertical (Base)
The student:

	Procedure		Repeat		Competency	
	Yes	No	Yes	No	Yes	No
35. Places the patient in the supine position, approximately 6–12 inches away from the Bucky/receptor, and sets a decreased technique from the normal SMV technique before positioning the patient.	☐	☐	☐	☐	☐	☐
36. Selects the appropriate receptor. For conventional cassettes, the flash must be away from any anatomy.	☐	☐	☐	☐	☐	☐
37. Ensures that the midsagittal line is perpendicular to the cassette/receptor.	☐	☐	☐	☐	☐	☐
38. Instructs the patient to extend his or her head back to rest it on the vertex and ensures that the infraorbitomeatal line is parallel to the cassette/receptor.	☐	☐	☐	☐	☐	☐
39. Ensures that the head is not tilted or rotated.	☐	☐	☐	☐	☐	☐
40. Centers the central ray to the midsagittal plane.	☐	☐	☐	☐	☐	☐
41. Directs the central ray perpendicularly, centered midway between the zygomatic arches, passing a coronal plane lying approximately 1 inch posteriorly to the outer canthi.	☐	☐	☐	☐	☐	☐

Parieto-Orbital Oblique (Rhese Method)
The student:

	Procedure		Repeat		Competency	
	Yes	No	Yes	No	Yes	No
42. Places the patient in the prone position against the Bucky/receptor.	☐	☐	☐	☐	☐	☐
43. Selects the appropriate receptor. For conventional cassettes, the flash must be away from any anatomy.	☐	☐	☐	☐	☐	☐
44. Instructs the patient to rest his or her head with the affected chin, cheek, and nose on the cassette/receptor, ensuring that the midsagittal plane forms a 53° angle with the cassette/receptor.	☐	☐	☐	☐	☐	☐
45. Ensures that the acanthiomeatal line is perpendicular to the cassette/receptor.	☐	☐	☐	☐	☐	☐
46. Centers the central ray so that it exits the lower outer quadrant of the affected orbit (the side down).	☐	☐	☐	☐	☐	☐
47. Directs the central ray perpendicularly to the affected orbit.	☐	☐	☐	☐	☐	☐

Comments:

_____

_____

IMPORTANT DETAILS
The student:

	Procedure		Repeat		Competency	
	Yes	No	Yes	No	Yes	No
48. Instills confidence in the patient by exhibiting self-confidence throughout the examination.	☐	☐	☐	☐	☐	☐
49. Places a lead marker in the appropriate area of the cassette/receptor (top/bottom/anteriorly/laterally), where it will be visualized on the finished radiograph, on the proper anatomical side (right/left), and in the appropriate position (face up/face down), depending on the patient's position.	☐	☐	☐	☐	☐	☐
50. Provides radiation protection (shield) for the patient, self, and others (closes doors).	☐	☐	☐	☐	☐	☐
51. Applies proper collimation and makes adjustments as necessary.	☐	☐	☐	☐	☐	☐
52. Properly measures the patient along the course of the central ray *for each projection.*	☐	☐	☐	☐	☐	☐

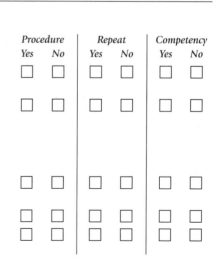

(continued)

	Procedure		Repeat		Competency	
	Yes	No	Yes	No	Yes	No
53. Sets the proper exposure techniques:	☐	☐	☐	☐	☐	☐

Conventional systems
- Sets the proper kVp, mA, and time and makes adjustments as necessary.

or

CR or DR systems
- Identifies the patient on the work-list (or manually types the patient information into the system).
- Selects appropriate body region, specific body part, and accurate view/ projection.
- Double-checks preset parameters:
  —Adult vs. pediatric patients
    ◦ Small, medium, or large
  —Bucky/receptor (upright vs. table) *or* non-Bucky
  —AEC vs. fixed
    ◦ If AEC, checks ion chambers
    ◦ Density setting
  —kVp and mA; adjusts if necessary
  —Focal spot/filament size

	Procedure		Repeat		Competency	
54. Exposes the cassette/receptor after telling the patient to hold still and after giving him or her proper breathing instructions (suspended) *for each projection.*	☐	☐	☐	☐	☐	☐
55. Provides each radiograph with the proper identification (flash) and/or processes each cassette (image) without difficulty (regardless of technology—film, CR, or DR).	▦	▦	▦	▦	☐	☐
56. Properly completes the examination by filling out all necessary paperwork, entering the examination in the computer, having the images checked by the appropriate staff members, answering any last-minute questions, and informing the patient that he or she is finished.	▦	▦	▦	▦	☐	☐
57. Exhibits the ability to adapt to new and difficult situations if and when necessary.	▦	▦	▦	▦	☐	☐
58. Accepts constructive criticism and uses it to his or her advantage.	☐	☐	☐	☐	☐	☐
59. Leaves the radiographic room neat and clean for the next examination.	▦	▦	▦	▦	☐	☐
60. Completes the examination within a reasonable time frame.	☐	☐	☐	☐	☐	☐

Comments:

_____

_____

RADIOGRAPHIC IMAGE QUALITY
The student is able to critique his or her radiographs as to whether they demonstrate:

	Procedure		Repeat		Competency	
	Yes	No	Yes	No	Yes	No
61. Proper technique/optimal density	▦	▦	▦	▦	☐	☐
62. Enhanced detail, without evidence of motion and without any visible artifacts	▦	▦	▦	▦	☐	☐
63. Proper positioning (all anatomy included, evidence of proper centering/ alignment, etc.)	▦	▦	▦	▦	☐	☐
64. Proper marker placement	▦	▦	▦	▦	☐	☐
65. Evidence of proper collimation and radiation protection	▦	▦	▦	▦	☐	☐
66. Long vs. short scale of contrast	▦	▦	▦	▦	☐	☐

Comments:

_____

_____

ORBIT ANATOMY
The student is able to identify:

	Procedure Yes	Procedure No	Repeat Yes	Repeat No	Competency Yes	Competency No
67. Frontal sinus	☐	☐	☐	☐	☐	☐
68. Ethmoid sinus	☐	☐	☐	☐	☐	☐
69. Maxillary sinus	☐	☐	☐	☐	☐	☐
70. Frontal bone	☐	☐	☐	☐	☐	☐
71. Nasal septum	☐	☐	☐	☐	☐	☐
72. Superior and inferior orbital margins	☐	☐	☐	☐	☐	☐
73. Optic foramen	☐	☐	☐	☐	☐	☐
74. Zygoma	☐	☐	☐	☐	☐	☐
75. Obvious pathology	☐	☐	☐	☐	☐	☐

Comments:

_____

_____

_____ _____ _____
Procedure Evaluator Signature   Repeat Evaluator Signature   Competency Evaluator Signature

_____ _____ _____
Date   Date   Date

END ORBITS AND OPTIC FORAMINA (RHESE) EVALUATION

The objective of this evaluation is to determine the student's competency level when performing specific radiographic examinations.

Student Name:_____

Procedure Grade	Repeat Grade	Competency Grade

PATIENT INFORMATION OR SIMULATED PROCEDURE *(circle if simulated)*

	Procedure	Repeat	Competency
Age			
Medical Record No.			
Ability to Cooperate			
Condition/Pathology			
Technical Factors Used			
Exposure Index			

FACILITY PREPARATION
The student:

	Procedure Yes	No	Repeat Yes	No	Competency Yes	No
1. Examines the radiographic room and cleans/straightens it before escorting the patient in.	☐	☐	☐	☐	☐	☐
2. Has all equipment and supplies (shield, markers, supplies to clean the upright Bucky/receptor and table, etc.) readily available before escorting the patient in.	☐	☐	☐	☐	☐	☐
3. Is able to manipulate all radiographic equipment with ease, and centers the central ray to the cassette/receptor *for all projections.*	☐	☐	☐	☐	☐	☐
4. Adjusts the tube to the proper SID *for each projection.*	☐	☐	☐	☐	☐	☐
5. Selects cassettes/receptor of the appropriate sizes *for all projections,* according to the patient's size and examination.	☐	☐	☐	☐	☐	☐

Comments:

_____

_____

PATIENT PREPARATION
The student:

	Procedure Yes	No	Repeat Yes	No	Competency Yes	No
6. Identifies the correct patient and examination according to the requisition while establishing a good rapport with him or her.	☐	☐	☐	☐	☐	☐
7. Obtains and documents the patient's history before the examination.	▣	▣	▣	▣	☐	☐
8. Explains the examination in terms the patient fully understands and properly communicates with the patient throughout the examination.	☐	☐	☐	☐	☐	☐
9. Asks female patients of childbearing age the date of their last menstrual period and documents this; inquires about the possibility of pregnancy and has them sign pregnancy consent forms.	☐	☐	☐	☐	☐	☐
10. Removes all obscuring objects (hair pins, jewelry, dentures, etc.) so as *not* to produce radiographic artifacts.	☐	☐	☐	☐	☐	☐

(continued)

	Procedure		Repeat		Competency	
	Yes	No	Yes	No	Yes	No
11. Respects the patient's modesty and provides ample comfort for his or her, and *cleans the Bucky/receptor in front of the patient.*	☐	☐	☐	☐	☐	☐

Comments:

_____

_____

PATIENT POSITIONING FOR ERECT SINUSES
Parietoacanthial (Waters)
The student:

	Procedure		Repeat		Competency	
	Yes	No	Yes	No	Yes	No
12. Places the patient in the prone position against the Bucky/receptor.	☐	☐	☐	☐	☐	☐
13. Selects the appropriate receptor. For conventional cassettes, the flash must be away from any anatomy.	☐	☐	☐	☐	☐	☐
14. Instructs the patient to extend his or her neck and rest his or her head with the tip of the chin on the cassette/receptor.	☐	☐	☐	☐	☐	☐
15. Ensures that the orbitomeatal line forms a 37° angle to the cassette/receptor.	☐	☐	☐	☐	☐	☐
16. Ensures that the midsagittal line is perpendicular to the cassette/receptor.	☐	☐	☐	☐	☐	☐
17. Ensures that the head is not tilted or rotated.	☐	☐	☐	☐	☐	☐
18. Centers the central ray to the midsagittal plane.	☐	☐	☐	☐	☐	☐
19. Directs the central ray perpendicularly to the acanthion, entering at the vertex and exiting at the anterior nasal spine.	☐	☐	☐	☐	☐	☐

Affected Lateral
The student:

	Procedure		Repeat		Competency	
	Yes	No	Yes	No	Yes	No
20. Places the patient in the semiprone position.	☐	☐	☐	☐	☐	☐
21. Selects the appropriate receptor. For conventional cassettes, the flash must be away from any anatomy.	☐	☐	☐	☐	☐	☐
22. Places the patient's affected side against the Bucky/receptor.	☐	☐	☐	☐	☐	☐
23. Ensures that the infraorbitomeatal line is parallel to the transverse axis of the cassette/receptor.	☐	☐	☐	☐	☐	☐
24. Ensures that the head is not tilted and that the interpupillary line is perpendicular and the midsagittal line is parallel to the cassette/receptor.	☐	☐	☐	☐	☐	☐
25. Centers the central ray 1/2–1 inch posteriorly to the outer canthus.	☐	☐	☐	☐	☐	☐
26. Directs the central ray perpendicularly.	☐	☐	☐	☐	☐	☐

PA Axial (Caldwell)
The student:

	Procedure		Repeat		Competency	
	Yes	No	Yes	No	Yes	No
27. Places the patient in the prone position against the Bucky/receptor.	☐	☐	☐	☐	☐	☐
28. Selects the appropriate receptor or places the cassette so that the upper border of the cassette/receptor is 2 inches above the vertex. For conventional cassettes, the flash must be away from any anatomy.	☐	☐	☐	☐	☐	☐
29. Places the patient's nose and forehead in contact with the Bucky/receptor.	☐	☐	☐	☐	☐	☐
30. Ensures that the orbitomeatal line is perpendicular to the cassette/receptor.	☐	☐	☐	☐	☐	☐
31. Ensures that the midsagittal line is perpendicular to the cassette/receptor.	☐	☐	☐	☐	☐	☐
32. Ensures that the head is not tilted or rotated.	☐	☐	☐	☐	☐	☐
33. Centers the central ray to the midsagittal plane.	☐	☐	☐	☐	☐	☐
34. Directs the central ray at an angle of 15° caudad to the nasion.	☐	☐	☐	☐	☐	☐

Submentovertical (Base)
The student:

	Procedure		Repeat		Competency	
	Yes	No	Yes	No	Yes	No
35. Places the patient in the supine position, approximately 6–12 inches away from the Bucky/receptor, and sets the technique before positioning the patient.	☐	☐	☐	☐	☐	☐
36. Selects the appropriate receptor. For conventional cassettes, the flash must be away from any anatomy.	☐	☐	☐	☐	☐	☐
37. Ensures that the midsagittal line is perpendicular to the cassette/receptor.	☐	☐	☐	☐	☐	☐
38. Instructs the patient to extend his or her head back to rest it on the vertex and ensures that the infraorbitomeatal line is parallel to the cassette/receptor.	☐	☐	☐	☐	☐	☐
39. Ensures that the head is not tilted or rotated.	☐	☐	☐	☐	☐	☐
40. Centers the central ray to the midsagittal plane.	☐	☐	☐	☐	☐	☐
41. Directs the central ray perpendicularly to the IOML, centered midway between the angles of the mandible, 3/4 inch anteriorly from the EAM, passing through the sella turcica.	☐	☐	☐	☐	☐	☐

Comments:

IMPORTANT DETAILS
The student:

	Procedure		Repeat		Competency	
	Yes	No	Yes	No	Yes	No
42. Instills confidence in the patient by exhibiting self-confidence throughout the examination.	☐	☐	☐	☐	☐	☐
43. Places a lead marker in the appropriate area of the cassette/receptor (top/bottom/anteriorly/laterally), where it will be visualized on the finished radiograph, on the proper anatomical side (right/left), and in the appropriate position (face up/face down), depending on the patient's position.	☐	☐	☐	☐	☐	☐
44. Provides radiation protection (shield) for the patient, self, and others (closes doors).	☐	☐	☐	☐	☐	☐
45. Applies proper collimation and makes adjustments as necessary.	☐	☐	☐	☐	☐	☐
46. Properly measures the patient along the course of the central ray *for each projection.*	☐	☐	☐	☐	☐	☐
47. Sets the proper exposure techniques:	☐	☐	☐	☐	☐	☐

Conventional systems
- Sets the proper kVp, mA, and time and makes adjustments as necessary.

or

CR or DR systems
- Identifies the patient on the work-list (or manually types the patient information into the system).
- Selects appropriate body region, specific body part, and accurate view/projection.
- Double-checks preset parameters:
  - Adult vs. pediatric patients
    - Small, medium, or large
  - Bucky/receptor (upright vs. table) *or* non-Bucky
  - AEC vs. fixed
    - If AEC, checks ion chambers
    - Density setting

(continued)

	Procedure		Repeat		Competency	
	Yes	No	Yes	No	Yes	No

—kVp and mA; adjusts if necessary
—Focal spot/filament size

	Procedure		Repeat		Competency	
48. Exposes the cassette/receptor after telling the patient to hold still and after giving him or her proper breathing instructions (suspended) *for each projection.*	☐	☐	☐	☐	☐	☐
49. Provides each radiograph with the proper identification (flash) and/or processes each cassette (image) without difficulty (regardless of technology—film, CR, or DR).	☐	☐	☐	☐	☐	☐
50. Properly completes the examination by filling out all necessary paperwork, entering the examination in the computer, having the images checked by the appropriate staff members, answering any last-minute questions, and informing the patient that he or she is finished.	☐	☐	☐	☐	☐	☐
51. Exhibits the ability to adapt to new and difficult situations if and when necessary.	☐	☐	☐	☐	☐	☐
52. Accepts constructive criticism and uses it to his or her advantage.	☐	☐	☐	☐	☐	☐
53. Leaves the radiographic room neat and clean for the next examination.	☐	☐	☐	☐	☐	☐
54. Completes the examination within a reasonable time frame.	☐	☐	☐	☐	☐	☐

Comments:

_____

_____

RADIOGRAPHIC IMAGE QUALITY
The student is able to critique his or her radiographs as to whether they demonstrate:

	Procedure		Repeat		Competency	
	Yes	No	Yes	No	Yes	No
55. Proper technique/optimal density	☐	☐	☐	☐	☐	☐
56. Enhanced detail, without evidence of motion and without any visible artifacts	☐	☐	☐	☐	☐	☐
57. Proper positioning (all anatomy included, evidence of proper centering/alignment, etc.)	☐	☐	☐	☐	☐	☐
58. Proper marker placement	☐	☐	☐	☐	☐	☐
59. Evidence of proper collimation and radiation protection	☐	☐	☐	☐	☐	☐
60. Long vs. short scale of contrast	☐	☐	☐	☐	☐	☐

Comments:

_____

_____

SINUS ANATOMY
The student is able to identify:

	Procedure		Repeat		Competency	
	Yes	No	Yes	No	Yes	No
61. Anterior and posterior clinoid processes	☐	☐	☐	☐	☐	☐
62. Sella turcica	☐	☐	☐	☐	☐	☐
63. Dorsum sellae	☐	☐	☐	☐	☐	☐
64. Mandibular rami	☐	☐	☐	☐	☐	☐
65. Frontal sinus	☐	☐	☐	☐	☐	☐
66. Ethmoid sinus	☐	☐	☐	☐	☐	☐
67. Sphenoid sinus	☐	☐	☐	☐	☐	☐
68. Maxillary sinus	☐	☐	☐	☐	☐	☐

	Procedure		Repeat		Competency	
	Yes	No	Yes	No	Yes	No
69. Parietal bone	☐	☐	☐	☐	☐	☐
70. Temporal bone	☐	☐	☐	☐	☐	☐
71. Frontal bone	☐	☐	☐	☐	☐	☐
72. Occipital bone	☐	☐	☐	☐	☐	☐
73. Foramen magnum	☐	☐	☐	☐	☐	☐
74. Nasal septum	☐	☐	☐	☐	☐	☐
75. Petrous ridge	☐	☐	☐	☐	☐	☐
76. Mastoid air cells	☐	☐	☐	☐	☐	☐
77. Obvious pathology	☐	☐	☐	☐	☐	☐

Comments:

_____

_____

Procedure Evaluator Signature	Repeat Evaluator Signature	Competency Evaluator Signature

Date	Date	Date

END PARANASAL SINUSES EVALUATION

Student Name:_____

Procedure Grade	Repeat Grade	Competency Grade

PATIENT INFORMATION OR SIMULATED PROCEDURE *(circle if simulated)*

	Procedure	Repeat	Competency
Age			
Medical Record No.			
Ability to Cooperate			
Condition/Pathology			
Technical Factors Used			
Exposure Index			

FACILITY PREPARATION
The student:

	Procedure Yes	Procedure No	Repeat Yes	Repeat No	Competency Yes	Competency No
1. Examines the radiographic room and cleans/straightens it before escorting the patient in.	☐	☐	☐	☐	☐	☐
2. Has all equipment and supplies (shield, markers, supplies to clean the upright Bucky/receptor and table, etc.) readily available before escorting the patient in.	☐	☐	☐	☐	☐	☐
3. Is able to manipulate all radiographic equipment with ease, and centers the central ray to the cassette/receptor *for all projections.*	☐	☐	☐	☐	☐	☐
4. Adjusts the tube to the proper SID *for each projection.*	☐	☐	☐	☐	☐	☐
5. Selects cassettes/receptor of the appropriate sizes *for all projections,* according to the patient's size and examination.	☐	☐	☐	☐	☐	☐

Comments:

_____

_____

PATIENT PREPARATION
The student:

	Procedure Yes	Procedure No	Repeat Yes	Repeat No	Competency Yes	Competency No
6. Identifies the correct patient and examination according to the requisition while establishing a good rapport with him or her.	☐	☐	☐	☐	☐	☐
7. Obtains and documents the patient's history before the examination.	▨	▨	▨	▨	☐	☐
8. Explains the examination in terms the patient fully understands and properly communicates with the patient throughout the examination.	☐	☐	☐	☐	☐	☐
9. Asks female patients of childbearing age the date of their last menstrual period and documents this; inquires about the possibility of pregnancy and has them sign pregnancy consent forms.	☐	☐	☐	☐	☐	☐
10. Removes all obscuring objects (hair pins, jewelry, dentures, etc.) so as *not* to produce radiographic artifacts.	☐	☐	☐	☐	☐	☐

(continued)

	Procedure		Repeat		Competency	
	Yes	No	Yes	No	Yes	No
11. Respects the patient's modesty and provides ample comfort for him or her, and *cleans the Bucky/receptor in front of the patient.*	☐	☐	☐	☐	☐	☐

Comments:

_____

_____

PATIENT POSITIONING FOR NASAL BONES
Parietoacanthial (Waters)
The student:

	Procedure		Repeat		Competency	
	Yes	No	Yes	No	Yes	No
12. Places the patient in the prone position against the Bucky/receptor.	☐	☐	☐	☐	☐	☐
13. Selects the appropriate receptor. For conventional cassettes, the flash must be away from any anatomy.	☐	☐	☐	☐	☐	☐
14. Instructs the patient to extend his or her neck and rest his or her head with the tip of the chin on the cassette/receptor.	☐	☐	☐	☐	☐	☐
15. Ensures that the mentomeatal line is perpendicular to the cassette/receptor and the orbitomeatal line forms a 37° angle to the cassette/receptor.	☐	☐	☐	☐	☐	☐
16. Ensures that the midsagittal line is perpendicular to the cassette/receptor.	☐	☐	☐	☐	☐	☐
17. Ensures that the head is not tilted or rotated.	☐	☐	☐	☐	☐	☐
18. Centers the central ray to the midsagittal plane.	☐	☐	☐	☐	☐	☐
19. Directs the central ray perpendicularly to the acanthion.	☐	☐	☐	☐	☐	☐

Left Lateral
The student:

	Procedure		Repeat		Competency	
	Yes	No	Yes	No	Yes	No
20. Places the patient in the semiprone position.	☐	☐	☐	☐	☐	☐
21. Selects the appropriate receptor or places the cassette on the table. For conventional cassettes, the flash must be away from any anatomy.	☐	☐	☐	☐	☐	☐
22. Places the patient's left side against the cassette/receptor.	☐	☐	☐	☐	☐	☐
23. Ensures that the infraorbitomeatal line is parallel to the transverse axis of the cassette/receptor.	☐	☐	☐	☐	☐	☐
24. Ensures that the head is not tilted and that the interpupillary line is perpendicular and the midsagittal line is parallel to the cassette/receptor.	☐	☐	☐	☐	☐	☐
25. Centers the central ray 1/2 inch distal to the nasion.	☐	☐	☐	☐	☐	☐
26. Directs the central ray perpendicularly to the bridge of the nose.	☐	☐	☐	☐	☐	☐

Right Lateral
The student:

	Procedure		Repeat		Competency	
	Yes	No	Yes	No	Yes	No
27. Places the patient in the semiprone position.	☐	☐	☐	☐	☐	☐
28. Selects the appropriate receptor or places the cassette on the table. For conventional cassettes, the flash must be away from any anatomy.	☐	☐	☐	☐	☐	☐
29. Places the patient's right side against the cassette/receptor.	☐	☐	☐	☐	☐	☐
30. Ensures that the infraorbitomeatal line is parallel to the transverse axis of the cassette/receptor.	☐	☐	☐	☐	☐	☐
31. Ensures that the head is not tilted and that the interpupillary line is perpendicular and the midsagittal line is parallel to the cassette/receptor.	☐	☐	☐	☐	☐	☐
32. Centers the central ray 1/2 inch distal to the nasion.	☐	☐	☐	☐	☐	☐
33. Directs the central ray perpendicularly to the bridge of the nose.	☐	☐	☐	☐	☐	☐

Comments:

_____

_____

IMPORTANT DETAILS
The student:

	Procedure Yes	Procedure No	Repeat Yes	Repeat No	Competency Yes	Competency No
34. Instills confidence in the patient by exhibiting self-confidence throughout the examination.	☐	☐	☐	☐	☐	☐
35. Places a lead marker in the appropriate area of the cassette/receptor (top/bottom/anteriorly/laterally), where it will be visualized on the finished radiograph, on the proper anatomical side (right/left), and in the appropriate position (face up/face down), depending on the patient's position.	☐	☐	☐	☐	☐	☐
36. Provides radiation protection (shield) for the patient, self, and others (closes doors).	☐	☐	☐	☐	☐	☐
37. Applies proper collimation and makes adjustments as necessary.	☐	☐	☐	☐	☐	☐
38. Properly measures the patient along the course of the central ray *for each projection.*	☐	☐	☐	☐	☐	☐
39. Sets the proper exposure techniques:	☐	☐	☐	☐	☐	☐

39. Sets the proper exposure techniques:

Conventional systems
- Sets the proper kVp, mA, and time and makes adjustments as necessary.

or

CR or DR systems
- Identifies the patient on the work-list (or manually types the patient information into the system).
- Selects appropriate body region, specific body part, and accurate view/projection.
- Double-checks preset parameters:
  —Adult vs. pediatric patients
    ○ Small, medium, or large
  —Bucky/receptor (upright vs. table) *or* non-Bucky
  —AEC vs. fixed
    ○ If AEC, checks ion chambers
    ○ Density setting
  —kVp and mA; adjusts if necessary
  —Focal spot/filament size

	Procedure Yes	Procedure No	Repeat Yes	Repeat No	Competency Yes	Competency No
40. Exposes the cassette/receptor after telling the patient to hold still and after giving him or her proper breathing instructions (suspended) *for each projection.*	☐	☐	☐	☐	☐	☐
41. Provides each radiograph with the proper identification (flash) and/or processes each cassette (image) without difficulty (regardless of technology—film, CR, or DR).	▩	▩	▩	▩	☐	☐
42. Properly completes the examination by filling out all necessary paperwork, entering the examination in the computer, having the images checked by the appropriate staff members, answering any last-minute questions, and informing the patient that he or she is finished.	▩	▩	▩	▩	☐	☐
43. Exhibits the ability to adapt to new and difficult situations if and when necessary.	▩	▩	▩	▩	☐	☐
44. Accepts constructive criticism and uses it to his or her advantage.	☐	☐	☐	☐	☐	☐
45. Leaves the radiographic room neat and clean for the next examination.	▩	▩	▩	▩	☐	☐

(continued)

	Procedure		Repeat		Competency	
	Yes	No	Yes	No	Yes	No
46. Completes the examination within a reasonable time frame.	☐	☐	☐	☐	☐	☐

Comments:

_____

_____

RADIOGRAPHIC IMAGE QUALITY
The student is able to critique his or her radiographs as to whether they demonstrate:

	Procedure		Repeat		Competency	
	Yes	No	Yes	No	Yes	No
47. Proper technique/optimal density	☐	☐	☐	☐	☐	☐
48. Enhanced detail, without evidence of motion and without any visible artifacts	☐	☐	☐	☐	☐	☐
49. Proper positioning (all anatomy included, evidence of proper centering/ alignment, etc.)	☐	☐	☐	☐	☐	☐
50. Proper marker placement	☐	☐	☐	☐	☐	☐
51. Evidence of proper collimation and radiation protection	☐	☐	☐	☐	☐	☐
52. Long vs. short scale of contrast	☐	☐	☐	☐	☐	☐

Comments:

_____

_____

NASAL BONE ANATOMY
The student is able to identify:

	Procedure		Repeat		Competency	
	Yes	No	Yes	No	Yes	No
53. Frontal sinus	☐	☐	☐	☐	☐	☐
54. Ethmoid sinus	☐	☐	☐	☐	☐	☐
55. Maxillary sinus	☐	☐	☐	☐	☐	☐
56. Frontal bone	☐	☐	☐	☐	☐	☐
57. Nasal bones	☐	☐	☐	☐	☐	☐
58. Nasal septum	☐	☐	☐	☐	☐	☐
59. Nasofrontal suture	☐	☐	☐	☐	☐	☐
60. Anterior nasal spine of maxilla	☐	☐	☐	☐	☐	☐
61. Obvious pathology	☐	☐	☐	☐	☐	☐

Comments:

_____

_____

_____   _____   _____
Procedure Evaluator Signature   Repeat Evaluator Signature   Competency Evaluator Signature

_____   _____   _____
Date   Date   Date

END NASAL BONES EVALUATION

Student Name:_____

Procedure Grade	Repeat Grade	Competency Grade

PATIENT INFORMATION OR SIMULATED PROCEDURE *(circle if simulated)*

	Procedure	Repeat	Competency
Age			
Medical Record No.			
Ability to Cooperate			
Condition/Pathology			
Technical Factors Used			
Exposure Index			

FACILITY PREPARATION
The student:

	Procedure Yes No	Repeat Yes No	Competency Yes No
1. Examines the radiographic room and cleans/straightens it before escorting the patient in.	☐ ☐	☐ ☐	☐ ☐
2. Has all equipment and supplies (shield, markers, supplies to clean the upright Bucky/receptor and table, etc.) readily available before escorting the patient in.	☐ ☐	☐ ☐	☐ ☐
3. Is able to manipulate all radiographic equipment with ease, and centers the central ray to the cassette/receptor *for all projections*.	☐ ☐	☐ ☐	☐ ☐
4. Adjusts the tube to the proper SID *for each projection*.	☐ ☐	☐ ☐	☐ ☐
5. Selects cassettes/receptor of the appropriate sizes *for all projections*, according to the patient's size and examination.	☐ ☐	☐ ☐	☐ ☐

Comments:

_____

_____

PATIENT PREPARATION
The student:

	Procedure Yes No	Repeat Yes No	Competency Yes No
6. Identifies the correct patient and examination according to the requisition while establishing a good rapport with him or her.	☐ ☐	☐ ☐	☐ ☐
7. Obtains and documents the patient's history before the examination.	▨ ▨	▨ ▨	☐ ☐
8. Explains the examination in terms the patient fully understands and properly communicates with the patient throughout the examination.	☐ ☐	☐ ☐	☐ ☐
9. Asks female patients of childbearing age the date of their last menstrual period and documents this; inquires about the possibility of pregnancy and has them sign pregnancy consent forms.	☐ ☐	☐ ☐	☐ ☐
10. Removes all obscuring objects (hair pins, jewelry, dentures, etc.) so as *not* to produce radiographic artifacts.	☐ ☐	☐ ☐	☐ ☐

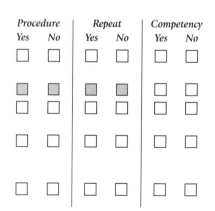

(continued)

	Procedure		Repeat		Competency	
	Yes	No	Yes	No	Yes	No
11. Respects the patient's modesty and provides ample comfort for his or her, and *cleans the Bucky/receptor in front of the patient.*	☐	☐	☐	☐	☐	☐

Comments:

_____

_____

PATIENT POSITIONING FOR A MANDIBLE
AP Axial (Towne)
The student:

	Procedure		Repeat		Competency	
	Yes	No	Yes	No	Yes	No
12. Places the patient in the supine position.	☐	☐	☐	☐	☐	☐
13. Selects the appropriate receptor or places the cassette so that the upper border of the cassette/receptor is at the vertex. For conventional cassettes, the flash must be away from any anatomy.	☐	☐	☐	☐	☐	☐
14. Instructs the patient to tuck his or her chin and ensures that the infraorbitomeatal line is perpendicular to the cassette/receptor.	☐	☐	☐	☐	☐	☐
15. Ensures that the midsagittal plane is perpendicular to the cassette/receptor.	☐	☐	☐	☐	☐	☐
16. Ensures that the head is not tilted or rotated.	☐	☐	☐	☐	☐	☐
17. Centers the central ray to the midsagittal plane.	☐	☐	☐	☐	☐	☐
18. Directs the central ray at an angle of 30° caudad to the glabella and so that it passes just below the TMJs.	☐	☐	☐	☐	☐	☐

PA or PA Axial Mandibular Body
The student:

	Procedure		Repeat		Competency	
	Yes	No	Yes	No	Yes	No
19. Places the patient in the prone position against the Bucky/receptor.	☐	☐	☐	☐	☐	☐
20. Selects the appropriate receptor. For conventional cassettes, the flash must be away from any anatomy.	☐	☐	☐	☐	☐	☐
21. Places the patient's nose and chin in contact with the Bucky/receptor.	☐	☐	☐	☐	☐	☐
22. Ensures that the midsagittal line is perpendicular to the cassette/receptor.	☐	☐	☐	☐	☐	☐
23. Ensures that the head is not tilted or rotated.	☐	☐	☐	☐	☐	☐
24. Centers the central ray to the midsagittal plane.	☐	☐	☐	☐	☐	☐
25. Directs the central ray in one of the following ways:	☐	☐	☐	☐	☐	☐

   a. PA—For the mandibular body, perpendicularly to the lips

   b. PA axial—For the mandibular body and TMJ, at an angle of 30° cephalad midway between the TMJs

PA or PA Axial Mandibular Rami
The student:

	Procedure		Repeat		Competency	
	Yes	No	Yes	No	Yes	No
26. Places the patient in the prone position against the Bucky/receptor.	☐	☐	☐	☐	☐	☐
27. Selects the appropriate receptor. For conventional cassettes, the flash must be away from any anatomy.	☐	☐	☐	☐	☐	☐
28. Places the patient's nose and forehead in contact with the Bucky/receptor.	☐	☐	☐	☐	☐	☐
29. Ensures that the midsagittal line is perpendicular to the cassette/receptor.	☐	☐	☐	☐	☐	☐
30. Ensures that the head is not tilted or rotated.	☐	☐	☐	☐	☐	☐
31. Centers the central ray to the midsagittal plane.	☐	☐	☐	☐	☐	☐
32. Directs the central ray in one of the following ways:	☐	☐	☐	☐	☐	☐

   a. PA—For the mandibular rami, perpendicularly to the acanthion

   b. PA axial—For the condylar processes, at an angle of 20–25° cephalad to the acanthion

Right Axiolateral (for Delineation of One of the Following)
The Mandibular Body
The student:

	Procedure		Repeat		Competency	
	Yes	No	Yes	No	Yes	No
33. Places the patient in the semiprone position.	☐	☐	☐	☐	☐	☐
34. Selects the appropriate receptor. For conventional cassettes, the flash must be away from any anatomy.	☐	☐	☐	☐	☐	☐
35. Places the patient's right side against the Bucky/receptor.	☐	☐	☐	☐	☐	☐
36. Ensures that the long axis of the mandibular body is parallel to the transverse axis of the cassette/receptor, with the head rotated 30° toward the cassette/receptor.	☐	☐	☐	☐	☐	☐
37. Centers the central ray to the center of the mandibular body.	☐	☐	☐	☐	☐	☐
38. Directs the central ray 25° cephalad.	☐	☐	☐	☐	☐	☐

Or

The Mandibular Symphysis
The student:

	Procedure		Repeat		Competency	
	Yes	No	Yes	No	Yes	No
39. Places the patient in the semiprone position.	☐	☐	☐	☐	☐	☐
40. Selects the appropriate receptor. For conventional cassettes, the flash must be away from any anatomy.	☐	☐	☐	☐	☐	☐
41. Places the patient's right side against the Bucky/receptor.	☐	☐	☐	☐	☐	☐
42. Extends the patient's head and instructs the patient to rest his or her head, rotated 45° toward the cassette/receptor, with the chin, cheek, and nose on the cassette/receptor.	☐	☐	☐	☐	☐	☐
43. Centers the central ray to the occlusal surface of the canine region (lips).	☐	☐	☐	☐	☐	☐
44. Directs the central ray 25° cephalad.	☐	☐	☐	☐	☐	☐

Or

The Mandibular Ramus
The student:

	Procedure		Repeat		Competency	
	Yes	No	Yes	No	Yes	No
45. Places the patient in the semiprone position.	☐	☐	☐	☐	☐	☐
46. Selects the appropriate receptor. For conventional cassettes, the flash must be away from any anatomy.	☐	☐	☐	☐	☐	☐
47. Places the patient's right side against the Bucky/receptor and extends the patient's chin to prevent the spine from superimposing over the ramus.	☐	☐	☐	☐	☐	☐
48. Instructs the patient to rest his or her head on the cheek, in the true lateral position.	☐	☐	☐	☐	☐	☐
49. Ensures that the broad axis of the mandibular ramus is parallel to the transverse axis of the cassette/receptor.	☐	☐	☐	☐	☐	☐
50. Ensures that the head is not tilted or rotated.	☐	☐	☐	☐	☐	☐
51. Centers the central ray to a point 1/2 inch anteriorly and 1 inch inferiorly to the EAM.	☐	☐	☐	☐	☐	☐
52. Directs the central ray 25° cephalad.	☐	☐	☐	☐	☐	☐

Left Axiolateral (for Delineation of One of the Following)
The Mandibular Body
The student:

	Procedure		Repeat		Competency	
	Yes	No	Yes	No	Yes	No
53. Places the patient in the semiprone position.	☐	☐	☐	☐	☐	☐
54. Selects the appropriate receptor. For conventional cassettes, the flash must be away from any anatomy.	☐	☐	☐	☐	☐	☐
55. Places the patient's left side against the Bucky/receptor.	☐	☐	☐	☐	☐	☐

(continued)

	Procedure		Repeat		Competency	
	Yes	No	Yes	No	Yes	No
56. Ensures that the long axis of the mandibular body is parallel to the transverse axis of the cassette/receptor, with the head rotated 30° toward the cassette/receptor.	☐	☐	☐	☐	☐	☐
57. Centers the central ray to the center of the mandibular body.	☐	☐	☐	☐	☐	☐
58. Directs the central ray 25° cephalad.	☐	☐	☐	☐	☐	☐

The Mandibular Symphysis
The student:

	Procedure		Repeat		Competency	
	Yes	No	Yes	No	Yes	No
59. Places the patient in the semiprone position.	☐	☐	☐	☐	☐	☐
60. Selects the appropriate receptor. For conventional cassettes, the flash must be away from any anatomy.	☐	☐	☐	☐	☐	☐
61. Places the patient's left side against the Bucky/receptor.	☐	☐	☐	☐	☐	☐
62. Extends the patient's head and instructs the patient to rest his or her head, rotated 45° toward the cassette/receptor, with the chin, cheek, and nose on the cassette/receptor.	☐	☐	☐	☐	☐	☐
63. Centers the central ray to the occlusal surface of the canine region (lips).	☐	☐	☐	☐	☐	☐
64. Directs the central ray 25° cephalad.	☐	☐	☐	☐	☐	☐

The Mandibular Ramus
The student:

	Procedure		Repeat		Competency	
	Yes	No	Yes	No	Yes	No
65. Places the patient in the semiprone position.	☐	☐	☐	☐	☐	☐
66. Selects the appropriate receptor. For conventional cassettes, the flash must be away from any anatomy.	☐	☐	☐	☐	☐	☐
67. Places the patient's left side against the Bucky/receptor and extends the patient's chin to prevent the spine from superimposing over the ramus.	☐	☐	☐	☐	☐	☐
68. Instructs the patient to rest his or her head on the cheek, in the true lateral position.	☐	☐	☐	☐	☐	☐
69. Ensures that the broad axis of the mandibular ramus is parallel to the transverse axis of the cassette/receptor.	☐	☐	☐	☐	☐	☐
70. Ensures that the head is not tilted or rotated.	☐	☐	☐	☐	☐	☐
71. Centers the central ray to a point 1/2 inch anteriorly and 1 inch inferiorly to the EAM.	☐	☐	☐	☐	☐	☐
72. Directs the central ray 25° cephalad.	☐	☐	☐	☐	☐	☐

Submentovertical (Base)
The student:

	Procedure		Repeat		Competency	
	Yes	No	Yes	No	Yes	No
73. Places the patient in the supine position, approximately 6–12 inches away from the Bucky/receptor and sets the technique before positioning the patient.	☐	☐	☐	☐	☐	☐
74. Selects the appropriate receptor. For conventional cassettes, the flash must be away from any anatomy.	☐	☐	☐	☐	☐	☐
75. Ensures that the midsagittal line is perpendicular to the cassette/receptor.	☐	☐	☐	☐	☐	☐
76. Instructs the patient to extend his or her head back to rest it on the vertex and ensures that the infraorbitomeatal line is parallel to the cassette/receptor.	☐	☐	☐	☐	☐	☐
77. Ensures that the head is not tilted or rotated.	☐	☐	☐	☐	☐	☐
78. Centers the central ray to the midsagittal plane.	☐	☐	☐	☐	☐	☐
79. Directs the central ray perpendicularly to the IOML, centered midway between the EAMs.	☐	☐	☐	☐	☐	☐

Comments:

_____

_____

IMPORTANT DETAILS
The student:

	Procedure		Repeat		Competency	
	Yes	No	Yes	No	Yes	No
80. Instills confidence in the patient by exhibiting self-confidence throughout the examination.	☐	☐	☐	☐	☐	☐
81. Places a lead marker in the appropriate area of the cassette/receptor (top/bottom/anteriorly/laterally), where it will be visualized on the finished radiograph, on the proper anatomical side (right/left), and in the appropriate position (face up/face down), depending on the patient's position.	☐	☐	☐	☐	☐	☐
82. Provides radiation protection (shield) for the patient, self, and others (closes doors).	☐	☐	☐	☐	☐	☐
83. Applies proper collimation and makes adjustments as necessary.	☐	☐	☐	☐	☐	☐
84. Properly measures the patient along the course of the central ray *for each projection.*	☐	☐	☐	☐	☐	☐
85. Sets the proper exposure techniques:	☐	☐	☐	☐	☐	☐

Conventional systems
- Sets the proper kVp, mA, and time and makes adjustments as necessary.

or

CR or DR systems
- Identifies the patient on the work-list (or manually types the patient information into the system).
- Selects appropriate body region, specific body part, and accurate view/projection.
- Double-checks preset parameters:
  —Adult vs. pediatric patients
  ○ Small, medium, or large
  —Bucky/receptor (upright vs. table) *or* non-Bucky
  —AEC vs. fixed
  ○ If AEC, checks ion chambers
  ○ Density setting
  —kVp and mA; adjusts if necessary
  —Focal spot/filament size

	Procedure		Repeat		Competency	
86. Exposes the cassette/receptor after telling the patient to hold still and after giving him or her proper breathing instructions (suspended) *for each projection.*	☐	☐	☐	☐	☐	☐
87. Provides each radiograph with the proper identification (flash) and/or processes each cassette (image) without difficulty (regardless of technology—film, CR, or DR).	☐	☐	☐	☐	☐	☐
88. Properly completes the examination by filling out all necessary paperwork, entering the examination in the computer, having the images checked by the appropriate staff members, answering any last-minute questions, and informing the patient that he or she is finished.	☐	☐	☐	☐	☐	☐
89. Exhibits the ability to adapt to new and difficult situations if and when necessary.	☐	☐	☐	☐	☐	☐
90. Accepts constructive criticism and uses it to his or her advantage.	☐	☐	☐	☐	☐	☐
91. Leaves the radiographic room neat and clean for the next examination.	☐	☐	☐	☐	☐	☐
92. Completes the examination within a reasonable time frame.	☐	☐	☐	☐	☐	☐

(continued)

Comments:

_____

_____

RADIOGRAPHIC IMAGE QUALITY

The student is able to critique his or her radiographs as to whether they demonstrate:

	Procedure Yes	Procedure No	Repeat Yes	Repeat No	Competency Yes	Competency No
93. Proper technique/optimal density	☐	☐	☐	☐	☐	☐
94. Enhanced detail, without evidence of motion and without any visible artifacts	☐	☐	☐	☐	☐	☐
95. Proper positioning (all anatomy included, evidence of proper centering/ alignment, etc.)	☐	☐	☐	☐	☐	☐
96. Proper marker placement	☐	☐	☐	☐	☐	☐
97. Evidence of proper collimation and radiation protection	☐	☐	☐	☐	☐	☐
98. Long vs. short scale of contrast	☐	☐	☐	☐	☐	☐

Comments:

_____

_____

MANDIBLE ANATOMY

The student is able to identify:

	Procedure Yes	Procedure No	Repeat Yes	Repeat No	Competency Yes	Competency No
99. TMJ	☐	☐	☐	☐	☐	☐
100. Mandibular body	☐	☐	☐	☐	☐	☐
101. Mandibular rami	☐	☐	☐	☐	☐	☐
102. Mandibular angle	☐	☐	☐	☐	☐	☐
103. Mandibular symphysis	☐	☐	☐	☐	☐	☐
104. Mandibular condyle	☐	☐	☐	☐	☐	☐
105. Coronoid process of mandible	☐	☐	☐	☐	☐	☐
106. Mental foramen	☐	☐	☐	☐	☐	☐
107. Obvious pathology	☐	☐	☐	☐	☐	☐

Comments:

_____

_____

Procedure Evaluator Signature	Repeat Evaluator Signature	Competency Evaluator Signature

Date	Date	Date

END MANDIBLE (OR PANOREX) EVALUATION

Student Name:_____

Procedure Grade	Repeat Grade	Competency Grade

PATIENT INFORMATION OR SIMULATED PROCEDURE *(circle if simulated)*

	Procedure	Repeat	Competency
Age			
Medical Record No.			
Ability to Cooperate			
Condition/Pathology			
Technical Factors Used			
Exposure Index			

FACILITY PREPARATION
The student:

	Procedure Yes / No	Repeat Yes / No	Competency Yes / No
1. Examines the radiographic room and cleans/straightens it before escorting the patient in.	☐ ☐	☐ ☐	☐ ☐
2. Has all equipment and supplies (shield, markers, supplies to clean the upright Bucky/receptor and table, etc.) readily available before escorting the patient in.	☐ ☐	☐ ☐	☐ ☐
3. Is able to manipulate all radiographic equipment with ease, and centers the central ray to the cassette/receptor *for all projections*.	☐ ☐	☐ ☐	☐ ☐
4. Adjusts the tube to the proper SID *for each projection*.	☐ ☐	☐ ☐	☐ ☐
5. Selects cassettes/receptor of the appropriate sizes *for all projections*, according to the patient's size and examination.	☐ ☐	☐ ☐	☐ ☐

Comments:

_____

_____

PATIENT PREPARATION
The student:

	Procedure Yes / No	Repeat Yes / No	Competency Yes / No
6. Identifies the correct patient and examination according to the requisition while establishing a good rapport with him or her.	☐ ☐	☐ ☐	☐ ☐
7. Obtains and documents the patient's history before the examination.	☐ ☐	☐ ☐	☐ ☐
8. Explains the examination in terms the patient fully understands and properly communicates with the patient throughout the examination.	☐ ☐	☐ ☐	☐ ☐
9. Asks female patients of childbearing age the date of their last menstrual period and documents this; inquires about the possibility of pregnancy and has them sign pregnancy consent forms.	☐ ☐	☐ ☐	☐ ☐
10. Removes all obscuring objects (hair pins, jewelry, dentures, etc.) so as *not* to produce radiographic artifacts.	☐ ☐	☐ ☐	☐ ☐

(continued)

	Procedure		Repeat		Competency	
	Yes	No	Yes	No	Yes	No
11. Respects the patient's modesty and provides ample comfort for him or her, and *cleans the Bucky/receptor in front of the patient.*	☐	☐	☐	☐	☐	☐

Comments:

_____

_____

PATIENT POSITIONING FOR THE TEMPOROMANDIBULAR JOINTS
AP Axial Closed Mouth
The student:

	Procedure		Repeat		Competency	
	Yes	No	Yes	No	Yes	No
12. Places the patient in the supine position.	☐	☐	☐	☐	☐	☐
13. Selects the appropriate receptor. For conventional cassettes, the flash must be away from any anatomy.	☐	☐	☐	☐	☐	☐
14. Ensures that the orbitomeatal line is perpendicular to the cassette/receptor.	☐	☐	☐	☐	☐	☐
15. Ensures that the midsagittal plane is perpendicular to the cassette/receptor.	☐	☐	☐	☐	☐	☐
16. Ensures that the head is not tilted or rotated.	☐	☐	☐	☐	☐	☐
17. Instructs the patient to tuck his or her chin and instructs the patient to close his or her mouth (occluding the posterior teeth rather than the incisors).	☐	☐	☐	☐	☐	☐
18. Centers the central ray to the midsagittal plane.	☐	☐	☐	☐	☐	☐
19. Directs the central ray at an angle of 35° caudad so that it passes just below the TMJs, entering approximately 3 inches above the nasion.	☐	☐	☐	☐	☐	☐

AP Axial Open Mouth
The student:

	Procedure		Repeat		Competency	
	Yes	No	Yes	No	Yes	No
20. Places the patient in the supine position.	☐	☐	☐	☐	☐	☐
21. Selects the appropriate receptor. For conventional cassettes, the flash must be away from any anatomy.	☐	☐	☐	☐	☐	☐
22. Ensures that the orbitomeatal line is perpendicular to the cassette/receptor.	☐	☐	☐	☐	☐	☐
23. Ensures that the midsagittal plane is perpendicular to the cassette/receptor.	☐	☐	☐	☐	☐	☐
24. Ensures that the head is not tilted or rotated.	☐	☐	☐	☐	☐	☐
25. Instructs the patient to tuck his or her chin and, only when not contraindicated, instructs the patient to open his or her mouth as wide as possible.	☐	☐	☐	☐	☐	☐
26. Centers the central ray to the midsagittal plane.	☐	☐	☐	☐	☐	☐
27. Directs the central ray at an angle of 35° caudad so that it passes just below the TMJs, entering approximately 3 inches above the nasion.	☐	☐	☐	☐	☐	☐

Right Closed Mouth Lateral
The student:

	Procedure		Repeat		Competency	
	Yes	No	Yes	No	Yes	No
28. Places the patient in the semiprone position.	☐	☐	☐	☐	☐	☐
29. Selects the appropriate receptor. For conventional cassettes, the flash must be away from any anatomy.	☐	☐	☐	☐	☐	☐
30. Places the patient's right side against the Bucky/receptor.	☐	☐	☐	☐	☐	☐
31. Ensures that the infraorbitomeatal line is parallel to the transverse axis of the cassette/receptor.	☐	☐	☐	☐	☐	☐
32. Ensures that the head is not tilted and that the interpupillary line is perpendicular and the midsagittal line is parallel to the cassette/receptor.	☐	☐	☐	☐	☐	☐
33. Instructs the patient to close his or her mouth (occluding the posterior teeth rather than the incisors).	☐	☐	☐	☐	☐	☐

	Procedure		Repeat		Competency	
	Yes	No	Yes	No	Yes	No
34. Centers the central ray to 1/2 inch anteriorly and 1 inch inferiorly to the right EAM (for 2 inches superiorly to the left/up EAM).	☐	☐	☐	☐	☐	☐
35. Directs the central ray 25–30° caudad (entering the left upper parietal region and passing through the right lower TMJ).	☐	☐	☐	☐	☐	☐

Right Open Mouth Lateral
The student:

	Procedure		Repeat		Competency	
	Yes	No	Yes	No	Yes	No
36. Places the patient in the semiprone position.	☐	☐	☐	☐	☐	☐
37. Selects the appropriate receptor. For conventional cassettes, the flash must be away from any anatomy.	☐	☐	☐	☐	☐	☐
38. Places the patient's right side against the Bucky/receptor.	☐	☐	☐	☐	☐	☐
39. Ensures that the infraorbitomeatal line is parallel to the transverse axis of the cassette/receptor.	☐	☐	☐	☐	☐	☐
40. Ensures that the head is not tilted and that the interpupillary line is perpendicular and the midsagittal line is parallel to the cassette/receptor.	☐	☐	☐	☐	☐	☐
41. Instructs the patient only when not contraindicated to open his or her mouth as wide as possible.	☐	☐	☐	☐	☐	☐
42. Centers the central ray to 1/2 inch anteriorly and 1 inch inferiorly to the right EAM (or 2 inches superiorly to the left/up EAM).	☐	☐	☐	☐	☐	☐
43. Directs the central ray 25–30° caudad, entering the left upper parietal region and passing through the right lower TMJ.	☐	☐	☐	☐	☐	☐

Left Closed Mouth Lateral
The student:

	Procedure		Repeat		Competency	
	Yes	No	Yes	No	Yes	No
44. Places the patient in the semiprone position.	☐	☐	☐	☐	☐	☐
45. Selects the appropriate receptor. For conventional cassettes, the flash must be away from any anatomy.	☐	☐	☐	☐	☐	☐
46. Places the patient's left side against the Bucky/receptor.	☐	☐	☐	☐	☐	☐
47. Ensures that the infraorbitomeatal line is parallel to the transverse axis of the cassette/receptor.	☐	☐	☐	☐	☐	☐
48. Ensures that the head is not tilted and that the interpupillary line is perpendicular and the midsagittal line is parallel to the cassette/receptor.	☐	☐	☐	☐	☐	☐
49. Instructs the patient to close his or her mouth (occluding the posterior teeth rather than the incisors).	☐	☐	☐	☐	☐	☐
50. Centers the central ray to 1/2 inch anteriorly and 1 inch inferiorly to the left EAM (or 2 inches superiorly to the right/up EAM).	☐	☐	☐	☐	☐	☐
51. Directs the central ray 25–30° caudad (entering the left upper parietal region and passing through the right lower TMJ).	☐	☐	☐	☐	☐	☐

Left Open Mouth Lateral
The student:

	Procedure		Repeat		Competency	
	Yes	No	Yes	No	Yes	No
52. Places the patient in the semiprone position.	☐	☐	☐	☐	☐	☐
53. Selects the appropriate receptor. For conventional cassettes, the flash must be away from any anatomy.	☐	☐	☐	☐	☐	☐
54. Places the patient's left side against the Bucky/receptor.	☐	☐	☐	☐	☐	☐
55. Ensures that the infraorbitomeatal line is parallel to the transverse axis of the cassette/receptor.	☐	☐	☐	☐	☐	☐

(continued)

	Procedure		Repeat		Competency	
	Yes	No	Yes	No	Yes	No
56. Ensures that the head is not tilted and that the interpupillary line is perpendicular and the midsagittal line is parallel to the cassette/receptor.	☐	☐	☐	☐	☐	☐
57. Instructs the patient, only when not contraindicated, to open his or her mouth as wide as possible.	☐	☐	☐	☐	☐	☐
58. Centers the central ray to 1/2 inch anteriorly and 1 inch inferiorly to the left EAM (or 2 inches superiorly to the right/up EAM).	☐	☐	☐	☐	☐	☐
59. Directs the central ray 25–30° caudad (entering the left upper parietal region and passing through the right lower TMJ).	☐	☐	☐	☐	☐	☐

Comments:

_____

_____

IMPORTANT DETAILS
The student:

	Procedure		Repeat		Competency	
	Yes	No	Yes	No	Yes	No
60. Instills confidence in the patient by exhibiting self-confidence throughout the examination.	☐	☐	☐	☐	☐	☐
61 Places a lead marker in the appropriate area of the cassette/receptor (top/bottom/anteriorly/laterally), where it will be visualized on the finished radiograph, on the proper anatomical side (right/left), and in the appropriate position (face up/face down), depending on the patient's position.	☐	☐	☐	☐	☐	☐
62. Provides radiation protection (shield) for the patient, self, and others (closes doors).	☐	☐	☐	☐	☐	☐
63. Applies proper collimation and makes adjustments as necessary.	☐	☐	☐	☐	☐	☐
64. Properly measures the patient along the course of the central ray *for each projection.*	☐	☐	☐	☐	☐	☐
65. Sets the proper exposure techniques:	☐	☐	☐	☐	☐	☐

Conventional systems
• Sets the proper kVp, mA, and time and makes adjustments as necessary.

or

CR or DR systems
• Identifies the patient on the work-list (or manually types the patient information into the system).
• Selects appropriate body region, specific body part, and accurate view/projection.
• Double-checks preset parameters:
  —Adult vs. pediatric patients
    ○ Small, medium, or large
  —Bucky/receptor (upright vs. table) *or* non-Bucky
  —AEC vs. fixed
    ○ If AEC, checks ion chambers
    ○ Density setting
  —kVp and mA; adjusts if necessary
  —Focal spot/filament size

	Procedure		Repeat		Competency	
66. Exposes the cassette/receptor after telling the patient to hold still and after giving him or her proper breathing instructions (suspended) *for each projection.*	☐	☐	☐	☐	☐	☐
67. Provides each radiograph with the proper identification (flash) and/or processes each cassette (image) without difficulty (regardless of technology—film, CR, or DR).	▨	▨	▨	▨	☐	☐

	Procedure		Repeat		Competency	
	Yes	No	Yes	No	Yes	No
68. Properly completes the examination by filling out all necessary paperwork, entering the examination in the computer, having the images checked by the appropriate staff members, answering any last-minute questions, and informing the patient that he or she is finished.	☐	☐	☐	☐	☐	☐
69. Exhibits the ability to adapt to new and difficult situations if and when necessary.	☐	☐	☐	☐	☐	☐
70. Accepts constructive criticism and uses it to his or her advantage.	☐	☐	☐	☐	☐	☐
71. Leaves the radiographic room neat and clean for the next examination.	☐	☐	☐	☐	☐	☐
72. Completes the examination within a reasonable time frame.	☐	☐	☐	☐	☐	☐

Comments:

_____

_____

RADIOGRAPHIC IMAGE QUALITY
The student is able to critique his or her radiographs as to whether they demonstrate:

	Procedure		Repeat		Competency	
	Yes	No	Yes	No	Yes	No
73. Proper technique/optimal density	☐	☐	☐	☐	☐	☐
74. Enhanced detail, without evidence of motion and without any visible artifacts	☐	☐	☐	☐	☐	☐
75. Proper positioning (all anatomy included, evidence of proper centering/alignment, etc.)	☐	☐	☐	☐	☐	☐
76. Proper marker placement	☐	☐	☐	☐	☐	☐
77. Evidence of proper collimation and radiation protection	☐	☐	☐	☐	☐	☐
78. Long vs. short scale of contrast	☐	☐	☐	☐	☐	☐

Comments:

_____

_____

TEMPOROMANDIBULAR JOINT ANATOMY
The student is able to identify:

	Procedure		Repeat		Competency	
	Yes	No	Yes	No	Yes	No
79. Mandibular fossa	☐	☐	☐	☐	☐	☐
80. TMJ	☐	☐	☐	☐	☐	☐
81. Mandibular rami	☐	☐	☐	☐	☐	☐
82. Mandibular angle	☐	☐	☐	☐	☐	☐
83. Mandibular condyle	☐	☐	☐	☐	☐	☐
84. Obvious pathology	☐	☐	☐	☐	☐	☐

Comments:

_____

_____

Procedure Evaluator Signature	Repeat Evaluator Signature	Competency Evaluator Signature
Date	Date	Date

END TEMPOROMANDIBULAR JOINTS EVALUATION

Student Name:_____

Procedure Grade	Repeat Grade	Competency Grade

PATIENT INFORMATION OR SIMULATED PROCEDURE *(circle if simulated)*

	Procedure	Repeat	Competency
Age			
Medical Record No.			
Ability to Cooperate			
Condition/Pathology			
Technical Factors Used			
Exposure Index			

FACILITY PREPARATION
The student:

	Procedure Yes No	Repeat Yes No	Competency Yes No
1. Examines the radiographic room and cleans/straightens it before escorting the patient in.	☐ ☐	☐ ☐	☐ ☐
2. Has all equipment and supplies (shield, markers, supplies to clean the upright Bucky/receptor and table, etc.) readily available before escorting the patient in.	☐ ☐	☐ ☐	☐ ☐
3. Is able to manipulate all radiographic equipment with ease, and centers the central ray to the cassette/receptor *for all projections*.	☐ ☐	☐ ☐	☐ ☐
4. Adjusts the tube to the proper SID *for each projection*.	☐ ☐	☐ ☐	☐ ☐
5. Selects cassettes/receptor of the appropriate sizes *for all projections,* according to the patient's size and examination.	☐ ☐	☐ ☐	☐ ☐

Comments:

_____

_____

PATIENT PREPARATION
The student:

	Procedure Yes No	Repeat Yes No	Competency Yes No
6. Identifies the correct patient and examination according to the requisition while establishing a good rapport with him or her.	☐ ☐	☐ ☐	☐ ☐
7. Obtains and documents the patient's history before the examination.	■ ■	■ ■	☐ ☐
8. Explains the examination in terms the patient fully understands and properly communicates with the patient throughout the examination.	☐ ☐	☐ ☐	☐ ☐
9. Asks female patients of childbearing age the date of their last menstrual period and documents this; inquires about the possibility of pregnancy and has them sign pregnancy consent forms.	☐ ☐	☐ ☐	☐ ☐
10. Removes all obscuring objects (hair pins, jewelry, dentures, etc.) so as *not* to produce radiographic artifacts.	☐ ☐	☐ ☐	☐ ☐

(continued)

	Procedure		Repeat		Competency	
	Yes	No	Yes	No	Yes	No
11. Respects the patient's modesty and provides ample comfort for his or her, and *cleans the Bucky/receptor in front of the patient.*	☐	☐	☐	☐	☐	☐

Comments:

_____

_____

PATIENT POSITIONING FOR BILATERAL MASTOIDS
Posterior Profile (Stenvers Method)
The student:

	Procedure		Repeat		Competency	
	Yes	No	Yes	No	Yes	No
12. Places the patient in the semiprone position.	☐	☐	☐	☐	☐	☐
13. Selects the appropriate receptor. For conventional cassettes, the flash must be away from any anatomy.	☐	☐	☐	☐	☐	☐
14. Places the patient's side against the cassette/receptor in the true lateral position.	☐	☐	☐	☐	☐	☐
15. Ensures that the infraorbitomeatal line is parallel to the transverse axis of the cassette/receptor.	☐	☐	☐	☐	☐	☐
16. Ensures that the head is not tilted and that the interpupillary line is perpendicular to the cassette/receptor.	☐	☐	☐	☐	☐	☐
17. Rotates the patient's head 45° toward the cassette/receptor from the lateral position, resting it on the forehead, nose, and cheek (midsagittal plane is at an angle of 45° to the cassette/receptor).	☐	☐	☐	☐	☐	☐
18. Centers the center of the cassette/receptor 1 inch directly anterior from the EAM against the cassette/receptor.	☐	☐	☐	☐	☐	☐
19. Directs the central ray 12° cephalad, entering approximately 2 inches posteriorly to the EAM away from the cassette/receptor.	☐	☐	☐	☐	☐	☐
20. Positions the patient for the opposite mastoid using the Stenvers method.	☐	☐	☐	☐	☐	☐

Axiolateral Oblique (Mayer Method)
The student:

	Procedure		Repeat		Competency	
	Yes	No	Yes	No	Yes	No
21. Places the patient in the AP/semi-supine position.	☐	☐	☐	☐	☐	☐
22. Selects the appropriate receptor. For conventional cassettes, the flash must be away from any anatomy.	☐	☐	☐	☐	☐	☐
23. Places the patient's side against the cassette/receptor in the true lateral position.	☐	☐	☐	☐	☐	☐
24. Ensures that the infraorbitomeatal line is parallel to the transverse axis of the cassette/receptor.	☐	☐	☐	☐	☐	☐
25. Ensures that the head is not tilted and that the interpupillary line is perpendicular to the cassette/receptor.	☐	☐	☐	☐	☐	☐
26. Rotates the patient's head 45° toward the cassette/receptor from the lateral position.	☐	☐	☐	☐	☐	☐
27. Centers the center of the cassette/receptor directly posterior from the EAM against the cassette/receptor, at the junction where the auricle and the head meet.	☐	☐	☐	☐	☐	☐
28. Directs the central ray 45° caudad to the EAM against the cassette/receptor.	☐	☐	☐	☐	☐	☐
29. Positions the patient for the opposite mastoid, using the Mayer method.	☐	☐	☐	☐	☐	☐

Axiolateral (Single-Tube Angle/Law Method)
The student:

	Procedure		Repeat		Competency	
	Yes	No	Yes	No	Yes	No
30. Places the patient in the semiprone position.	☐	☐	☐	☐	☐	☐
31. Selects the appropriate receptor. For conventional cassettes, the flash must be away from any anatomy.	☐	☐	☐	☐	☐	☐
32. Places the patient's side against the cassette/receptor, in the true lateral position.	☐	☐	☐	☐	☐	☐
33. Ensures that the infraorbitomeatal line is parallel to the transverse axis of the cassette/receptor.	☐	☐	☐	☐	☐	☐
34. Ensures that the head is not tilted and that the interpupillary line is perpendicular to the cassette/receptor.	☐	☐	☐	☐	☐	☐
35. Rotates the patient's head 15° toward the cassette/receptor from the lateral position.	☐	☐	☐	☐	☐	☐
36. Centers the center of the cassette/receptor 1 inch directly posterior from the EAM against the cassette/receptor.	☐	☐	☐	☐	☐	☐
37. Directs the central ray 15° caudad, entering approximately 2 inches posteriorly and 2 inches superiorly to the EAM away from the cassette/receptor.	☐	☐	☐	☐	☐	☐
38. Positions the patient for the opposite mastoid, using the Law method.	☐	☐	☐	☐	☐	☐

Comments:

_____

_____

IMPORTANT DETAILS
The student:

	Procedure		Repeat		Competency	
	Yes	No	Yes	No	Yes	No
39. Instills confidence in the patient by exhibiting self-confidence throughout the examination.	☐	☐	☐	☐	☐	☐
40. Places a lead marker in the appropriate area of the cassette/receptor (top/bottom/anteriorly/laterally), where it will be visualized on the finished radiograph, on the proper anatomical side (right/left), and in the appropriate position (face up/face down), depending on the patient's position.	☐	☐	☐	☐	☐	☐
41. Provides radiation protection (shield) for the patient, self, and others (closes doors).	☐	☐	☐	☐	☐	☐
42. Applies proper collimation and makes adjustments as necessary.	☐	☐	☐	☐	☐	☐
43. Properly measures the patient along the course of the central ray *for each projection.*	☐	☐	☐	☐	☐	☐
44. Sets the proper exposure techniques:	☐	☐	☐	☐	☐	☐

Conventional systems
• Sets the proper kVp, mA, and time and makes adjustments as necessary.

or

CR or DR systems
• Identifies the patient on the work-list (or manually types the patient information into the system).
• Selects appropriate body region, specific body part, and accurate view/projection.
• Double-checks preset parameters:
 —Adult vs. pediatric patients
  ○ Small, medium, or large
 —Bucky/receptor (upright vs. table) *or* non-Bucky

(continued)

	Procedure		Repeat		Competency	
	Yes	No	Yes	No	Yes	No

—AEC vs. fixed
- ○ If AEC, checks ion chambers
- ○ Density setting
—kVp and mA; adjusts if necessary
—Focal spot/filament size

	Procedure		Repeat		Competency	
	Yes	No	Yes	No	Yes	No
45. Exposes the cassette/receptor after telling the patient to hold still and after giving him or her proper breathing instructions (suspended) *for each projection.*	☐	☐	☐	☐	☐	☐
46. Provides each radiograph with the proper identification (flash) and/or processes each cassette (image) without difficulty (regardless of technology—film, CR, or DR).	▨	▨	▨	▨	☐	☐
47. Properly completes the examination by filling out all necessary paperwork, entering the examination in the computer, having the images checked by the appropriate staff members, answering any last-minute questions, and informing the patient that he or she is finished.	▨	▨	▨	▨	☐	☐
48. Exhibits the ability to adapt to new and difficult situations if and when necessary.	▨	▨	▨	▨	☐	☐
49. Accepts constructive criticism and uses it to his or her advantage.	☐	☐	☐	☐	☐	☐
50. Leaves the radiographic room neat and clean for the next examination.	▨	▨	▨	▨	☐	☐
51. Completes the examination within a reasonable time frame.	☐	☐	☐	☐	☐	☐

Comments:

_____

_____

RADIOGRAPHIC IMAGE QUALITY
The student is able to critique his or her radiographs as to whether they demonstrate:

	Procedure		Repeat		Competency	
	Yes	No	Yes	No	Yes	No
52. Proper technique/optimal density	▨	▨	▨	▨	☐	☐
53. Enhanced detail, without evidence of motion and without any visible artifacts	▨	▨	▨	▨	☐	☐
54. Proper positioning (all anatomy included, evidence of proper centering/ alignment, etc.)	▨	▨	▨	▨	☐	☐
55. Proper marker placement	▨	▨	▨	▨	☐	☐
56. Evidence of proper collimation and radiation protection	▨	▨	▨	▨	☐	☐
57. Long vs. short scale of contrast	▨	▨	▨	▨	☐	☐

Comments:

_____

_____

MASTOID ANATOMY
The student is able to identify:

	Procedure		Repeat		Competency	
	Yes	No	Yes	No	Yes	No
58. Mandibular condyle	▨	▨	▨	▨	☐	☐
59. Occipital bone	▨	▨	▨	▨	☐	☐
60. Mastoid air cells	▨	▨	▨	▨	☐	☐
61. Mastoid process	▨	▨	▨	▨	☐	☐
62. Obvious pathology	▨	▨	▨	▨	☐	☐

Comments:

_____

_____

Procedure Evaluator Signature	Repeat Evaluator Signature	Competency Evaluator Signature
Date	Date	Date

END MASTOIDS/TEMPORAL BONES EVALUATION

Student Name:_____

	Procedure Grade	Repeat Grade	Competency Grade

PATIENT INFORMATION OR SIMULATED PROCEDURE *(circle if simulated)*

	Procedure	Repeat	Competency
Age			
Medical Record No.			
Ability to Cooperate			
Condition/Pathology			
Technical Factors Used			
Exposure Index			

FACILITY PREPARATION
The student:

	Procedure Yes / No	Repeat Yes / No	Competency Yes / No
1. Examines the radiographic room and cleans/straightens it before escorting the patient in.	☐ ☐	☐ ☐	☐ ☐
2. Has all equipment and supplies (shield, markers, supplies to clean the upright Bucky/receptor and table, etc.) readily available before escorting the patient in.	☐ ☐	☐ ☐	☐ ☐
3. Is able to manipulate all radiographic equipment with ease, and centers the central ray to the cassette/receptor *for all projections*.	☐ ☐	☐ ☐	☐ ☐
4. Adjusts the tube to the proper SID *for each projection*.	☐ ☐	☐ ☐	☐ ☐
5. Selects cassettes/receptor of the appropriate sizes *for all projections*, according to the patient's size and examination.	☐ ☐	☐ ☐	☐ ☐

Comments:

_____

_____

PATIENT PREPARATION
The student:

	Procedure Yes / No	Repeat Yes / No	Competency Yes / No
6. Identifies the correct patient and examination according to the requisition while establishing a good rapport with him or her.	☐ ☐	☐ ☐	☐ ☐
7. Obtains and documents the patient's history before the examination.	☐ ☐	☐ ☐	☐ ☐
8. Explains the examination in terms the patient fully understands and properly communicates with the patient throughout the examination.	☐ ☐	☐ ☐	☐ ☐
9. Asks female patients of childbearing age the date of their last menstrual period and documents this; inquires about the possibility of pregnancy and has them sign pregnancy consent forms.	☐ ☐	☐ ☐	☐ ☐
10. Removes all obscuring objects (hair pins, jewelry, dentures, etc.) so as *not* to produce radiographic artifacts.	☐ ☐	☐ ☐	☐ ☐

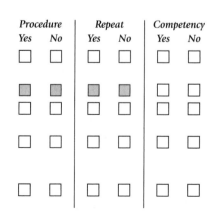

(continued)

	Procedure		Repeat		Competency	
	Yes	No	Yes	No	Yes	No
11. Respects the patient's modesty and provides ample comfort for his or her, and *cleans the Bucky/receptor in front of the patient.*	☐	☐	☐	☐	☐	☐

Comments:

_____

_____

PATIENT POSITIONING FOR A ZYGOMA
AP Axial (Towne)
The student:

	Procedure		Repeat		Competency	
	Yes	No	Yes	No	Yes	No
12. Places the patient in the supine position.	☐	☐	☐	☐	☐	☐
13. Selects the appropriate receptor or places the cassette so that the upper border of the cassette/receptor is at the vertex. For conventional cassettes, the flash must be away from any anatomy.	☐	☐	☐	☐	☐	☐
14. Instructs the patient to tuck his or her chin and ensures that the orbitomeatal line is perpendicular to the cassette/receptor.	☐	☐	☐	☐	☐	☐
15. Ensures that the midsagittal plane is perpendicular to the cassette/receptor.	☐	☐	☐	☐	☐	☐
16. Ensures that the head is not tilted or rotated.	☐	☐	☐	☐	☐	☐
17. Centers the central ray to the midsagittal plane.	☐	☐	☐	☐	☐	☐
18. Directs the central ray at an angle of 30° caudad to the glabella, approximately 1 inch above the nasion, passing through the mandibular condyles.	☐	☐	☐	☐	☐	☐

Parietoacanthial Axial (Superoinferior/Modified Titterington Method)
The student:

	Procedure		Repeat		Competency	
	Yes	No	Yes	No	Yes	No
19. Places the patient in the prone position against the Bucky/receptor.	☐	☐	☐	☐	☐	☐
20. Selects the appropriate receptor. For conventional cassettes, the flash must be away from any anatomy.	☐	☐	☐	☐	☐	☐
21. Instructs the patient to extend his or her neck and rest his or her head on the tip with the chin and tip of the nose on the cassette/receptor.	☐	☐	☐	☐	☐	☐
22. Ensures that the mentomeatal line is perpendicular to the cassette/receptor, and the orbitomeatal line forms a 37° angle to the cassette/receptor.	☐	☐	☐	☐	☐	☐
23. Ensures that the midsagittal line is perpendicular to the cassette/receptor.	☐	☐	☐	☐	☐	☐
24. Centers the central ray to the midsagittal plane.	☐	☐	☐	☐	☐	☐
25. Directs the central ray 23–38° caudad to the tip of the chin.	☐	☐	☐	☐	☐	☐

Right Axial Oblique (Tangential)
The student:

	Procedure		Repeat		Competency	
	Yes	No	Yes	No	Yes	No
26. Places the patient in the supine position, approximately 6–12 inches away from the Bucky/receptor, and sets a decreased technique from the normal SMV technique before positioning the patient.	☐	☐	☐	☐	☐	☐
27. Selects the appropriate receptor. For conventional cassettes, the flash must be away from any anatomy.	☐	☐	☐	☐	☐	☐
28. Instructs the patient to extend his or her head back to rest it on the vertex and ensures that the infraorbitomeatal line is parallel to the cassette/receptor.	☐	☐	☐	☐	☐	☐
29. Rotates the patient's head approximately 15° toward the right side.	☐	☐	☐	☐	☐	☐
30. Centers the central ray to the right zygomatic arch.	☐	☐	☐	☐	☐	☐
31. Directs the central ray perpendicularly to the IOML.	☐	☐	☐	☐	☐	☐

Left Axial Oblique (Tangential)
The student:

	Procedure		Repeat		Competency	
	Yes	No	Yes	No	Yes	No
32. Places the patient in the supine position, approximately 6–12 inches away from the Bucky/receptor, and sets a decreased technique from the normal SMV technique before positioning the patient.	☐	☐	☐	☐	☐	☐
33. Selects the appropriate receptor. For conventional cassettes, the flash must be away from any anatomy.	☐	☐	☐	☐	☐	☐
34. Instructs the patient to extend his or her head back to rest it on the vertex and ensures that the infraorbitomeatal line is parallel to the cassette/receptor.	☐	☐	☐	☐	☐	☐
35. Rotates the patient's head approximately 15° toward the left side.	☐	☐	☐	☐	☐	☐
36. Centers the central ray to the left zygomatic arch.	☐	☐	☐	☐	☐	☐
37. Directs the central ray perpendicularly to the IOML.	☐	☐	☐	☐	☐	☐

Submentovertical (Base)
The student:

	Procedure		Repeat		Competency	
	Yes	No	Yes	No	Yes	No
38. Places the patient in the supine position, approximately 6–12 inches away from the Bucky/receptor, and sets a decreased technique from the normal SMV technique before positioning the patient.	☐	☐	☐	☐	☐	☐
39. Selects the appropriate receptor. For conventional cassettes, the flash must be away from any anatomy.	☐	☐	☐	☐	☐	☐
40. Ensures that the midsagittal line is perpendicular to the cassette/receptor.	☐	☐	☐	☐	☐	☐
41. Instructs the patient to extend his or her head back to rest it on the vertex and ensures that the infraorbitomeatal line is parallel to the cassette/receptor.	☐	☐	☐	☐	☐	☐
42. Ensures that the head is not tilted or rotated.	☐	☐	☐	☐	☐	☐
43. Centers the central ray to the midsagittal plane.	☐	☐	☐	☐	☐	☐
44. Directs the central ray perpendicularly to the IOML, centered midway between the zygomatic arches, passing a coronal plane lying approximately 1 inch posteriorly to the outer canthi.	☐	☐	☐	☐	☐	☐

Comments:

_____

_____

IMPORTANT DETAILS
The student:

	Procedure		Repeat		Competency	
	Yes	No	Yes	No	Yes	No
45. Instills confidence in the patient by exhibiting self-confidence throughout the examination.	☐	☐	☐	☐	☐	☐
46. Places a lead marker in the appropriate area of the cassette/receptor (top/bottom/anteriorly/laterally), where it will be visualized on the finished radiograph, on the proper anatomical side (right/left), and in the appropriate position (face up/face down), depending on the patient's position.	☐	☐	☐	☐	☐	☐
47. Provides radiation protection (shield) for the patient, self, and others (closes doors).	☐	☐	☐	☐	☐	☐
48. Applies proper collimation and makes adjustments as necessary.	☐	☐	☐	☐	☐	☐
49. Properly measures the patient along the course of the central ray *for each projection.*	☐	☐	☐	☐	☐	☐
50. Sets the proper exposure techniques: *Conventional systems* • Sets the proper kVp, mA, and time and makes adjustments as necessary.	☐	☐	☐	☐	☐	☐

(continued)

	Procedure		Repeat		Competency	
	Yes	No	Yes	No	Yes	No

or

CR or DR systems
- Identifies the patient on the work-list (or manually types the patient information into the system).
- Selects appropriate body region, specific body part, and accurate view/ projection.
- Double-checks preset parameters:
  —Adult vs. pediatric patients
  ○ Small, medium, or large
  —Bucky/receptor (upright vs. table) *or* non-Bucky
  —AEC vs. fixed
  ○ If AEC, checks ion chambers
  ○ Density setting
  —kVp and mA; adjusts if necessary
  —Focal spot/filament size

	Procedure		Repeat		Competency	
	Yes	No	Yes	No	Yes	No
51. Exposes the cassette/receptor after telling the patient to hold still and after giving him or her proper breathing instructions (suspended) *for each projection.*	☐	☐	☐	☐	☐	☐
52. Provides each radiograph with the proper identification (flash) and/or processes each cassette (image) without difficulty (regardless of technology—film, CR, or DR).	☑	☑	☑	☑	☐	☐
53. Properly completes the examination by filling out all necessary paperwork, entering the examination in the computer, having the images checked by the appropriate staff members, answering any last-minute questions, and informing the patient that he or she is finished.	☑	☑	☑	☑	☐	☐
54. Exhibits the ability to adapt to new and difficult situations if and when necessary.	☑	☑	☑	☑	☐	☐
55. Accepts constructive criticism and uses it to his or her advantage.	☐	☐	☐	☐	☐	☐
56. Leaves the radiographic room neat and clean for the next examination.	☑	☑	☑	☑	☐	☐
57. Completes the examination within a reasonable time frame.	☑	☑	☑	☑	☐	☐

Comments:

_____

_____

RADIOGRAPHIC IMAGE QUALITY
The student is able to critique his or her radiographs as to whether they demonstrate:

	Procedure		Repeat		Competency	
	Yes	No	Yes	No	Yes	No
58. Proper technique/optimal density	☑	☑	☑	☑	☐	☐
59. Enhanced detail, without evidence of motion and without any visible artifacts	☑	☑	☑	☑	☐	☐
60. Proper positioning (all anatomy included, evidence of proper centering/ alignment, etc.)	☑	☑	☑	☑	☐	☐
61. Proper marker placement	☑	☑	☑	☑	☐	☐
62. Evidence of proper collimation and radiation protection	☑	☑	☑	☑	☐	☐
63. Long vs. short scale of contrast	☑	☑	☑	☑	☐	☐

Comments:

_____

_____

ZYGOMA ANATOMY
The student is able to identify:

	Procedure		Repeat		Competency	
	Yes	No	Yes	No	Yes	No
64. Mandible	☐	☐	☐	☐	☐	☐
65. Maxillary sinus	☐	☐	☐	☐	☐	☐
66. Temporal bone	☐	☐	☐	☐	☐	☐
67. Occipital bone	☐	☐	☐	☐	☐	☐
68. Orbit	☐	☐	☐	☐	☐	☐
69. Zygoma	☐	☐	☐	☐	☐	☐
70. Zygomatic arches	☐	☐	☐	☐	☐	☐
71. Obvious pathology	☐	☐	☐	☐	☐	☐

Comments:

_____

_____

_____ _____ _____
Procedure Evaluator Signature   Repeat Evaluator Signature   Competency Evaluator Signature

_____ _____ _____
Date   Date   Date

END ZYGOMA AND ARCHES EVALUATION

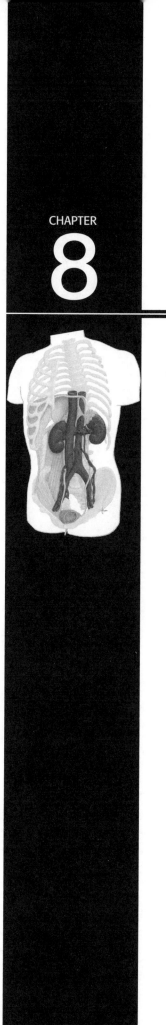

Student Name:_____

Procedure Grade	Repeat Grade	Competency Grade

PATIENT INFORMATION OR SIMULATED PROCEDURE *(circle if simulated)*

	Procedure	Repeat	Competency
Age			
Medical Record No.			
Ability to Cooperate			
Condition/Pathology			
Technical Factors Used			
Exposure Index			

FACILITY PREPARATION
The student:

	Procedure Yes	Procedure No	Repeat Yes	Repeat No	Competency Yes	Competency No
1. Identifies the correct patient and examination according to the requisition.	☐	☐	☐	☐	☐	☐
2. Locates and drives the mobile unit to the patient's room.	☐	☐	☐	☐	☐	☐
3. Politely asks the patient's visitors to wait outside the room until the examination is complete.	☐	☐	☐	☐	☐	☐
4. Explains the examination in terms the patient fully understands and properly communicates with the patient throughout the examination.	☐	☐	☐	☐	☐	☐
5. Obtains and documents the patient's history before the examination.	☐	☐	☐	☐	☐	☐
6. Asks female patients of childbearing age the date of their last menstrual period and documents this; inquires about the possibility of pregnancy and has them sign pregnancy consent forms.	☐	☐	☐	☐	☐	☐
7. Removes all obscuring objects (snaps, jewelry, personal belongings, etc.) so as *not* to produce radiographic artifacts.	☐	☐	☐	☐	☐	☐
8. Respects the patient's modesty and provides ample comfort for the patient.	☐	☐	☐	☐	☐	☐
9. Examines the room and adjusts any furniture before bringing in the mobile unit.	☐	☐	☐	☐	☐	☐
10. Examines the patient and selects the appropriate cassette, according to the patient's size and examination.	☐	☐	☐	☐	☐	☐
11. Adjusts the patient into the erect or supine position, as appropriate.	☐	☐	☐	☐	☐	☐
12. Is able to manipulate mobile radiographic equipment with ease, positions it at the patient's bedside, and centers the central ray to the cassette.	☐	☐	☐	☐	☐	☐
13. Adjusts the tube to the proper SID.	☐	☐	☐	☐	☐	☐

Comments:

_____

_____

(continued)

PATIENT POSITIONING FOR A MOBILE CHEST
The student:

	Procedure		Repeat		Competency	
	Yes	No	Yes	No	Yes	No
14. Places the cassette behind the patient lengthwise or crosswise, depending on the patient's build, adjusts it so that the image will include all the necessary anatomy, and ensures that the upper border of the cassette is 1–2 inches above the patient's shoulders. For conventional cassettes, the flash must be at the top and away from any anatomy.	☐	☐	☐	☐	☐	☐
15. Centers the central ray to the midsagittal plane.	☐	☐	☐	☐	☐	☐
16. Directs the central ray perpendicularly to the level of the sixth thoracic vertebra, unless it is necessary to angle according to the patient's position.	☐	☐	☐	☐	☐	☐

Comments:

_____

_____

IMPORTANT DETAILS
The student:

	Procedure		Repeat		Competency	
	Yes	No	Yes	No	Yes	No
17. Instills confidence in the patient by exhibiting self-confidence throughout the examination.	☐	☐	☐	☐	☐	☐
18. Places a lead marker in the appropriate area of the cassette (top/bottom/anteriorly/laterally), where it will be visualized on the finished radiograph, on the proper anatomical side (right/left), and in the appropriate position (face up/face down), depending on the patient's position.	☐	☐	☐	☐	☐	☐
19. Provides radiation protection (shield) for the patient, self, and others.	☐	☐	☐	☐	☐	☐
20. Applies proper collimation and makes adjustments as necessary.	☐	☐	☐	☐	☐	☐
21. Sets the proper technique (kVp, mA, time) and makes adjustments as necessary.	☐	☐	☐	☐	☐	☐
22. While standing at least 6 feet away, exposes the cassette, telling the patient to hold still and giving him or her proper breathing instructions (inspiration) *for each projection.*	☐	☐	☐	☐	☐	☐
23. Provides each radiograph with the proper identification (flash) and/or processes each cassette (image) without difficulty (regardless of technology: film or CR).	☐	☐	☐	☐	☐	☐
24. Properly completes the examination by filling out all necessary paperwork and entering the examination in the computer.	☐	☐	☐	☐	☐	☐
25. Exhibits the ability to adapt to new and difficult situations if and when necessary.	☐	☐	☐	☐	☐	☐
26. Accepts constructive criticism and uses it to his or her advantage.	☐	☐	☐	☐	☐	☐
27. Leaves the room neat and puts things back the way they were before he or she entered.	☐	☐	☐	☐	☐	☐
28. Completes the examination within a reasonable time frame.	☐	☐	☐	☐	☐	☐
29. Returns the mobile unit to the proper location and charges it as needed.	☐	☐	☐	☐	☐	☐

Comments:

_____

_____

RADIOGRAPHIC IMAGE QUALITY
The student is able to critique his or her radiographs as to whether they demonstrate:

	Procedure		Repeat		Competency	
	Yes	No	Yes	No	Yes	No
30. Proper technique/optimal density	☐	☐	☐	☐	☐	☐
31. Enhanced detail, without evidence of motion and without any visible artifacts	☐	☐	☐	☐	☐	☐
32. Proper positioning (all anatomy included, evidence of proper centering/alignment, etc.)	☐	☐	☐	☐	☐	☐
33. Proper marker placement	☐	☐	☐	☐	☐	☐
34. Evidence of proper collimation and radiation protection	☐	☐	☐	☐	☐	☐
35. Long vs. short scale of contrast	☐	☐	☐	☐	☐	☐

Comments:

CHEST ANATOMY
The student is able to identify:

	Procedure		Repeat		Competency	
	Yes	No	Yes	No	Yes	No
36. Apices	☐	☐	☐	☐	☐	☐
37. Scapula	☐	☐	☐	☐	☐	☐
38. Ribs	☐	☐	☐	☐	☐	☐
39. Thoracic spine	☐	☐	☐	☐	☐	☐
40. Diaphragm	☐	☐	☐	☐	☐	☐
41. Bases	☐	☐	☐	☐	☐	☐
42. Costophrenic angles	☐	☐	☐	☐	☐	☐
43. Acromioclavicular joints	☐	☐	☐	☐	☐	☐
44. Trachea	☐	☐	☐	☐	☐	☐
45. Hilum	☐	☐	☐	☐	☐	☐
46. Heart	☐	☐	☐	☐	☐	☐
47. Mediastinum	☐	☐	☐	☐	☐	☐
48. Clavicles	☐	☐	☐	☐	☐	☐
49. Sternoclavicular joints	☐	☐	☐	☐	☐	☐
50. Aortic knob/arch	☐	☐	☐	☐	☐	☐
51. Humeral head	☐	☐	☐	☐	☐	☐
52. Distal cervical spine	☐	☐	☐	☐	☐	☐
53. Obvious pathology	☐	☐	☐	☐	☐	☐

Comments:

Procedure Evaluator Signature	Repeat Evaluator Signature	Competency Evaluator Signature
Date	Date	Date

END MOBILE CHEST EVALUATION

Student Name:_____

Procedure Grade	Repeat Grade	Competency Grade

PATIENT INFORMATION OR SIMULATED PROCEDURE *(circle if simulated)*

	Procedure	Repeat	Competency
Age			
Medical Record No.			
Ability to Cooperate			
Condition/Pathology			
Technical Factors Used			
Exposure Index			

FACILITY PREPARATION
The student:

	Procedure Yes	No	Repeat Yes	No	Competency Yes	No
1. Identifies the correct patient and examination according to the requisition.	▪	▪	▪	▪	☐	☐
2. Locates and drives the mobile unit to the patient's room.	▪	▪	▪	▪	☐	☐
3. Politely asks the patient's visitors to wait outside the room until the examination is complete.	▪	▪	▪	▪	☐	☐
4. Explains the examination in terms the patient fully understands and properly communicates with the patient throughout the examination.	▪	▪	▪	▪	☐	☐
5. Obtains and documents the patient's history before the examination.	▪	▪	▪	▪	☐	☐
6. Asks female patients of childbearing age the date of their last menstrual period and documents this; inquires about the possibility of pregnancy and has them sign pregnancy consent forms.	▪	▪	▪	▪	☐	☐
7. Removes all obscuring objects (snaps, jewelry, personal belongings, etc.) so as *not* to produce radiographic artifacts.	▪	▪	▪	▪	☐	☐
8. Respects the patient's modesty and provides ample comfort for the patient.	▪	▪	▪	▪	☐	☐
9. Examines the room and adjusts any furniture before bringing in the mobile unit.	▪	▪	▪	▪	☐	☐
10. Examines the patient and selects the appropriate cassette, according to the patient's size and examination.	▪	▪	▪	▪	☐	☐
11. Adjusts the patient into the erect or supine position, as appropriate.	▪	▪	▪	▪	☐	☐
12. Is able to manipulate mobile radiographic equipment with ease, positions it at the patient's bedside, and centers the central ray to the cassette.	▪	▪	▪	▪	☐	☐
13. Adjusts the tube to the proper SID.	▪	▪	▪	▪	☐	☐

Comments:

_____

_____

(continued)

PATIENT POSITIONING FOR A MOBILE ABDOMEN
Right Anterior Oblique
The student:

	Procedure		Repeat		Competency	
	Yes	No	Yes	No	Yes	No
14. Places the cassette behind the patient lengthwise and adjusts it so that the image will include all the necessary anatomy. For conventional cassettes, the flash must be at the bottom and away from any anatomy.	☐	☐	☐	☐	☐	☐
15. Centers the central ray to the midsagittal plane.	☐	☐	☐	☐	☐	☐
16. Directs the central ray perpendicular to the level of the iliac crest.	☐	☐	☐	☐	☐	☐

Comments:

_____

_____

IMPORTANT DETAILS
The student:

	Procedure		Repeat		Competency	
	Yes	No	Yes	No	Yes	No
17. Instills confidence in the patient by exhibiting self-confidence throughout the examination.	☐	☐	☐	☐	☐	☐
18. Places a lead marker in the appropriate area of the cassette (top/bottom/anteriorly/laterally), where it will be visualized on the finished radiograph, on the proper anatomical side (right/left), and in the appropriate position (face up/face down), depending on the patient's position.	☐	☐	☐	☐	☐	☐
19. Provides radiation protection (shield) for the patient, self, and others.	☐	☐	☐	☐	☐	☐
20. Applies proper collimation and makes adjustments as necessary.	☐	☐	☐	☐	☐	☐
21. Sets the proper kVp, mA, and time and makes adjustments as necessary.	☐	☐	☐	☐	☐	☐
22. While standing at least 6 feet away, exposes the cassette, telling the patient to hold still and giving him or her proper breathing instructions (expiration) *for each projection.*	☐	☐	☐	☐	☐	☐
23. Provides each radiograph with the proper identification (flash) and/or processes each cassette (image) without difficulty (regardless of technology: film or CR).	☐	☐	☐	☐	☐	☐
24. Properly completes the examination by filling out all necessary paperwork and entering the examination in the computer.	☐	☐	☐	☐	☐	☐
25. Exhibits the ability to adapt to new and difficult situations if and when necessary.	☐	☐	☐	☐	☐	☐
26. Accepts constructive criticism and uses it to his or her advantage.	☐	☐	☐	☐	☐	☐
27. Leaves the room neat and puts things back the way they were before he or she entered.	☐	☐	☐	☐	☐	☐
28. Completes the examination within a reasonable time frame.	☐	☐	☐	☐	☐	☐
29. Returns the mobile unit to the proper location and charges it as needed.	☐	☐	☐	☐	☐	☐

Comments:

_____

RADIOGRAPHIC IMAGE QUALITY
The student is able to critique his or her radiographs as to whether they demonstrate:

	Procedure		Repeat		Competency	
	Yes	No	Yes	No	Yes	No
30. Proper technique/optimal density	☐	☐	☐	☐	☐	☐
31. Enhanced detail, without evidence of motion and without any visible artifacts	☐	☐	☐	☐	☐	☐

	Procedure		Repeat		Competency	
	Yes	No	Yes	No	Yes	No
32. Proper positioning (all anatomy included, evidence of proper centering/alignment, etc.)	☑	☑	☑	☑	☐	☐
33. Proper marker placement	☑	☑	☑	☑	☐	☐
34. Evidence of proper collimation and radiation protection	☑	☑	☑	☑	☐	☐
35. Long vs. short scale of contrast	☑	☑	☑	☑	☐	☐

Comments:

_____

_____

ABDOMEN ANATOMY
The student is able to identify:

	Procedure		Repeat		Competency	
	Yes	No	Yes	No	Yes	No
36. Kidneys	☑	☑	☑	☑	☐	☐
37. Psoas muscles	☑	☑	☑	☑	☐	☐
38. Bladder	☑	☑	☑	☑	☐	☐
39. Diaphragm	☑	☑	☑	☑	☐	☐
40. Symphysis pubis	☑	☑	☑	☑	☐	☐
41. Iliac crest	☑	☑	☑	☑	☐	☐
42. Hips	☑	☑	☑	☑	☐	☐
43. Stomach	☑	☑	☑	☑	☐	☐
44. Liver	☑	☑	☑	☑	☐	☐
45. Bowel gas	☑	☑	☑	☑	☐	☐
46. Obvious pathology	☑	☑	☑	☑	☐	☐

Comments:

_____

_____

_____   _____   _____
Procedure Evaluator Signature   Repeat Evaluator Signature   Competency Evaluator Signature

_____   _____   _____
Date   Date   Date

END MOBILE ABDOMEN (KUB) EVALUATION

Student Name:_____

Procedure Grade	Repeat Grade	Competency Grade

PATIENT INFORMATION OR SIMULATED PROCEDURE *(circle if simulated)*

	Procedure	Repeat	Competency
Age			
Medical Record No.			
Ability to Cooperate			
Condition/Pathology			
Technical Factors Used			
Exposure Index			

FACILITY PREPARATION
The student:

	Procedure Yes	Procedure No	Repeat Yes	Repeat No	Competency Yes	Competency No
1. Identifies the correct patient and examination according to the requisition.	☐	☐	☐	☐	☐	☐
2. Locates and drives the mobile unit to the patient's room.	☐	☐	☐	☐	☐	☐
3. Politely asks the patient's visitors to wait outside the room until the examination is complete.	☐	☐	☐	☐	☐	☐
4. Explains the examination in terms the patient fully understands and properly communicates with the patient throughout the examination.	☐	☐	☐	☐	☐	☐
5. Obtains and documents the patient's history before the examination.	☐	☐	☐	☐	☐	☐
6. Asks female patients of childbearing age the date of their last menstrual period and documents this; inquires about the possibility of pregnancy and has them sign pregnancy consent forms.	☐	☐	☐	☐	☐	☐
7. Removes all obscuring objects (snaps, jewelry, personal belongings, etc.) so as *not* to produce radiographic artifacts.	☐	☐	☐	☐	☐	☐
8. Respects the patient's modesty and provides ample comfort for the patient.	☐	☐	☐	☐	☐	☐
9. Examines the room and adjusts any furniture before bringing in the mobile unit.	☐	☐	☐	☐	☐	☐
10. Examines the patient and selects the appropriate cassette, according to the patient's size and examination.	☐	☐	☐	☐	☐	☐
11. Adjusts the patient into the erect or supine position, as appropriate.	☐	☐	☐	☐	☐	☐
12. Is able to manipulate mobile radiographic equipment with ease, positions it at the patient's bedside, and centers the central ray to the cassette.	☐	☐	☐	☐	☐	☐
13. Adjusts the tube to the proper SID.	☐	☐	☐	☐	☐	☐

Comments:

_____

_____

(continued)

PATIENT POSITIONING FOR A MOBILE ORTHOPAEDICS/EXTREMITY
AP or PA
The student:

	Procedure		Repeat		Competency	
	Yes	No	Yes	No	Yes	No
14. Places the cassette behind the patient lengthwise and adjusts the cassette so that the image includes all the necessary anatomy. For conventional cassettes, the flash must be away from any anatomy.	▣	▣	▣	▣	☐	☐
15. Places the appropriate surface (anterior/posterior) of the extremity on the appropriate area of the cassette.	▣	▣	▣	▣	☐	☐
16. Centers the anatomy of interest to the center of the cassette, including appropriate joints.	▣	▣	▣	▣	☐	☐
17. Centers the central ray perpendicularly to the middle of the extremity.	▣	▣	▣	▣	☐	☐

Lateral
The student:

	Procedure		Repeat		Competency	
	Yes	No	Yes	No	Yes	No
18. Selects a new, clean cassette, places it behind the patient lengthwise, and adjusts it so that the image includes all the necessary anatomy. For conventional cassettes, the flash must be anterior and away from any anatomy.	▣	▣	▣	▣	☐	☐
19. While instructing the patient, rotates the extremity to the true lateral position, or if necessary positions the equipment and cassette for cross-table/horizontal beam projection.	▣	▣	▣	▣	☐	☐
20. Centers the anatomy of interest to the center of the cassette, including appropriate joints.	▣	▣	▣	▣	☐	☐
21. Centers the central ray perpendicularly to the middle of the extremity.	▣	▣	▣	▣	☐	☐

Comments:

_____

_____

IMPORTANT DETAILS
The student:

	Procedure		Repeat		Competency	
	Yes	No	Yes	No	Yes	No
22. Instills confidence in the patient by exhibiting self-confidence throughout the examination.	▣	▣	▣	▣	☐	☐
23. Places a lead marker in the appropriate area of the cassette (top/bottom/anteriorly/laterally), where it will be visualized on the finished radiograph, on the proper anatomical side (right/left), and in the appropriate position (face up/face down), depending on the patient's position.	▣	▣	▣	▣	☐	☐
24. Provides radiation protection (shield) for the patient, self, and others.	▣	▣	▣	▣	☐	☐
25. Applies proper collimation and makes adjustments as necessary.	▣	▣	▣	▣	☐	☐
26. Sets the proper kVp, mA, and time and makes adjustments as necessary.	▣	▣	▣	▣	☐	☐
27. While standing at least 6 feet away, exposes the cassette, telling the patient to hold still and giving him or her proper breathing instructions *for each projection.*	▣	▣	▣	▣	☐	☐
28. Provides each radiograph with the proper identification (flash) and/or processes each cassette (image) without difficulty (regardless of technology: film or CR).	▣	▣	▣	▣	☐	☐
29. Properly completes the examination by filling out all necessary paperwork and entering the examination in the computer.	▣	▣	▣	▣	☐	☐
30. Exhibits the ability to adapt to new and difficult situations if and when necessary.	▣	▣	▣	▣	☐	☐
31. Accepts constructive criticism and uses it to his or her advantage.	▣	▣	▣	▣	☐	☐

	Procedure		Repeat		Competency	
	Yes	No	Yes	No	Yes	No
32. Leaves the room neat and puts things back the way they were before he or she entered.	☐	☐	☐	☐	☐	☐
33. Completes the examination within a reasonable time frame.	☐	☐	☐	☐	☐	☐
34. Returns the mobile unit to the proper location and charges it as needed.	☐	☐	☐	☐	☐	☐

Comments:

_____

_____

RADIOGRAPHIC IMAGE QUALITY
The student is able to critique his or her radiographs as to whether they demonstrate:

	Procedure		Repeat		Competency	
	Yes	No	Yes	No	Yes	No
35. Proper technique/optimal density	☐	☐	☐	☐	☐	☐
36. Enhanced detail, without evidence of motion and without any visible artifacts	☐	☐	☐	☐	☐	☐
37. Proper positioning (all anatomy included, evidence of proper centering/alignment, etc.)	☐	☐	☐	☐	☐	☐
38. Proper marker placement	☐	☐	☐	☐	☐	☐
39. Evidence of proper collimation and radiation protection	☐	☐	☐	☐	☐	☐
40. Long vs. short scale of contrast	☐	☐	☐	☐	☐	☐

Comments:

_____

_____

ORTHOPEDIC/EXTREMITY ANATOMY
The student is able to identify:

	Procedure		Repeat		Competency	
	Yes	No	Yes	No	Yes	No
41. _____	☐	☐	☐	☐	☐	☐
42. _____	☐	☐	☐	☐	☐	☐
43. _____	☐	☐	☐	☐	☐	☐
44. _____	☐	☐	☐	☐	☐	☐
45. _____	☐	☐	☐	☐	☐	☐
46. _____	☐	☐	☐	☐	☐	☐
47. _____	☐	☐	☐	☐	☐	☐
48. Obvious pathology	☐	☐	☐	☐	☐	☐

Comments:

_____

_____

Procedure Evaluator Signature	Repeat Evaluator Signature	Competency Evaluator Signature
Date	Date	Date

END MOBILE ORTHOPEDICS/EXTREMITIES EVALUATION

Student Name:_____

Procedure Grade	Repeat Grade	Competency Grade

PATIENT INFORMATION OR SIMULATED PROCEDURE *(circle if simulated)*

	Procedure	Repeat	Competency
Age			
Medical Record No.			
Ability to Cooperate			
Condition/Pathology			
Technical Factors Used			
Exposure Index			

FACILITY PREPARATION
The student:

	Procedure Yes No	Repeat Yes No	Competency Yes No
1. Identifies the correct patient and examination according to the requisition.	☐ ☐	☐ ☐	☐ ☐
2. Examines the room and adjusts any obstacles before bringing in the mobile unit.	☐ ☐	☐ ☐	☐ ☐
3. Locates and drives the mobile unit to the appropriate operating room, using the brakes when needed.	☐ ☐	☐ ☐	☐ ☐

Comments:

_____

_____

MANIPULATION OF C-ARM EQUIPMENT DURING A PROCEDURE
The student:

	Procedure Yes No	Repeat Yes No	Competency Yes No
4. Switches the unit on and off.	☐ ☐	☐ ☐	☐ ☐
5. Connects the monitor to the C-arm.	☐ ☐	☐ ☐	☐ ☐
6. Connects the monitor to the outlet.	☐ ☐	☐ ☐	☐ ☐
7. Selects the appropriate mode:	☐ ☐	☐ ☐	☐ ☐
a. Fluoroscopy			
b. Pulsed fluoroscopy			
c. Digital—single image			
d. Digital—serial images			
8. Uses collimators.	☐ ☐	☐ ☐	☐ ☐
9. Manipulates the images:	☐ ☐	☐ ☐	☐ ☐
a. Reverse			
b. Rotated			
c. With contrast adjustment on either monitor (A or B)			

(continued)

	Procedure		Repeat		Competency	
	Yes	No	Yes	No	Yes	No

10. Uses program functions: ☐ ☐ | ☐ ☐ | ☐ ☐

   a. Timer

   b. Recall or forward

   c. Part programs, including:

   (1) Chest

   (2) Abdomen

   (3) Hip/spine

   (4) Extremity

   (5) Standard

11. Captures the images: ☐ ☐ | ☐ ☐ | ☐ ☐

   a. "Freezes" live images on Monitor A, and is able to transfer the images to Monitor B for printing/filming.

   b. Inserts cassettes.

   c. Removes the darkslide and makes an exposure.

   d. Unloads, processes, and fills cassettes.

12. Manipulates the C-arm by operating all locks: ☐ ☐ | ☐ ☐ | ☐ ☐

   a. Up and down

   b. Lateral and oblique

   c. In, out, and swivel

Comments:

_____

_____

IMPORTANT DETAILS

The student:

	Procedure		Repeat		Competency	
	Yes	No	Yes	No	Yes	No
13. Observes and does not interfere with the sterile field.	☐	☐	☐	☐	☐	☐
14. Provides each radiograph with the proper patient identification by using the computer, and processes each cassette (image) without difficulty.	☐	☐	☐	☐	☐	☐
15. Properly completes the examination by filling out all necessary paperwork.	☐	☐	☐	☐	☐	☐
16. Exhibits the ability to adapt to new and difficult situations if and when necessary.	☐	☐	☐		☐	☐
17. Accepts constructive criticism and uses it to his or her advantage.	☐	☐	☐	☐	☐	☐
18. Completes the examination within a reasonable time frame.	☐	☐	☐	☐	☐	☐
19. Returns the mobile unit to the proper location and charges it as needed.	☐	☐	☐	☐	☐	☐

Comments:

_____

_____

_____ | _____ | _____
Procedure Evaluator Signature   Repeat Evaluator Signature   Competency Evaluator Signature

_____ | _____ | _____
Date   Date   Date

END C-ARM PROCEDURE EVALUATION

Student Name:_____

	Procedure Grade	Repeat Grade	Competency Grade

PATIENT INFORMATION OR SIMULATED PROCEDURE *(circle if simulated)*

	Procedure	Repeat	Competency
Age			
Medical Record No.			
Ability to Cooperate			
Condition/Pathology			
Technical Factors Used			
Exposure Index			

FACILITY PREPARATION
The student:

	Procedure Yes No	Repeat Yes No	Competency Yes No
1. Examines the room and adjusts any obstacles before bringing in the mobile unit.	▢ ▢	▢ ▢	☐ ☐
2. Locates and drives the mobile unit to the appropriate room and engages the brakes.	▢ ▢	▢ ▢	☐ ☐

Comments:

_____

_____

PATIENT POSITIONING AND EQUIPMENT MANIPULATION FOR A NERVE BLOCK PROCEDURE
The student:

	Procedure Yes No	Repeat Yes No	Competency Yes No
3. Examines the patient and selects the appropriate cassette, according to the patient's size and examination.	▢ ▢	▢ ▢	☐ ☐
4. Ensures that the patient's position is appropriate for the requested radiographs.	▢ ▢	▢ ▢	☐ ☐
5. Ensures that there are no obscuring objects (snaps, jewelry, personal belongings, etc.) over the area of interest so as not to produce radiographic artifacts.	▢ ▢	▢ ▢	☐ ☐
6. Respects the patient's modesty and provides ample comfort for the patient.	▢ ▢	▢ ▢	☐ ☐
7. Is able to manipulate mobile radiographic equipment with ease, positions it, and centers the central ray to the cassette.	▢ ▢	▢ ▢	☐ ☐
8. Adjusts the tube to the proper SID.			
9. Places a lead marker in the appropriate area of the cassette (top/bottom/anteriorly/laterally), where it will be visualized on the finished radiograph, on the proper anatomical side (right/left), and in the appropriate position (face up/face down), depending on the patient's position.	▢ ▢	▢ ▢	☐ ☐

(continued)

	Procedure		Repeat		Competency	
	Yes	No	Yes	No	Yes	No
10. Provides radiation protection (shield) for the patient, self, and others.	☐	☐	☐	☐	☐	☐
11. Applies proper collimation and makes adjustments as necessary.	☐	☐	☐	☐	☐	☐
12. Sets the proper kVp, mA, and time and makes adjustments as necessary.	☐	☐	☐	☐	☐	☐

Comments:

IMPORTANT DETAILS
The student:

	Procedure		Repeat		Competency	
	Yes	No	Yes	No	Yes	No
13. Provides each radiograph with the proper patient identification by using the computer, and processes each cassette (image) without difficulty.	☐	☐	☐	☐	☐	☐
14. Properly completes the examination by filling out all necessary paperwork.	☐	☐	☐	☐	☐	☐
15. Exhibits the ability to adapt to new and difficult situations if and when necessary.	☐	☐	☐	☐	☐	☐
16. Accepts constructive criticism and uses it to his or her advantage.	☐	☐	☐	☐	☐	☐
17. Completes the examination within a reasonable time frame.	☐	☐	☐	☐	☐	☐
18. Returns the mobile unit to the proper location and charges it as needed.	☐	☐	☐	☐	☐	☐

Comments:

RADIOGRAPHIC IMAGE QUALITY
The student is able to critique his or her radiographs as to whether they demonstrate:

	Procedure		Repeat		Competency	
	Yes	No	Yes	No	Yes	No
19. Proper technique/optimal density	☐	☐	☐	☐	☐	☐
20. Enhanced detail, without evidence of motion and without any visible artifacts	☐	☐	☐	☐	☐	☐
21. Proper positioning (all anatomy included, evidence of proper centering/alignment, etc.)	☐	☐	☐	☐	☐	☐
22. Proper marker placement	☐	☐	☐	☐	☐	☐
23. Evidence of proper collimation and radiation protection	☐	☐	☐	☐	☐	☐
24. Long vs. short scale of contrast	☐	☐	☐	☐	☐	☐

Comments:

Procedure Evaluator Signature   Repeat Evaluator Signature   Competency Evaluator Signature

Date   Date   Date

END NERVE BLOCK EVALUATION

The objective of
specific radiogr   orming

Student Name:_____

	Procedure Grade	Repeat Grade	Competency Grade

PATIENT INFORMATION OR SIMULATED PROCEDURE *(circle if simulated)*

	Procedure	Repeat	Competency
Age			
Medical Record No.			
Ability to Cooperate			
Condition/Pathology			
Technical Factors Used			
Exposure Index			

FACILITY PREPARATION
The student:

	Procedure Yes	No	Repeat Yes	No	Competency Yes	No
1. Identifies the correct patient and examination according to the requisition.	☐	☐	☐	☐	☐	☐
2. Locates and drives the mobile unit to the patient's room.	☐	☐	☐	☐	☐	☐
3. Politely asks the patient's visitors to wait outside the room until the examination is complete.	☐	☐	☐	☐	☐	☐
4. Explains the examination in terms the parent/guardian fully understands, and properly communicates with the patient and parent/guardian throughout the examination.	☐	☐	☐	☐	☐	☐
5. Obtains and documents the patient's history before the examination.	☐	☐	☐	☐	☐	☐
6. If she intends to stay in the room during the exposure, asks the patient's mother/female guardian of childbearing age the date of her last menstrual period and documents this; inquires about the possibility of pregnancy and has her sign a pregnancy consent form.	☐	☐	☐	☐	☐	☐
7. Removes all obscuring objects (snaps, jewelry, personal belongings, etc.) so as *not* to produce radiographic artifacts.	☐	☐	☐	☐	☐	☐
8. Respects the patient's modesty and provides ample comfort for the patient.	☐	☐	☐	☐	☐	☐
9. Examines the room and adjusts any furniture before bringing in the mobile unit.	☐	☐	☐	☐	☐	☐
10. Examines the patient and selects the appropriate cassette, according to the patient's size and examination.	☐	☐	☐	☐	☐	☐
11. Adjusts the patient into the erect or supine position, as appropriate.	☐	☐	☐	☐	☐	☐
12. Is able to manipulate mobile radiographic equipment with ease, positions it at the patient's bedside, and centers the central ray to the cassette.	☐	☐	☐	☐	☐	☐
13. Adjusts the tube to the proper SID.	☐	☐	☐	☐	☐	☐

Comments:

_____

_____

(continued)

PATIENT POSITIONING FOR A PEDIATRIC MOBILE STUDY
The student:

	Procedure		Repeat		Competency	
	Yes	No	Yes	No	Yes	No
14. Places the appropriate size cassette behind the patient lengthwise or crosswise, depending on the part being radiographed and adjusts the cassette so that the image includes all the necessary anatomy. For conventional cassettes, the flash must be away from any anatomy.	☐	☐	☐	☐	☐	☐
15. Centers the central ray to the midline of the affected area.	☐	☐	☐	☐	☐	☐
16. Directs the central ray perpendicularly or with the appropriate angle relative to the part being radiographed..	☐	☐	☐	☐	☐	☐

Comments:

IMPORTANT DETAILS
The student:

	Procedure		Repeat		Competency	
	Yes	No	Yes	No	Yes	No
17. Instills confidence in the patient by exhibiting self-confidence throughout the examination.	☐	☐	☐	☐	☐	☐
18. Places a lead marker in the appropriate area of the cassette (top/bottom/anteriorly/laterally), where it will be visualized on the finished radiograph, on the proper anatomical side (right/left), and in the appropriate position (face up/face down), depending on the patient's position.	☐	☐	☐	☐	☐	☐
19. Provides radiation protection (shield) for the patient, self, and others.	☐	☐	☐	☐	☐	☐
20. Applies proper collimation and makes adjustments as necessary.	☐	☐	☐	☐	☐	☐
21. Sets the proper kVp, mA, and time and makes adjustments as necessary.	☐	☐	☐	☐	☐	☐
22. While standing at least 6 feet away, exposes the cassette while watching for proper inspiration or expiration, especially if the child is crying or there is other motion, *for each projection.*	☐	☐	☐	☐	☐	☐
23. Provides each radiograph with the proper identification (flash) and/or processes each cassette (image) without difficulty (regardless of technology: film or CR).	☐	☐	☐	☐	☐	☐
24. Properly completes the examination by filling out all necessary paperwork and entering the examination in the computer.	☐	☐	☐	☐	☐	☐
25. Exhibits the ability to adapt to new and difficult situations if and when necessary.	☐	☐	☐	☐	☐	☐
26. Accepts constructive criticism and uses it to his or her advantage.	☐	☐	☐	☐	☐	☐
27. Leaves the room neat and puts things back the way they were before he or she entered.	☐	☐	☐	☐	☐	☐
28. Completes the examination within a reasonable time frame.	☐	☐	☐	☐	☐	☐
29. Returns the mobile unit to the proper location and charges it as needed.	☐	☐	☐	☐	☐	☐

Comments:

RADIOGRAPHIC IMAGE QUALITY
The student is able to critique his or her radiographs as to whether they demonstrate:

	Procedure		Repeat		Competency	
	Yes	No	Yes	No	Yes	No
30. Proper technique/optimal density	☐	☐	☐	☐	☐	☐
31. Enhanced detail, without evidence of motion and without any visible artifacts	☐	☐	☐	☐	☐	☐

	Procedure		Repeat		Competency	
	Yes	No	Yes	No	Yes	No
32. Proper positioning (all anatomy included, evidence of proper centering/alignment, etc.)	☐	☐	☐	☐	☐	☐
33. Proper marker placement	☐	☐	☐	☐	☐	☐
34. Evidence of proper collimation and radiation protection	☐	☐	☐	☐	☐	☐
35. Long vs. short scale of contrast	☐	☐	☐	☐	☐	☐

Comments:

_____

_____

PEDIATRIC ANATOMY
The student is able to identify:

	Procedure		Repeat		Competency	
	Yes	No	Yes	No	Yes	No
36. _____	☐	☐	☐	☐	☐	☐
37. _____	☐	☐	☐	☐	☐	☐
38. _____	☐	☐	☐	☐	☐	☐
39. _____	☐	☐	☐	☐	☐	☐
40. _____	☐	☐	☐	☐	☐	☐
41. _____	☐	☐	☐	☐	☐	☐
42. _____	☐	☐	☐	☐	☐	☐
43. Obvious pathology	☐	☐	☐	☐	☐	☐

Comments:

_____

_____

_____   _____   _____
Procedure Evaluator Signature   Repeat Evaluator Signature   Competency Evaluator Signature

_____   _____   _____
Date   Date   Date

END PEDIATRIC MOBILE STUDY (AGE 6 OR YOUNGER) EVALUATION

Gastrointestinal/Urinary

Single-Contrast Barium Enema

The objective of this evaluation is to determine the student's competency level when performing specific radiographic examinations.

Student Name: _____

Procedure Grade	Repeat Grade	Competency Grade

PATIENT INFORMATION OR SIMULATED PROCEDURE *(circle if simulated)*

	Procedure	Repeat	Competency
Age			
Medical Record No.			
Ability to Cooperate			
Condition/Pathology			
Technical Factors Used			
Exposure Index			

FACILITY PREPARATION
The student:

	Procedure Yes / No	Repeat Yes / No	Competency Yes / No
1. Examines the radiographic room and cleans/straightens it before escorting the patient in.	☐ ☐	☐ ☐	☐ ☐
2. Has all equipment and supplies (patient gown, shield, markers, tape, cassettes, lead aprons, blockers, hemostats, compression paddle, lubricant, proper contrast material, etc.) readily available before escorting the patient in, the Bucky drawer in the proper position, the monitor by the table, and the fluoro on.	☐ ☐	☐ ☐	☐ ☐

Additional supplies:

_____
_____
_____
_____

	Procedure Yes / No	Repeat Yes / No	Competency Yes / No
3. Selects and prepares the contrast material without difficulty.	▨ ▨	▨ ▨	☐ ☐
4. Is able to manipulate all radiographic equipment with ease, and centers the central ray to the cassette/receptor *for all projections.*	☐ ☐	☐ ☐	☐ ☐
5. Adjusts the tube to the proper SID *for all projections.*	☐ ☐	☐ ☐	☐ ☐
6. Selects cassettes/receptor of the appropriate sizes *for all projections,* according to the patient's size and examination.	☐ ☐	☐ ☐	☐ ☐

Comments:

_____

_____

PATIENT PREPARATION
The student:

	Procedure Yes / No	Repeat Yes / No	Competency Yes / No
7. Identifies the correct patient and examination according to the requisition while establishing a good rapport with him or her.	☐ ☐	☐ ☐	☐ ☐

(continued)

	Procedure		Repeat		Competency	
	Yes	No	Yes	No	Yes	No
8. Obtains and documents the patient's history before the examination, including whether the patient ate before the examination and preparation instructions.	☑	☑	☑	☑	☐	☐
9. Thoroughly explains the examination in terms the patient fully understands and properly communicates with the patient throughout the examination.	☐	☐	☐	☐	☐	☐
10. Asks female patients of childbearing age the date of their last menstrual period and documents this; inquires about the possibility of pregnancy and has them sign pregnancy consent forms.	☐	☐	☐	☐	☐	☐
11. Removes all obscuring objects (snaps, zippers, jewelry, belts, etc.) so as *not* to produce radiographic artifacts.	☐	☐	☐	☐	☐	☐
12. Places the patient in the Sims' position, inserts the enema tip, and secures it with a reasonable amount of tape.	☑	☑	☑	☑	☐	☐
13. Respects the patient's modesty and provides ample comfort for the patient while positioning him or her prone to begin the examination.	☐	☐	☐	☐	☐	☐
14. Performs a scout radiograph when indicated.	☐	☐	☐	☐	☐	☐

Comments:

_____

_____

TASKS DURING FLUOROSCOPY
The student:

	Procedure		Repeat		Competency	
	Yes	No	Yes	No	Yes	No
15. Relays the patient's history to the radiologist.	☑	☑	☑	☑	☐	☐
16. Assists the radiologist throughout the examination.	☑	☑	☑	☑	☐	☐
17. Monitors, communicates with, and assists the patient throughout the examination.	☑	☑	☑	☑	☐	☐
18. Takes charge of the examination after the radiologist departs.	☑	☑	☑	☑	☐	☐

Comments:

_____

_____

PATIENT POSITIONING FOR A SINGLE-CONTRAST BARIUM ENEMA
Supine Abdomen
The student:

	Procedure		Repeat		Competency	
	Yes	No	Yes	No	Yes	No
19. Places the patient in the supine position on the radiographic table, with arms at sides and without rotation.	☐	☐	☐	☐	☐	☐
20. Selects the appropriate receptor or places the cassette lengthwise. For conventional cassettes, the flash must be at the bottom and away from any anatomy.	☐	☐	☐	☐	☐	☐
21. Centers the central ray to the midsagittal plane of the body.	☐	☐	☐	☐	☐	☐
22. Directs the central ray perpendicularly at the level of the iliac crest.	☐	☐	☐	☐	☐	☐

Axial (Sigmoid)
The student:

	Procedure		Repeat		Competency	
	Yes	No	Yes	No	Yes	No
23. Places the patient in the supine or prone position on the radiographic table, with arms at sides and without rotation.	☐	☐	☐	☐	☐	☐
24. Selects the appropriate receptor or places the cassette lengthwise. For conventional cassettes, the flash must be at the bottom and away from any anatomy.	☐	☐	☐	☐	☐	☐

	Procedure		Repeat		Competency	
	Yes	No	Yes	No	Yes	No
25. Centers the central ray to the midsagittal plane of the body.	☐	☐	☐	☐	☐	☐
26. Directs the central ray at an angle of 30–40° cephalad if supine, or 30–40° caudad if prone, centered at the level of the anterosuperior iliac spine (ASIS).	☐	☐	☐	☐	☐	☐

RPO or LAO
The student:

	Procedure		Repeat		Competency	
	Yes	No	Yes	No	Yes	No
27. Places the patient in the oblique position, at a 35–45° angle.	☐	☐	☐	☐	☐	☐
28. Selects the appropriate receptor or places the cassette lengthwise. For conventional cassettes, the flash must be at the bottom and away from any anatomy.	☐	☐	☐	☐	☐	☐
29. Centers the central ray midway between the lateral surfaces of the abdomen, making sure both flexures will be fully demonstrated on the radiograph.	☐	☐	☐	☐	☐	☐
30. Centers the central ray perpendicularly at the level of the iliac crest.	☐	☐	☐	☐	☐	☐

LPO or RAO
The student:

	Procedure		Repeat		Competency	
	Yes	No	Yes	No	Yes	No
31. Places the patient in the oblique position, at a 35–45° angle.	☐	☐	☐	☐	☐	☐
32. Selects the appropriate receptor or places the cassette lengthwise. For conventional cassettes, the flash must be at the bottom and away from any anatomy.	☐	☐	☐	☐	☐	☐
33. Centers the central ray midway between the lateral surfaces of the abdomen, making sure both flexures will be fully demonstrated on the radiograph.	☐	☐	☐	☐	☐	☐
34. Centers the central ray perpendicularly at the level of the iliac crest.	☐	☐	☐	☐	☐	☐

Left Lateral Rectum
The student:

	Procedure		Repeat		Competency	
	Yes	No	Yes	No	Yes	No
35. Places the patient in the left lateral position on the radiographic table, without rotation.	☐	☐	☐	☐	☐	☐
36. Selects the appropriate receptor or places the cassette lengthwise. For conventional cassettes, the flash must be at the bottom and away from any anatomy.	☐	☐	☐	☐	☐	☐
37. Raises the patient's arms up above the area of the abdomen.	☐	☐	☐	☐	☐	☐
38. Directs the central ray perpendicularly at the level of the rectum.	☐	☐	☐	☐	☐	☐

Comments:

_____

_____

IMPORTANT DETAILS
The student:

	Procedure		Repeat		Competency	
	Yes	No	Yes	No	Yes	No
39. Instills confidence in the patient by exhibiting self-confidence throughout the examination.	☐	☐	☐	☐	☐	☐

(continued)

	Procedure		Repeat		Competency	
	Yes	No	Yes	No	Yes	No
40. Places a lead marker in the appropriate area of the cassette/receptor (top/bottom/anteriorly/laterally), where it will be visualized on the finished radiograph, on the proper anatomical side (right/left), and in the appropriate position (face up/face down), depending on the patient's position.	☐	☐	☐	☐	☐	☐
41. Provides radiation protection (shield) for the patient (when appropriate), self, and others (closes doors).	☐	☐	☐	☐	☐	☐
42. Applies proper collimation and makes adjustments as necessary.	☐	☐	☐	☐	☐	☐
43. Properly measures the patient along the course of the central ray *for each projection.*	☐	☐	☐	☐	☐	☐
44. Sets the proper technique *for fluoroscopy* (kVp, mA, time).	☐	☐	☐	☐	☐	☐

And all projections/spot images:

Conventional systems

- Sets the proper kVp, mA, and time and makes adjustments as necessary.

or

CR or DR systems
- Identifies the patient on the work-list (or manually types the patient information into the system).
- Selects appropriate body region, specific body part, and accurate view/projection.
- Double-checks preset parameters:
  —Adult vs. pediatric patients
  ○ Small, medium, or large
  —Bucky/receptor (upright vs. table) or non-Bucky
  —AEC vs. fixed
  ○ If AEC, checks ion chambers
  ○ Density setting
  —kVp and mA; adjusts if necessary
  —Focal spot/filament size

	Procedure		Repeat		Competency	
45. Exposes the cassette/receptor after telling the patient to hold still and after giving him or her proper breathing instructions (expiration) *for each projection.*	☐	☐	☐	☐	☐	☐
46. Provides each radiograph with the proper identification (flash) and/or processes each cassette (image) without difficulty (regardless of technology—film, CR, or DR).	▨	▨	▨	▨	☐	☐
47. Properly completes the examination by filling out all necessary paperwork, entering the examination in the computer, having the images checked by the appropriate staff members, answering any last-minute questions, and informing the patient that he or she is finished. Provides proper post-exam instructions as required.	▨	▨	▨	▨	☐	☐
48. Exhibits the ability to adapt to new and difficult situations if and when necessary.	▨	▨	▨	▨	☐	☐
49. Accepts constructive criticism and uses it to his or her advantage.	☐	☐	☐	☐	☐	☐
50. Leaves the radiographic room neat and clean for the next examination.	▨	▨	▨	▨	☐	☐
51. Completes the examination within a reasonable time frame.	☐	☐	☐	☐	☐	☐

Comments:

RADIOGRAPHIC IMAGE QUALITY
The student is able to critique his or her radiographs as to whether they demonstrate:

	Procedure Yes	No	Repeat Yes	No	Competency Yes	No
52. Proper technique/optimal density	☑	☑	☑	☑	☐	☐
53. Enhanced detail, without evidence of motion and without any visible artifacts	☑	☑	☑	☑	☐	☐
54. Proper positioning (all anatomy included, evidence of proper centering/alignment, etc.)	☑	☑	☑	☑	☐	☐
55. Proper marker placement						
56. Evidence of proper collimation and radiation protection	☑	☑	☑	☑	☐	☐
57. Long vs. short scale of contrast	☑	☑	☑	☑	☐	☐
58. Image/projection identification and/or other identification	☑	☑	☑	☑	☐	☐

Comments:

_____

_____

ABDOMEN ANATOMY
The student is able to identify:

	Procedure Yes	No	Repeat Yes	No	Competency Yes	No
59. Diaphragm	☑	☑	☑	☑	☐	☐
60. Symphysis pubis	☑	☑	☑	☑	☐	☐
61. Iliac crest	☑	☑	☑	☑	☐	☐
62. Bowel gas	☑	☑	☑	☑	☐	☐
63. Stomach	☑	☑	☑	☑	☐	☐
64. Liver	☑	☑	☑	☑	☐	☐
65. Ileum	☑	☑	☑	☑	☐	☐
66. Cecum/appendix (if applicable)	☑	☑	☑	☑	☐	☐
67. Appendix (if applicable)	☑	☑	☑	☑	☐	☐
68. Ascending colon	☑	☑	☑	☑	☐	☐
69. Hepatic flexure	☑	☑	☑	☑	☐	☐
70. Transverse colon	☑	☑	☑	☑	☐	☐
71. Splenic flexure	☑	☑	☑	☑	☐	☐
72. Descending colon	☑	☑	☑	☑	☐	☐
73. Sigmoid colon	☑	☑	☑	☑	☐	☐
74. Rectum	☑	☑	☑	☑	☐	☐
75. Obvious pathology	☑	☑	☑	☑	☐	☐

Comments:

_____

_____

_____	_____	_____
Procedure Evaluator Signature	Repeat Evaluator Signature	Competency Evaluator Signature
_____	_____	_____
Date	Date	Date

END SINGLE-CONTRAST BARIUM ENEMA EVALUATION

Student Name:_____

Procedure Grade	Repeat Grade	Competency Grade

PATIENT INFORMATION OR SIMULATED PROCEDURE *(circle if simulated)*

	Procedure	Repeat	Competency
Age			
Medical Record No.			
Ability to Cooperate			
Condition/Pathology			
Technical Factors Used			
Exposure Index			

FACILITY PREPARATION
The student:

	Procedure Yes	Procedure No	Repeat Yes	Repeat No	Competency Yes	Competency No
1. Examines the radiographic room and cleans/straightens it before escorting the patient in.	☐	☐	☐	☐	☐	☐
2. Has all equipment and supplies (patient gown, shield, markers, tape, cassettes, lead aprons, blockers, hemostats, compression paddle, lubricant, proper contrast material, etc.) readily available before escorting the patient in, the Bucky drawer in the proper position, the monitor by the table, and the fluoro on.	☐	☐	☐	☐	☐	☐

Additional supplies:

_____
_____
_____
_____

	Procedure Yes	Procedure No	Repeat Yes	Repeat No	Competency Yes	Competency No
3. Selects and prepares the contrast material without difficulty.	▨	▨	▨	▨	☐	☐
4. Is able to manipulate all radiographic equipment with ease, and centers the central ray to the cassette/receptor *for all projections.*	☐	☐	☐	☐	☐	☐
5. Adjusts the tube to the proper SID *for all projections.*	☐	☐	☐	☐	☐	☐
6. Selects cassettes/receptor/receptor of the appropriate sizes *for all projections,* according to the patient's size and examination.	☐	☐	☐	☐	☐	☐

Comments:

_____

_____

PATIENT PREPARATION
The student:

	Procedure Yes	Procedure No	Repeat Yes	Repeat No	Competency Yes	Competency No
7. Identifies the correct patient and examination according to the requisition while establishing a good rapport with him or her.	☐	☐	☐	☐	☐	☐

(continued)

	Procedure		Repeat		Competency	
	Yes	No	Yes	No	Yes	No
8. Obtains and documents the patient's history before the examination, including whether the patient ate before the examination and preparation instructions.	▣	▣	▣	▣	☐	☐
9. Thoroughly explains the examination in terms the patient fully understands and properly communicates with the patient throughout the examination.	☐	☐	☐	☐	☐	☐
10. Asks female patients of childbearing age the date of their last menstrual period and documents this; inquires about the possibility of pregnancy and has them sign pregnancy consent forms.	☐	☐	☐	☐	☐	☐
11. Removes all obscuring objects (snaps, zippers, jewelry, belts, etc.) so as *not* to produce radiographic artifacts.	☐	☐	☐	☐	☐	☐
12. Places the patient in the Sims' position, inserts enema tip, and secures it with a reasonable amount of tape.	▣	▣	▣	▣	☐	☐
13. Respects the patient's modesty and provides ample comfort for the patient while positioning him or her prone to begin the examination.	☐	☐	☐	☐	☐	☐
14. Performs a scout radiograph when indicated.	☐	☐	☐	☐	☐	☐

Comments:

_____

_____

TASKS DURING FLUOROSCOPY
The student:

	Procedure		Repeat		Competency	
	Yes	No	Yes	No	Yes	No
15. Relays the patient's history to the radiologist.	▣	▣	▣	▣	☐	☐
16. Assists the radiologist throughout the examination.	▣	▣	▣	▣	☐	☐
17. Monitors, communicates with, and assists the patient throughout the examination.	▣	▣	▣	▣	☐	☐
18. Takes charge of the examination after the radiologist departs.	▣	▣	▣	▣	☐	☐

Comments:

_____

_____

PATIENT POSITIONING FOR A DOUBLE-CONTRAST BARIUM ENEMA
Supine Abdomen
The student:

	Procedure		Repeat		Competency	
	Yes	No	Yes	No	Yes	No
19. Places the patient in the supine position on the radiographic table, with arms at sides and without rotation.	☐	☐	☐	☐	☐	☐
20. Selects the appropriate receptor or places the cassette lengthwise. For conventional cassettes, the flash must be at the bottom and away from any anatomy.	☐	☐	☐	☐	☐	☐
21. Centers the central ray to the midsagittal plane of the body.	☐	☐	☐	☐	☐	☐
22. Directs the central ray perpendicularly at the level of the iliac crest.	☐	☐	☐	☐	☐	☐

Axial (Sigmoid)
The student:

	Procedure		Repeat		Competency	
	Yes	No	Yes	No	Yes	No
23. Places the patient in the supine or prone position on the radiographic table, with arms at sides and without rotation.	☐	☐	☐	☐	☐	☐

	Procedure		Repeat		Competency	
	Yes	No	Yes	No	Yes	No
24. Selects the appropriate receptor or places the cassette lengthwise. For conventional cassettes, the flash must be at the bottom and away from any anatomy.	☐	☐	☐	☐	☐	☐
25. Centers the central ray to the midsagittal plane of the body.	☐	☐	☐	☐	☐	☐
26. Directs the central ray perpendicularly at the level of the iliac crest.	☐	☐	☐	☐	☐	☐

RPO or LAO
The student:

	Procedure		Repeat		Competency	
	Yes	No	Yes	No	Yes	No
27. Places the patient in the oblique position, at a 35–45° angle.	☐	☐	☐	☐	☐	☐
28. Selects the appropriate receptor or places the cassette lengthwise. For conventional cassettes, the flash must be at the bottom and away from any anatomy.	☐	☐	☐	☐	☐	☐
29. Centers the central ray midway between the lateral surfaces of the abdomen, making sure both flexures will be fully demonstrated on the radiograph.	☐	☐	☐	☐	☐	☐
30. Centers the central ray perpendicularly at the level of the iliac crest.	☐	☐	☐	☐	☐	☐

LPO or RAO
The student:

	Procedure		Repeat		Competency	
	Yes	No	Yes	No	Yes	No
31. Places the patient in the oblique position, at a 35–45° angle.	☐	☐	☐	☐	☐	☐
32. Selects the appropriate receptor or places the cassette lengthwise. For conventional cassettes, the flash must be at the bottom and away from any anatomy.	☐	☐	☐	☐	☐	☐
33. Centers the central ray midway between the lateral surfaces of the abdomen, making sure both flexures will be fully demonstrated on the radiograph.	☐	☐	☐	☐	☐	☐
34. Centers the central ray perpendicularly at the level of the iliac crest.	☐	☐	☐	☐	☐	☐

Cross-Table Lateral Rectum
The student:

	Procedure		Repeat		Competency	
	Yes	No	Yes	No	Yes	No
35. Places the patient in the prone position on the radiographic table, without rotation.	☐	☐	☐	☐	☐	☐
36. Selects the appropriate receptor or places the grid/cassette next to the patient's buttocks as close as possible. For conventional cassettes, the flash must be away from any anatomy.	☐	☐	☐	☐	☐	☐
37. Raises the patient's arms up above the area of the abdomen.	☐	☐	☐	☐	☐	☐
38. Horizontally directs the central ray perpendicularly at the level of the rectum.	☐	☐	☐	☐	☐	☐

Left Lateral Decubitus
The student:

	Procedure		Repeat		Competency	
	Yes	No	Yes	No	Yes	No
39. Places the patient in the left lateral recumbent position, with the patient "built up" to adequately demonstrate the left side.	☐	☐	☐	☐	☐	☐
40. Selects the appropriate receptor or places the grid/cassette lengthwise, as close to the patient as possible. For conventional cassettes, the flash must be at the bottom and away from any anatomy.	☐	☐	☐	☐	☐	☐
41. Instructs the patient to raise his or her arms above the area of the abdomen and adjusts the thorax to a true lateral position, making sure there is no rotation.	☐	☐	☐	☐	☐	☐

(continued)

	Procedure		Repeat		Competency	
	Yes	No	Yes	No	Yes	No
42. Centers the central ray to the midsagittal plane.	☐	☐	☐	☐	☐	☐
43. Directs the central ray perpendicularly at the level of the iliac crest.	☐	☐	☐	☐	☐	☐

Right Lateral Decubitus
The student:

	Procedure		Repeat		Competency	
	Yes	No	Yes	No	Yes	No
44. Places the patient in the right lateral recumbent position, with the patient "built up" to adequately demonstrate the right side.	☐	☐	☐	☐	☐	☐
45. Selects the appropriate receptor or places the grid/cassette lengthwise, as close to the patient as possible. For conventional cassettes, the flash must be at the bottom and away from any anatomy.	☐	☐	☐	☐	☐	☐
46. Instructs the patient to raise his or her arms above the area of the abdomen and adjusts the thorax to a true lateral position, making sure there is no rotation.	☐	☐	☐	☐	☐	☐
47. Centers the central ray to the midsagittal plane.	☐	☐	☐	☐	☐	☐
48. Directs the central ray perpendicularly at the level of the iliac crest.	☐	☐	☐	☐	☐	☐

Erect Abdomen
The student:

	Procedure		Repeat		Competency	
	Yes	No	Yes	No	Yes	No
49. Places the patient in the anteroposterior (AP) erect position against the upright Bucky/receptor, with arms at sides and without rotation.	☐	☐	☐	☐	☐	☐
50. Selects the appropriate receptor or places the cassette lengthwise. For conventional cassettes, the flash must be at the bottom and away from any anatomy.	☐	☐	☐	☐	☐	☐
51. Centers the central ray to the midsagittal plane of the body.	☐	☐	☐	☐	☐	☐
52. Directs the central ray perpendicularly at a level 1–3 inches above the iliac crest.	☐	☐	☐	☐	☐	☐

Prone Abdomen
The student:

	Procedure		Repeat		Competency	
	Yes	No	Yes	No	Yes	No
53. Places the patient in the prone position on the radiographic table, with arms at sides and without rotation.	☐	☐	☐	☐	☐	☐
54. Selects the appropriate receptor or places the cassette lengthwise. For conventional cassettes, the flash must be at the bottom and away from any anatomy.	☐	☐	☐	☐	☐	☐
55. Centers the central ray to the midsagittal plane of the body.	☐	☐	☐	☐	☐	☐
56. Directs the central ray perpendicularly at the level of the iliac crest.	☐	☐	☐	☐	☐	☐

Comments:

_____

_____

IMPORTANT DETAILS
The student:

	Procedure		Repeat		Competency	
	Yes	No	Yes	No	Yes	No
57. Instills confidence in the patient by exhibiting self-confidence throughout the examination.	☐	☐	☐	☐	☐	☐

	Procedure		Repeat		Competency	
	Yes	No	Yes	No	Yes	No
58. Places a lead marker in the appropriate area of the cassette/receptor (top/bottom/anteriorly/laterally), where it will be visualized on the finished radiograph, on the proper anatomical side (right/left), and in the appropriate position (face up/face down), depending on the patient's position.	☐	☐	☐	☐	☐	☐
59. Provides radiation protection (shield) for the patient (when appropriate), self, and others (closes doors).	☐	☐	☐	☐	☐	☐
60. Applies proper collimation and makes adjustments as necessary.	☐	☐	☐	☐	☐	☐
61. Properly measures the patient along the course of the central ray *for each projection.*	☐	☐	☐	☐	☐	☐
62. Sets the proper technique *for fluoroscopy* (kVp, mA, time).	☐	☐	☐	☐	☐	☐

62. *And all projections/spot images:*

Conventional systems

- Sets the proper kVp, mA, and time and makes adjustments as necessary.

or

CR or DR systems
- Identifies the patient on the work-list (or manually types the patient information into the system).
- Selects appropriate body region, specific body part, and accurate view/projection.
- Double-checks preset parameters:
  —Adult vs. pediatric patients
    ○ Small, medium, or large
  —Bucky/receptor (upright vs. table) *or* non-Bucky
  —AEC vs. fixed
    ○ If AEC, checks ion chambers
    ○ Density setting
  —kVp and mA; adjusts if necessary
  —Focal spot/filament size

	Procedure		Repeat		Competency	
63. Exposes the cassette/receptor after telling the patient to hold still and after giving him or her proper breathing instructions (expiration) *for each projection.*	☐	☐	☐	☐	☐	☐
64. Provides each radiograph with the proper identification (flash) and/or processes each cassette (image) without difficulty (regardless of technology—film, CR, or DR).	▨	▨	▨	▨	☐	☐
65. Properly completes the examination by filling out all necessary paperwork, entering the examination in the computer, having the images checked by the appropriate staff members, answering any last-minute questions, and informing the patient that he or she is finished. Provides proper post-exam instructions as required.	▨	▨	▨	▨	☐	☐
66. Exhibits the ability to adapt to new and difficult situations if and when necessary.	▨	▨	▨	▨	☐	☐
67. Accepts constructive criticism and uses it to his or her advantage.	☐	☐	☐	☐	☐	☐
68. Leaves the radiographic room neat and clean for the next examination.	▨	▨	▨	▨	☐	☐
69. Completes the examination within a reasonable time frame.	☐	☐	☐	☐	☐	☐

Comments:

_____

_____

(continued)

RADIOGRAPHIC IMAGE QUALITY
The student is able to critique his or her radiographs as to whether they demonstrate:

	Procedure		Repeat		Competency	
	Yes	No	Yes	No	Yes	No
70. Proper technique/optimal density	☐	☐	☐	☐	☐	☐
71. Enhanced detail, without evidence of motion and without any visible artifacts	☐	☐	☐	☐	☐	☐
72. Proper positioning (all anatomy included, evidence of proper centering/alignment, etc.)	☐	☐	☐	☐	☐	☐
73. Proper marker placement						
74. Evidence of proper collimation and radiation protection	☐	☐	☐	☐	☐	☐
75. Long vs. short scale of contrast	☐	☐	☐	☐	☐	☐
76. Image/projection identification and/or other identification	☐	☐	☐	☐	☐	☐

Comments:

_____

_____

ABDOMEN ANATOMY
The student is able to identify:

	Procedure		Repeat		Competency	
	Yes	No	Yes	No	Yes	No
77. Diaphragm	☐	☐	☐	☐	☐	☐
78. Symphysis pubis	☐	☐	☐	☐	☐	☐
79. Iliac crest	☐	☐	☐	☐	☐	☐
80. Bowel gas	☐	☐	☐	☐	☐	☐
81. Stomach	☐	☐	☐	☐	☐	☐
82. Liver	☐	☐	☐	☐	☐	☐
83. Ileum	☐	☐	☐	☐	☐	☐
84. Cecum/appendix (if applicable)	☐	☐	☐	☐	☐	☐
85. Appendix (if applicable)	☐	☐	☐	☐	☐	☐
86. Ascending colon	☐	☐	☐	☐	☐	☐
87. Hepatic flexure	☐	☐	☐	☐	☐	☐
88. Transverse colon	☐	☐	☐	☐	☐	☐
89. Splenic flexure	☐	☐	☐	☐	☐	☐
90. Descending colon	☐	☐	☐	☐	☐	☐
91. Sigmoid colon	☐	☐	☐	☐	☐	☐
92. Rectum	☐	☐	☐	☐	☐	☐
93. Obvious pathology	☐	☐	☐	☐	☐	☐

Comments:

_____

_____

Procedure Evaluator Signature	Repeat Evaluator Signature	Competency Evaluator Signature
Date	Date	Date

END DOUBLE-CONTRAST BARIUM ENEMA EVALUATION

Student Name:_____

PATIENT INFORMATION OR SIMULATED PROCEDURE *(circle if simulated)*

	Procedure	Repeat	Competency
Age			
Medical Record No.			
Ability to Cooperate			
Condition/Pathology			
Technical Factors Used			
Exposure Index			

FACILITY PREPARATION
The student:

	Procedure Yes	No	Repeat Yes	No	Competency Yes	No
1. Examines the radiographic room and cleans/straightens it before escorting the patient in.	☐	☐	☐	☐	☐	☐
2. Has all equipment and supplies (patient gown, shield, markers, tape, cassettes, lead aprons, blockers, hemostats, compression paddle, proper contrast material, etc.) readily available before escorting the patient in, the Bucky drawer in the proper position, the monitor by the table, and the fluoro on.	☐	☐	☐	☐	☐	☐

Additional supplies:

_____
_____
_____
_____

	Procedure Yes	No	Repeat Yes	No	Competency Yes	No
3. Selects and prepares the contrast material without difficulty.	▨	▨	▨	▨	☐	☐
4. Is able to manipulate all radiographic equipment with ease, and centers the central ray to the cassette/receptor *for all projections.*	☐	☐	☐	☐	☐	☐
5. Adjusts the tube to the proper SID *for all projections.*	☐	☐	☐	☐	☐	☐
6. Selects cassettes/receptor/receptor of the appropriate sizes *for all projections,* according to the patient's size and examination.	☐	☐	☐	☐	☐	☐

Comments:

_____
_____

PATIENT PREPARATION
The student:

	Procedure Yes	No	Repeat Yes	No	Competency Yes	No
7. Identifies the correct patient and examination according to the requisition while establishing a good rapport with him or her.	☐	☐	☐	☐	☐	☐

(continued)

	Procedure		Repeat		Competency	
	Yes	No	Yes	No	Yes	No
8. Obtains and documents the patient's history before the examination, including whether the patient ate before the examination and preparation instructions.	▣	▣	▣	▣	☐	☐
9. Thoroughly explains the examination in terms the patient fully understands and properly communicates with the patient throughout the examination.	☐	☐	☐	☐	☐	☐
10. Asks female patients of childbearing age the date of their last menstrual period and documents this; inquires about the possibility of pregnancy and has them sign pregnancy consent forms.	☐	☐	☐	☐	☐	☐
11. Removes all obscuring objects (snaps, zippers, jewelry, belts, etc.) so as *not* to produce radiographic artifacts.	☐	☐	☐	☐	☐	☐
12. Respects the patient's modesty and provides ample comfort for the patient while positioning him or her prone to begin the examination (RAO).	☐	☐	☐	☐	☐	☐
13. Performs a scout radiograph when indicated.	☐	☐	☐	☐	☐	☐

Comments:

_____

_____

TASKS DURING FLUOROSCOPY
The student:

	Procedure		Repeat		Competency	
	Yes	No	Yes	No	Yes	No
14. Relays the patient's history to the radiologist.	▣	▣	▣	▣	☐	☐
15. Assists the radiologist throughout the examination.	▣	▣	▣	▣	☐	☐
16. Monitors, communicates with, and assists the patient throughout the examination.	▣	▣	▣	▣	☐	☐
17. Takes charge of the examination after the radiologist departs.	▣	▣	▣	▣	☐	☐

Comments:

_____

_____

PATIENT POSITIONING FOR A SINGLE-CONSTRACT UPPER GI
Supine or Prone Abdomen
The student:

	Procedure		Repeat		Competency	
	Yes	No	Yes	No	Yes	No
18. Places the patient in the supine position on the radiographic table, with arms at sides and without rotation.	☐	☐	☐	☐	☐	☐
19. Selects the appropriate receptor or places the cassette lengthwise. For conventional cassettes, the flash must be at the bottom and away from any anatomy.	☐	☐	☐	☐	☐	☐
20. Centers the central ray to the midsagittal plane of the body.	☐	☐	☐	☐	☐	☐
21. Directs the central ray perpendicularly at a level 2–3 inches above the iliac crest.	☐	☐	☐	☐	☐	☐

LPO or RAO
The student:

	Procedure		Repeat		Competency	
	Yes	No	Yes	No	Yes	No
22. Places the patient in the oblique position at a 45° angle (30–70°, depending on body habitus).	☐	☐	☐	☐	☐	☐

	Procedure		Repeat		Competency	
	Yes	No	Yes	No	Yes	No
23. Selects the appropriate receptor or places the cassette lengthwise. For conventional cassettes, the flash must be at the bottom and away from any anatomy.	☐	☐	☐	☐	☐	☐
24. Centers the central ray between the spinous processes and the left lateral border so that the stomach will be fully demonstrated on the radiograph.	☐	☐	☐	☐	☐	☐
25. Centers the central ray perpendicularly at a level 2–3 inches above the iliac crest.	☐	☐	☐	☐	☐	☐

RIGHT LATERAL
The student:

	Procedure		Repeat		Competency	
	Yes	No	Yes	No	Yes	No
26. Places the patient in the right lateral position, without rotation.	☐	☐	☐	☐	☐	☐
27. Selects the appropriate receptor or places the cassette lengthwise. For conventional cassettes, the flash must be at the bottom and away from any anatomy.	☐	☐	☐	☐	☐	☐
28. Centers the central ray midway between the midcoronal plane and the anterior surface of the abdominal cavity.	☐	☐	☐	☐	☐	☐
29. Centers the central ray perpendicularly, to the level of L2, or if erect, to L3.	☐	☐	☐	☐	☐	☐

Comments:

_____

_____

IMPORTANT DETAILS
The student:

	Procedure		Repeat		Competency	
	Yes	No	Yes	No	Yes	No
30. Instills confidence in the patient by exhibiting self-confidence throughout the examination.	☐	☐	☐	☐	☐	☐
31. Places a lead marker in the appropriate area of the cassette/receptor (top/bottom/anteriorly/laterally), where it will be visualized on the finished radiograph, on the proper anatomical side (right/left), and in the appropriate position (face up/face down), depending on the patient's position.	☐	☐	☐	☐	☐	☐
32. Provides radiation protection (shield) for the patient (when appropriate), self, and others (closes doors).	☐	☐	☐	☐	☐	☐
33. Applies proper collimation and makes adjustments as necessary.	☐	☐	☐	☐	☐	☐
34. Properly measures the patient along the course of the central ray *for each projection.*	☐	☐	☐	☐	☐	☐
35. Sets the proper technique *for fluoroscopy* (kVp, mA, time).	☐	☐	☐	☐	☐	☐

And all projections/spot images:

Conventional systems

• Sets the proper kVp, mA, and time and makes adjustments as necessary.

or

CR or DR systems
• Identifies the patient on the work-list (or manually types the patient information into the system).
• Selects appropriate body region, specific body part, and accurate view/projection.
• Double-checks preset parameters:
  —Adult vs. pediatric patients
    ○ Small, medium, or large
  —Bucky/receptor (upright vs. table) or non-Bucky

(continued)

—AEC vs. fixed
  ○ If AEC, checks ion chambers
  ○ Density setting
—kVp and mA; adjusts if necessary
—Focal spot/filament size

	Procedure		Repeat		Competency	
	Yes	No	Yes	No	Yes	No
36. Exposes the cassette/receptor after telling the patient to hold still and after giving him or her proper breathing instructions (expiration) *for each projection.*	☐	☐	☐	☐	☐	☐
37. Provides each radiograph with the proper identification (flash) and/or processes each cassette (image) without difficulty (regardless of technology—film, CR, or DR).	☑	☑	☑	☑	☐	☐
38. Properly completes the examination by filling out all necessary paperwork, entering the examination in the computer, having the images checked by the appropriate staff members, answering any last-minute questions, and informing the patient that he or she is finished. Provides proper post-exam instructions as required.	☑	☑	☑	☑	☐	☐
39. Exhibits the ability to adapt to new and difficult situations if and when necessary.	☑	☑	☑	☑	☐	☐
40. Accepts constructive criticism and uses it to his or her advantage.	☐	☐	☐	☐	☐	☐
41. Leaves the radiographic room neat and clean for the next examination.	☑	☑	☑	☑	☐	☐
42. Completes the examination within a reasonable time frame.	☐	☐	☐	☐	☐	☐

Comments:

_____

_____

RADIOGRAPHIC IMAGE QUALITY
The student is able to critique his or her radiographs as to whether they demonstrate:

	Procedure		Repeat		Competency	
	Yes	No	Yes	No	Yes	No
43. Proper technique/optimal density	☑	☑	☑	☑	☐	☐
44. Enhanced detail, without evidence of motion and without any visible artifacts	☑	☑	☑	☑	☐	☐
45. Proper positioning (all anatomy included, evidence of proper centering/alignment, etc.)	☑	☑	☑	☑	☐	☐
46. Proper marker placement						
47. Evidence of proper collimation and radiation protection	☑	☑	☑	☑	☐	☐
48. Long vs. short scale of contrast	☑	☑	☑	☑	☐	☐
49. Image/projection identification and/or other identification	☑	☑	☑	☑	☐	☐

Comments:

_____

_____

ABDOMEN ANATOMY
The student is able to identify:

	Procedure		Repeat		Competency	
	Yes	No	Yes	No	Yes	No
50. Diaphragm	☑	☑	☑	☑	☐	☐
51. Symphysis pubis	☑	☑	☑	☑	☐	☐
52. Iliac crest	☑	☑	☑	☑	☐	☐
53. Small vs. large bowel (gas)	☑	☑	☑	☑	☐	☐

	Procedure		Repeat		Competency	
	Yes	No	Yes	No	Yes	No
54. Liver	☐	☐	☐	☐	☐	☐
55. Lesser and greater curvatures	☐	☐	☐	☐	☐	☐
56. Fundus	☐	☐	☐	☐	☐	☐
57. Body	☐	☐	☐	☐	☐	☐
58. Pylorus	☐	☐	☐	☐	☐	☐
59. Cardiac and pyloric antrums/sphincters	☐	☐	☐	☐	☐	☐
60. Duodenum	☐	☐	☐	☐	☐	☐
61. Rugal folds	☐	☐	☐	☐	☐	☐
62. Obvious pathology	☐	☐	☐	☐	☐	☐

Comments:

_____

_____

_____ _____ _____
Procedure Evaluator Signature   Repeat Evaluator Signature   Competency Evaluator Signature

_____ _____ _____
Date   Date   Date

END SINGLE-CONTRAST GASTROINTESTINAL SERIES EVALUATION

Double-Contrast Gastrointestinal Series

The objective of this evaluation is to determine the student's competency level when performing specific radiographic examinations.

Student Name:_____

	Procedure Grade	Repeat Grade	Competency Grade

PATIENT INFORMATION OR SIMULATED PROCEDURE *(circle if simulated)*

	Procedure	Repeat	Competency
Age			
Medical Record No.			
Ability to Cooperate			
Condition/Pathology			
Technical Factors Used			
Exposure Index			

FACILITY PREPARATION
The student:

	Procedure Yes	No	Repeat Yes	No	Competency Yes	No
1. Examines the radiographic room and cleans/straightens it before escorting the patient in.	☐	☐	☐	☐	☐	☐
2. Has all equipment and supplies (patient gown, shield, markers, tape, cassettes, lead aprons, blockers, hemostats, compression paddle, proper contrast material, etc.) readily available before escorting the patient in, the Bucky drawer in the proper position, the monitor by the table, and the fluoro on.	☐	☐	☐	☐	☐	☐

Additional supplies:

_____
_____
_____
_____

	Procedure Yes	No	Repeat Yes	No	Competency Yes	No
3. Selects and prepares the contrast material without difficulty.	▣	▣	▣	▣	☐	☐
4. Is able to manipulate all radiographic equipment with ease, and centers the central ray to the cassette/receptor *for all projections.*	☐	☐	☐	☐	☐	☐
5. Adjusts the tube to the proper SID *for each projections.*	☐	☐	☐	☐	☐	☐
6. Selects cassettes/receptor/receptor of the appropriate sizes *for all projections,* according to the patient's size and examination.	☐	☐	☐	☐	☐	☐

Comments:

_____
_____

PATIENT PREPARATION
The student:

	Procedure Yes	No	Repeat Yes	No	Competency Yes	No
7. Identifies the correct patient and examination according to the requisition while establishing a good rapport with him or her.	☐	☐	☐	☐	☐	☐

(continued)

	Procedure		Repeat		Competency	
	Yes	No	Yes	No	Yes	No
8. Obtains and documents the patient's history before the examination, including whether the patient ate before the examination and preparation instructions.	☑	☑	☑	☑	☐	☐
9. Thoroughly explains the examination in terms the patient fully understands and properly communicates with the patient throughout the examination.	☐	☐	☐	☐	☐	☐
10. Asks female patients of childbearing age the date of their last menstrual period and documents this; inquires about the possibility of pregnancy and has them sign pregnancy consent forms.	☐	☐	☐	☐	☐	☐
11. Removes all obscuring objects (snaps, zippers, jewelry, belts, etc.) so as *not* to produce radiographic artifacts.	☐	☐	☐	☐	☐	☐
12. Respects the patient's modesty and provides ample comfort for the patient while positioning him or her to begin the examination (double GI with or without small bowel series (SBS), and esophagrams and barium swallows—AP standing).	☐	☐	☐	☐	☐	☐
13. Performs a scout radiograph when indicated.	☐	☐	☐	☐	☐	☐

Comments:

_____

_____

TASKS DURING FLUOROSCOPY
The student:

	Procedure		Repeat		Competency	
	Yes	No	Yes	No	Yes	No
14. Relays the patient's history to the radiologist.	☑	☑	☑	☑	☐	☐
15. Assists the radiologist throughout the examination.	☑	☑	☑	☑	☐	☐
16. Monitors, communicates with, and assists the patient throughout the examination.	☑	☑	☑	☑	☐	☐
17. Takes charge of the examination after the radiologist departs.	☑	☑	☑	☑	☐	☐

Comments:

_____

_____

PATIENT POSITIONING FOR A DOUBLE-CONTRAST UPPER GI
Supine/Prone Abdomen
The student:

	Procedure		Repeat		Competency	
	Yes	No	Yes	No	Yes	No
18. Places the patient in the supine or prone position on the radiographic table, with arms at sides and without rotation.	☐	☐	☐	☐	☐	☐
19. Selects the appropriate receptor or places the cassette lengthwise. For conventional cassettes, the flash must be at the bottom and away from any anatomy.	☐	☐	☐	☐	☐	☐
20. Centers the central ray to the midsagittal plane of the body.	☐	☐	☐	☐	☐	☐
21. Directs the central ray perpendicularly at a level 2–3 inches above the iliac crest.	☐	☐	☐	☐	☐	☐

LPO or RAO
The student:

	Procedure		Repeat		Competency	
	Yes	No	Yes	No	Yes	No
22. Places the patient in the oblique position at a 45° angle (40–70° from prone).	☐	☐	☐	☐	☐	☐

	Procedure		Repeat		Competency	
	Yes	No	Yes	No	Yes	No
23. Selects the appropriate receptor or places the cassette lengthwise. For conventional cassettes, the flash must be at the bottom and away from any anatomy.	☐	☐	☐	☐	☐	☐
24. Centers the central ray between the spinous processes and the left lateral border so that the stomach will be fully demonstrated on the radiograph.	☐	☐	☐	☐	☐	☐
25. Centers the central ray perpendicularly at a level 2–3 inches above the iliac crest or 1–2 inches above the lowest level of the ribs (level of L1-L2).	☐	☐	☐	☐	☐	☐

Right Lateral
The student:

	Procedure		Repeat		Competency	
	Yes	No	Yes	No	Yes	No
26. Places the patient in the right lateral position, without rotation.	☐	☐	☐	☐	☐	☐
27. Selects the appropriate receptor or places the cassette lengthwise. For conventional cassettes, the flash must be at the bottom and away from any anatomy.	☐	☐	☐	☐	☐	☐
28. Centers the central ray midway between the midcoronal plane and the anterior surface of the abdominal cavity.	☐	☐	☐	☐	☐	☐
29. Centers the central ray perpendicularly, to the level of L2, or if erect, to L3.	☐	☐	☐	☐	☐	☐

Comments:

_____

_____

IMPORTANT DETAILS
The student:

	Procedure		Repeat		Competency	
	Yes	No	Yes	No	Yes	No
30. Instills confidence in the patient by exhibiting self-confidence throughout the examination.	☐	☐	☐	☐	☐	☐
31. Places a lead marker in the appropriate area of the cassette/receptor (top/bottom/anteriorly/laterally), where it will be visualized on the finished radiograph, on the proper anatomical side (right/left), and in the appropriate position (face up/face down), depending on the patient's position.	☐	☐	☐	☐	☐	☐
32. Provides radiation protection (shield) for the patient (when appropriate), self, and others (closes doors).	☐	☐	☐	☐	☐	☐
33. Applies proper collimation and makes adjustments as necessary.	☐	☐	☐	☐	☐	☐
34. Properly measures the patient along the course of the central ray *for each projection.*	☐	☐	☐	☐	☐	☐
35. Sets the proper technique *for fluoroscopy* (kVp, mA, time).	☐	☐	☐	☐	☐	☐

And all projections/spot images:

Conventional systems

- Sets the proper kVp, mA, and time and makes adjustments as necessary.

or

CR or DR systems
- Identifies the patient on the work-list (or manually types the patient information into the system).
- Selects appropriate body region, specific body part, and accurate view/projection.
- Double-checks preset parameters:
  —Adult vs. pediatric patients
    ○ Small, medium, or large

(continued)

	Procedure		Repeat		Competency	
	Yes	No	Yes	No	Yes	No

—Bucky/receptor (upright vs. table) *or* non-Bucky
—AEC vs. fixed
   ◦ If AEC, checks ion chambers
   ◦ Density setting
—kVp and mA; adjusts if necessary
—Focal spot/filament size

	Procedure		Repeat		Competency	
	Yes	No	Yes	No	Yes	No
36. Exposes the cassette/receptor after telling the patient to hold still and after giving him or her proper breathing instructions (expiration) *for each projection.*	☐	☐	☐	☐	☐	☐
37. Provides each radiograph with the proper identification (flash) and/or processes each cassette (image) without difficulty (regardless of technology—film, CR, or DR).	▣	▣	▣	▣	☐	☐
38. Properly completes the examination by filling out all necessary paperwork, entering the examination in the computer, having the images checked by the appropriate staff members, answering any last-minute questions, and informing the patient that he or she is finished. Provides proper post-exam instructions as required.	▣	▣	▣	▣	☐	☐
39. Exhibits the ability to adapt to new and difficult situations if and when necessary.	▣	▣	▣	▣	☐	☐
40. Accepts constructive criticism and uses it to his or her advantage.	☐	☐	☐	☐	☐	☐
41. Leaves the radiographic room neat and clean for the next examination.	▣	▣	▣	▣	☐	☐
42. Completes the examination within a reasonable time frame.	☐	☐	☐	☐	☐	☐

Comments:
_____
_____

RADIOGRAPHIC IMAGE QUALITY
The student is able to critique his or her radiographs as to whether they demonstrate:

	Procedure		Repeat		Competency	
	Yes	No	Yes	No	Yes	No
43. Proper technique/optimal density	▣	▣	▣	▣	☐	☐
44. Enhanced detail, without evidence of motion and without any visible artifacts	▣	▣	▣	▣	☐	☐
45. Proper positioning (all anatomy included, evidence of proper centering/alignment, etc.)	▣	▣	▣	▣	☐	☐
46. Proper marker placement						
47. Evidence of proper collimation and radiation protection	▣	▣	▣	▣	☐	☐
48. Long vs. short scale of contrast	▣	▣	▣	▣	☐	☐
49. Image/projection identification and/or other identification	▣	▣	▣	▣	☐	☐

Comments:
_____
_____

ABDOMEN ANATOMY
The student is able to identify:

	Procedure		Repeat		Competency	
	Yes	No	Yes	No	Yes	No
50. Diaphragm	▣	▣	▣	▣	☐	☐
51. Symphysis pubis	▣	▣	▣	▣	☐	☐
52. Iliac crest	▣	▣	▣	▣	☐	☐
53. Small vs. large bowel (gas)	▣	▣	▣	▣	☐	☐
54. Liver	▣	▣	▣	▣	☐	☐

	Procedure		Repeat		Competency	
	Yes	No	Yes	No	Yes	No
55. Lesser and greater curvatures	☐	☐	☐	☐	☐	☐
56. Fundus	☐	☐	☐	☐	☐	☐
57. Body	☐	☐	☐	☐	☐	☐
58. Pylorus	☐	☐	☐	☐	☐	☐
59. Cardiac and pyloric antrums/sphincters	☐	☐	☐	☐	☐	☐
60. Duodenum	☐	☐	☐	☐	☐	☐
61. Rugal folds	☐	☐	☐	☐	☐	☐
62. Obvious pathology	☐	☐	☐	☐	☐	☐

Comments:

_____

_____

_____   _____   _____
Procedure Evaluator Signature   Repeat Evaluator Signature   Competency Evaluator Signature

_____   _____   _____
Date   Date   Date

END DOUBLE-CONTRAST GASTROINTESTINAL SERIES EVALUATION

Student Name:_____

Procedure Grade	Repeat Grade	Competency Grade

PATIENT INFORMATION OR SIMULATED PROCEDURE *(circle if simulated)*

	Procedure	Repeat	Competency
Age			
Medical Record No.			
Ability to Cooperate			
Condition/Pathology			
Technical Factors Used			
Exposure Index			

FACILITY PREPARATION
The student:

	Procedure Yes No	Repeat Yes No	Competency Yes No
1. Examines the radiographic room and cleans/straightens it before escorting the patient in.	☐ ☐	☐ ☐	☐ ☐
2. Has all equipment and supplies (patient gown, shield, markers, tape, cassettes, lead aprons, blockers, hemostats, compression paddle, proper contrast material, etc.) readily available before escorting the patient in, the Bucky drawer in the proper position, the monitor by the table, and the fluoro on.	☐ ☐	☐ ☐	☐ ☐

Additional supplies:

_____
_____
_____
_____

	Procedure Yes No	Repeat Yes No	Competency Yes No
3. Selects and prepares the contrast material without difficulty.	▣ ▣	▣ ▣	☐ ☐
4. Is able to manipulate all radiographic equipment with ease, and centers the central ray to the cassette/receptor *for all projections.*	☐ ☐	☐ ☐	☐ ☐
5. Adjusts the tube to the proper SID *for each projections.*	☐ ☐	☐ ☐	☐ ☐
6. Selects cassettes/receptor/receptor of the appropriate sizes *for all projections,* according to the patient's size and examination.	☐ ☐	☐ ☐	☐ ☐

Comments:

_____
_____

PATIENT PREPARATION
The student:

	Procedure Yes No	Repeat Yes No	Competency Yes No
7. Identifies the correct patient and examination according to the requisition while establishing a good rapport with him or her.	☐ ☐	☐ ☐	☐ ☐

(continued)

	Procedure		Repeat		Competency	
	Yes	No	Yes	No	Yes	No
8. Obtains and documents the patient's history before the examination, including whether the patient ate before the examination and preparation instructions.	▣	▣	▣	▣	☐	☐
9. Thoroughly explains the examination in terms the patient fully understands and properly communicates with the patient throughout the examination.	☐	☐	☐	☐	☐	☐
10. Asks female patients of childbearing age the date of their last menstrual period and documents this; inquires about the possibility of pregnancy and has them sign pregnancy consent forms.	☐	☐	☐	☐	☐	☐
11. Removes all obscuring objects (snaps, zippers, jewelry, belts, etc.) so as *not* to produce radiographic artifacts.	☐	☐	☐	☐	☐	☐
12. Respects the patient's modesty and provides ample comfort for the patient while positioning him or her to begin the examination (AP standing).	☐	☐	☐	☐	☐	☐
13. Performs a scout radiograph when indicated.	☐	☐	☐	☐	☐	☐

Comments:

_____

_____

TASKS DURING FLUOROSCOPY
The student:

	Procedure		Repeat		Competency	
	Yes	No	Yes	No	Yes	No
14. Prepares the patient in the right PA oblique position (RAO: 35–40°).	▣	▣	▣	▣	☐	☐
15. Relays the patient's history to the radiologist.	▣	▣	▣	▣	☐	☐
16. Assists the radiologist throughout the examination.	▣	▣	▣	▣	☐	☐
17. Monitors, communicates with, and assists the patient throughout the examination.	▣	▣	▣	▣	☐	☐
18. Takes charge of the examination after the radiologist departs.	▣	▣	▣	▣	☐	☐

Comments:

_____

_____

IMPORTANT DETAILS
The student:

	Procedure		Repeat		Competency	
	Yes	No	Yes	No	Yes	No
19. Instills confidence in the patient by exhibiting self-confidence throughout the examination.	☐	☐	☐	☐	☐	☐
20. Places a lead marker in the appropriate area of the cassette/receptor (top/bottom/anteriorly/laterally), where it will be visualized on the finished radiograph, on the proper anatomical side (right/left), and in the appropriate position (face up/face down), depending on the patient's position.	☐	☐	☐	☐	☐	☐
21. Provides radiation protection (shield) for the patient (when appropriate), self, and others (closes doors).	☐	☐	☐	☐	☐	☐
22. Applies proper collimation and makes adjustments as necessary.	☐	☐	☐	☐	☐	☐
23. Properly measures the patient along the course of the central ray *for each projection.*	☐	☐	☐	☐	☐	☐
24. Sets the proper technique *for fluoroscopy* (kVp, mA, time).	☐	☐	☐	☐	☐	☐
And all projections/spot images:						

	Procedure		Repeat		Competency	
	Yes	No	Yes	No	Yes	No

Conventional systems

- Sets the proper kVp, mA, and time and makes adjustments as necessary.

or

CR or DR systems

- Identifies the patient on the work-list (or manually types the patient information into the system).
- Selects appropriate body region, specific body part, and accurate view/projection.
- Double-checks preset parameters:
  —Adult vs. pediatric patients
  ○ Small, medium, or large
  —Bucky/receptor (upright vs. table) *or* non-Bucky
  —AEC vs. fixed
  ○ If AEC, checks ion chambers
  ○ Density setting
  —kVp and mA; adjusts if necessary
  —Focal spot/filament size

	Procedure		Repeat		Competency	
	Yes	No	Yes	No	Yes	No
25. Exposes the cassette/receptor after telling the patient to hold still and after giving him or her proper breathing instructions (expiration) *for each projection*.	☐	☐	☐	☐	☐	☐
26. Provides each radiograph with the proper identification (flash) and/or processes each cassette (image) without difficulty (regardless of technology—film, CR, or DR).	▨	▨	▨	▨	☐	☐
27. Properly completes the examination by filling out all necessary paperwork, entering the examination in the computer, having the images checked by the appropriate staff members, answering any last-minute questions, and informing the patient that he or she is finished. Provides proper post-exam instructions as required.	▨	▨	▨	▨	☐	☐
28. Exhibits the ability to adapt to new and difficult situations if and when necessary.	▨	▨	▨	▨	☐	☐
29. Accepts constructive criticism and uses it to his or her advantage.	☐	☐	☐	☐	☐	☐
30. Leaves the radiographic room neat and clean for the next examination.	▨	▨	▨	▨	☐	☐
31. Completes the examination within a reasonable time frame.	☐	☐	☐	☐	☐	☐

Comments:

_____

_____

RADIOGRAPHIC IMAGE QUALITY

The student is able to critique his or her radiographs as to whether they demonstrate:

	Procedure		Repeat		Competency	
	Yes	No	Yes	No	Yes	No
32. Proper technique/optimal density	▨	▨	▨	▨	☐	☐
33. Enhanced detail, without evidence of motion and without any visible artifacts	▨	▨	▨	▨	☐	☐
34. Proper positioning (all anatomy included, evidence of proper centering/alignment, etc.)	▨	▨	▨	▨	☐	☐
35. Proper marker placement						
36. Evidence of proper collimation and radiation protection	▨	▨	▨	▨	☐	☐
37. Long vs. short scale of contrast	▨	▨	▨	▨	☐	☐
38. Image/projection identification and/or other identification	▨	▨	▨	▨	☐	☐

(continued)

Comments:

_____

_____

ABDOMEN ANATOMY
The student is able to identify:

	Procedure		Repeat		Competency	
	Yes	No	Yes	No	Yes	No
39. Proximal esophagus	☐	☐	☐	☐	☐	☐
40. Distal esophagus	☐	☐	☐	☐	☐	☐
41. Cardiac sphincter	☐	☐	☐	☐	☐	☐
42. Diaphragm	☐	☐	☐	☐	☐	☐
43. Heart shadows	☐	☐	☐	☐	☐	☐
44. Ribs	☐	☐	☐	☐	☐	☐
45. Vertebrae	☐	☐	☐	☐	☐	☐
46. Obvious pathology	☐	☐	☐	☐	☐	☐

Comments:

_____

_____

_____   _____   _____
Procedure Evaluator Signature   Repeat Evaluator Signature   Competency Evaluator Signature

_____   _____   _____
Date   Date   Date

END BARIUM SWALLOW OR ESOPHAGRAM EVALUATION

Small Bowel Series

The objective of this evaluation is to determine the student's competency level when performing specific radiographic examinations.

Student Name:_____

Procedure Grade	Repeat Grade	Competency Grade

PATIENT INFORMATION OR SIMULATED PROCEDURE *(circle if simulated)*

	Procedure	Repeat	Competency
Age			
Medical Record No.			
Ability to Cooperate			
Condition/Pathology			
Technical Factors Used			
Exposure Index			

FACILITY PREPARATION
The student:

	Procedure Yes No	Repeat Yes No	Competency Yes No
1. Examines the radiographic room and cleans/straightens it before escorting the patient in.	☐ ☐	☐ ☐	☐ ☐
2. Has all equipment and supplies (patient gown, shield, markers, tape, proper contrast material, etc.) readily available before escorting the patient in.	☐ ☐	☐ ☐	☐ ☐

Additional supplies:

_____

_____

_____

_____

	Procedure	Repeat	Competency
3. Selects and prepares the contrast material without difficulty.	☐ ☐	☐ ☐	☐ ☐
4. Is able to manipulate all radiographic equipment with ease, and centers the central ray to the cassette/receptor *for all projections.*	☐ ☐	☐ ☐	☐ ☐
5. Adjusts the tube to the proper SID *for each projection.*	☐ ☐	☐ ☐	☐ ☐
6. Selects cassettes/receptor of the appropriate sizes *for all projection,* according to the patient's size and examination.	☐ ☐	☐ ☐	☐ ☐

Comments:

_____

_____

PATIENT PREPARATION
The student:

	Procedure Yes No	Repeat Yes No	Competency Yes No
7. Identifies the correct patient and examination according to the requisition while establishing a good rapport with him or her.	☐ ☐	☐ ☐	☐ ☐
8. Obtains and documents the patient's history before the examination, including whether the patient ate before the examination and preparation instructions.	☐ ☐	☐ ☐	☐ ☐

(continued)

	Procedure		Repeat		Competency	
	Yes	No	Yes	No	Yes	No

9. Thoroughly explains the examination in terms the patient fully understands, *emphasizing the timing sequence for small bowel radiography,* and properly communicates with the patient throughout the examination. | ☐ | ☐ | ☐ | ☐ | ☐ | ☐ |
10. Asks female patients of childbearing age the date of their last menstrual period and documents this; inquires about the possibility of pregnancy and has them sign pregnancy consent forms. | ☐ | ☐ | ☐ | ☐ | ☐ | ☐ |
11. Removes all obscuring objects (snaps, zippers, jewelry, belts, etc.) so as *not* to produce radiographic artifacts. | ☐ | ☐ | ☐ | ☐ | ☐ | ☐ |
12. Respects the patient's modesty and provides ample comfort for the patient while positioning him or her to begin the examination. | ☐ | ☐ | ☐ | ☐ | ☐ | ☐ |
13. Performs a scout radiograph when indicated. | ☐ | ☐ | ☐ | ☐ | ☐ | ☐ |

Comments:

_____

_____

PATIENT POSITIONING FOR A SMALL-BOWEL SERIES
Immediate Supine or Prone Abdomen
The student:

	Procedure		Repeat		Competency	
	Yes	No	Yes	No	Yes	No

14. Places the patient in the supine or prone position on the radiographic table, with arms at sides and without rotation. | ☐ | ☐ | ☐ | ☐ | ☐ | ☐ |
15. Selects the appropriate receptor or places the cassette lengthwise. For conventional cassettes, the flash must be at the bottom and away from any anatomy. | ☐ | ☐ | ☐ | ☐ | ☐ | ☐ |
16. Centers the central ray to the midsagittal plane of the body. | ☐ | ☐ | ☐ | ☐ | ☐ | ☐ |
17. Directs the central ray perpendicularly at a level 3 inches above the iliac crest. | ☐ | ☐ | ☐ | ☐ | ☐ | ☐ |

Supine or Prone Abdomen at Specified Time Intervals
The student:

	Procedure		Repeat		Competency	
	Yes	No	Yes	No	Yes	No

18. Places the patient in the supine or prone position on the radiographic table, with arms at sides and without rotation. | ☐ | ☐ | ☐ | ☐ | ☐ | ☐ |
19. Selects the appropriate receptor or places the cassette lengthwise. For conventional cassettes, the flash must be at the bottom and away from any anatomy. | ☐ | ☐ | ☐ | ☐ | ☐ | ☐ |
20. Centers the central ray to the midsagittal plane of the body. | ☐ | ☐ | ☐ | ☐ | ☐ | ☐ |
21. Directs the central ray perpendicularly to the iliac crest. | ☐ | ☐ | ☐ | ☐ | ☐ | ☐ |
22. Is sure to accurately change markers indicating appropriate time intervals. | ☐ | ☐ | ☐ | ☐ | ☐ | ☐ |

Comments:

_____

_____

IMPORTANT DETAILS
The student:

	Procedure		Repeat		Competency	
	Yes	No	Yes	No	Yes	No

23. Instills confidence in the patient by exhibiting self-confidence throughout the examination. | ☐ | ☐ | ☐ | ☐ | ☐ | ☐ |
24. Places a lead marker in the appropriate area of the cassette/receptor (top/bottom/anteriorly/laterally), where it will be visualized on the finished radiograph, on the proper anatomical side (right/left), and in the appropriate position (face up/face down), depending on the patient's position. | ☐ | ☐ | ☐ | ☐ | ☐ | ☐ |

	Procedure		Repeat		Competency	
	Yes	No	Yes	No	Yes	No
25. Provides radiation protection (shield) for the patient (when appropriate), self, and others (closes doors).	☐	☐	☐	☐	☐	☐
26. Applies proper collimation and makes adjustments as necessary.	☐	☐	☐	☐	☐	☐
27. Properly measures the patient along the course of the central ray *for each projection.*	☐	☐	☐	☐	☐	☐
28. Sets the proper technique *for fluoroscopy* (kVp, mA, time).	☐	☐	☐	☐	☐	☐

And all projections/spot images:

Conventional systems

- Sets the proper kVp, mA, and time and makes adjustments as necessary.

or

CR or DR systems
- Identifies the patient on the work-list (or manually types the patient information into the system).
- Selects appropriate body region, specific body part, and accurate view/projection.
- Double-checks preset parameters:
  —Adult vs. pediatric patients
    ○ Small, medium, or large
  —Bucky/receptor (upright vs. table) *or* non-Bucky
  —AEC vs. fixed
    ○ If AEC, checks ion chambers
    ○ Density setting
  —kVp and mA; adjusts if necessary
  —Focal spot/filament size

	Procedure		Repeat		Competency	
29. Exposes the cassette/receptor after telling the patient to hold still and after giving him or her proper breathing instructions (expiration) *for each projection.*	☐	☐	☐	☐	☐	☐
30. Provides each radiograph with the proper identification (flash) and/or processes each cassette (image) without difficulty (regardless of technology—film, CR, or DR).	▨	▨	▨	▨	☐	☐
31. Properly completes the examination by filling out all necessary paperwork, entering the examination in the computer, having the images checked by the appropriate staff members, answering any last-minute questions, and informing the patient that he or she is finished. Provides proper post-exam instructions as required.	▨	▨	▨	▨	☐	☐
32. Exhibits the ability to adapt to new and difficult situations if and when necessary.	▨	▨	▨	▨	☐	☐
33. Accepts constructive criticism and uses it to his or her advantage.	☐	☐	☐	☐	☐	☐
34. Leaves the radiographic room neat and clean for the next examination.	▨	▨	▨	▨	☐	☐
35. Completes the examination within a reasonable time frame.	☐	☐	☐	☐	☐	☐

Comments:

_____

_____

RADIOGRAPHIC IMAGE QUALITY
The student is able to critique his or her radiographs as to whether they demonstrate:

	Procedure		Repeat		Competency	
	Yes	No	Yes	No	Yes	No
36. Proper technique/optimal density	▨	▨	▨	▨	☐	☐
37. Enhanced detail, without evidence of motion and without any visible artifacts	▨	▨	▨	▨	☐	☐

(continued)

	Procedure		Repeat		Competency	
	Yes	No	Yes	No	Yes	No
38. Proper positioning (all anatomy included, evidence of proper centering/alignment, etc.)	☐	☐	☐	☐	☐	☐
39. Proper marker placement						
40. Evidence of proper collimation and radiation protection	☐	☐	☐	☐	☐	☐
41. Long vs. short scale of contrast	☐	☐	☐	☐	☐	☐
42. Image/projection identification and/or other identification	☐	☐	☐	☐	☐	☐

Comments:

ABDOMEN ANATOMY
The student is able to identify:

	Procedure		Repeat		Competency	
	Yes	No	Yes	No	Yes	No
43. Duodenum	☐	☐	☐	☐	☐	☐
44. Jejunum	☐	☐	☐	☐	☐	☐
45. Ileum	☐	☐	☐	☐	☐	☐
46. Diaphragm	☐	☐	☐	☐	☐	☐
47. Symphysis pubis	☐	☐	☐	☐	☐	☐
48. Iliac crest	☐	☐	☐	☐	☐	☐
49. Small vs. large bowel (gas)	☐	☐	☐	☐	☐	☐
50. Liver	☐	☐	☐	☐	☐	☐
51. Lesser and greater curvatures	☐	☐	☐	☐	☐	☐
52. Fundus	☐	☐	☐	☐	☐	☐
53. Body	☐	☐	☐	☐	☐	☐
54. Pylorus	☐	☐	☐	☐	☐	☐
55. Cardiac and pyloric antrums/sphincters	☐	☐	☐	☐	☐	☐
56. Rugal folds	☐	☐	☐	☐	☐	☐
57. Obvious pathology	☐	☐	☐	☐	☐	☐

Comments:

Procedure Evaluator Signature   Repeat Evaluator Signature   Competency Evaluator Signature

Date   Date   Date

END SMALL BOWEL SERIES EVALUATION

Intravenous Urogram (IVU) or Tomographic Intravenous Pyelogram (IVP)

The objective of this evaluation is to determine the student's competency level when performing specific radiographic examinations.

Student Name:_____

Procedure Grade	Repeat Grade	Competency Grade

PATIENT INFORMATION OR SIMULATED PROCEDURE *(circle if simulated)*

	Procedure	Repeat	Competency
Age			
Medical Record No.			
Ability to Cooperate			
Condition/Pathology			
Technical Factors Used			
Exposure Index			

FACILITY PREPARATION
The student:

	Procedure Yes	Procedure No	Repeat Yes	Repeat No	Competency Yes	Competency No
1. Examines the radiographic room and cleans/straightens it before escorting the patient in.	☐	☐	☐	☐	☐	☐
2. Has all equipment and supplies (patient gown, shield, markers, tape, alcohol, tourniquet, needles, syringes, butterflies/angiocatheters, stopper, gauze, number markers, hemostats, stethoscope, blood pressure cuff, proper contrast material, etc.) readily available before escorting the patient in.	☐	☐	☐	☐	☐	☐

Additional supplies:

_____

_____

_____

_____

	Procedure Yes	Procedure No	Repeat Yes	Repeat No	Competency Yes	Competency No
3. Selects and prepares the contrast material without difficulty.	▨	▨	▨	▨	☐	☐
4. Checks the code box/code cart to be sure diphenhydramine and epinephrine are available and have not expired, and also knows how to call a code.	☐	☐	☐	☐	☐	☐
5. Is able to manipulate all radiographic equipment with ease, and centers the central ray to the cassette/receptor *for all projections.*	☐	☐	☐	☐	☐	☐
6. Adjusts the tube to the proper SID *for each projection.*	☐	☐	☐	☐	☐	☐
7. Selects cassettes/receptor of the appropriate sizes *for all projections,* according to the patient's size and examination.	☐	☐	☐	☐	☐	☐

Comments:

_____

_____

(continued)

PATIENT PREPARATION
The student:

	Procedure		Repeat		Competency	
	Yes	No	Yes	No	Yes	No
8. Identifies the correct patient and examination according to the requisition while establishing a good rapport with him or her.	☐	☐	☐	☐	☐	☐
9. Obtains and documents the patient's history before the examination (whether the patient ate before the examination, preparation instructions, reasons for the IVU/IVP, food and drug allergies, asthma, heart disease, diabetes, current medications, BUN, creatinine, and/or GFR, etc.), and asks the patient if he or she has had a contrast study before.	▣	▣	▣	▣	☐	☐
10. Asks female patients of childbearing age the date of their last menstrual period and documents this; inquires about the possibility of pregnancy and has them sign pregnancy consent forms.	☐	☐	☐	☐	☐	☐
11. Thoroughly explains the examination in terms the patient fully understands (how the study is performed/tube movement during tomography, possible reactions, such as itchiness, warmness, nausea, metallic taste, etc.), has the patient sign the consent form, and properly communicates with the patient throughout the examination.	☐	☐	☐	☐	☐	☐
12. Removes all obscuring objects (snaps, zippers, jewelry, belts, etc.) so as *not* to produce radiographic artifacts.	☐	☐	☐	☐	☐	☐
13. Respects the patient's modesty and provides ample comfort for the patient while positioning him or her to begin the examination.	☐	☐	☐	☐	☐	☐
14. Ensures that the patient's bladder is empty before performing the initial radiographs.	☐	☐	☐	☐	☐	☐

Comments:

_____

_____

TASKS DURING CONTRAST INJECTION OR ADMINISTRATION
The student:

	Procedure		Repeat		Competency	
	Yes	No	Yes	No	Yes	No
15. Relays the patient's history to the radiologist.	▣	▣	▣	▣	☐	☐
16. Assists the radiologist throughout the examination.	▣	▣	▣	▣	☐	☐
17. Monitors, communicates with, and assists the patient throughout the examination.	▣	▣	▣	▣	☐	☐
18. Takes charge of the examination after the radiologist departs.	▣	▣	▣	▣	☐	☐

Comments:

_____

_____

PATIENT POSITIONING FOR AN IVP
Scout AP Abdomen
The student:

	Procedure		Repeat		Competency	
	Yes	No	Yes	No	Yes	No
19. Places the patient in the supine position on the radiographic table, without rotation	☐	☐	☐	☐	☐	☐
20. Selects the appropriate receptor or places the cassette lengthwise. For conventional cassettes, the flash must be at the bottom and away from any anatomy.	☐	☐	☐	☐	☐	☐
21. Centers the central ray to the midsagittal plane of the body.	☐	☐	☐	☐	☐	☐
22. Directs the central ray perpendicularly to the iliac crest, making sure the symphysis pubis is included on the cassette/receptor.	☐	☐	☐	☐	☐	☐

Scout Tomogram
The student:

	Procedure		Repeat		Competency	
	Yes	No	Yes	No	Yes	No
23. Places the patient in the supine position on the radiographic table.	☐	☐	☐	☐	☐	☐
24. Selects the appropriate receptor or places the cassette crosswise. For conventional cassettes, the flash must be away from any anatomy.	☐	☐	☐	☐	☐	☐
25. Centers the central ray to the midsagittal plane of the body.	☐	☐	☐	☐	☐	☐
26. Directs the central ray perpendicularly, midway between the iliac crest and the xiphoid process.	☐	☐	☐	☐	☐	☐
27. Accurately sets the fulcrum level by utilizing patient measurement.	☐	☐	☐	☐	☐	☐

Tomograms at Appropriate Time Intervals and Fulcrum Levels
The student:

	Procedure		Repeat		Competency	
	Yes	No	Yes	No	Yes	No
28. Places the patient in the supine position on the radiographic table.	☐	☐	☐	☐	☐	☐
29. Selects the appropriate receptor or places the cassette crosswise. For conventional cassettes, the flash must be away from any anatomy.	☐	☐	☐	☐	☐	☐
30. Centers the central ray to the midsagittal plane of the body.	☐	☐	☐	☐	☐	☐
31. Directs the central ray perpendicularly, midway between the iliac crest and the xiphoid process.	☐	☐	☐	☐	☐	☐
32. Accurately adjusts the fulcrum levels for second and third postinjection tomograms.	☐	☐	☐	☐	☐	☐
33. Is sure to accurately change markers indicating appropriate fulcrum intervals (as well as time intervals/delayed imaging when required).	☐	☐	☐	☐	☐	☐

AP Abdomen
The student:

	Procedure		Repeat		Competency	
	Yes	No	Yes	No	Yes	No
34. Places the patient in the supine position on the radiographic table, without rotation.	☐	☐	☐	☐	☐	☐
35. Selects the appropriate receptor or places the cassette lengthwise. For conventional cassettes, the flash must be at the bottom and away from any anatomy.	☐	☐	☐	☐	☐	☐
36. Centers the central ray to the midsagittal plane of the body.	☐	☐	☐	☐	☐	☐
37. Directs the central ray perpendicularly to the iliac crest, making sure the symphysis pubis is included on the cassette/receptor.	☐	☐	☐	☐	☐	☐

Left Posterior Oblique
The student:

	Procedure		Repeat		Competency	
	Yes	No	Yes	No	Yes	No
38. Places the patient in the oblique position, at a 30° angle.	☐	☐	☐	☐	☐	☐
39. Selects the appropriate receptor or places the cassette lengthwise. For conventional cassettes, the flash must be at the bottom and away from any anatomy.	☐	☐	☐	☐	☐	☐
40. Centers the central ray midway between the lateral surfaces of the abdomen, making sure both kidneys will be fully demonstrated on the radiograph.	☐	☐	☐	☐	☐	☐
41. Centers the central ray perpendicularly at the level of the iliac crest.	☐	☐	☐	☐	☐	☐

Right Posterior Oblique
The student:

	Procedure		Repeat		Competency	
	Yes	No	Yes	No	Yes	No
42. Places the patient in the oblique position, at a 30° angle.	☐	☐	☐	☐	☐	☐

(continued)

	Procedure		Repeat		Competency	
	Yes	No	Yes	No	Yes	No
43. Selects the appropriate receptor or places the cassette lengthwise. For conventional cassettes, the flash must be at the bottom and away from any anatomy.	☐	☐	☐	☐	☐	☐
44. Centers the central ray midway between the lateral surfaces of the abdomen, making sure both kidneys will be fully demonstrated on the radiograph.	☐	☐	☐	☐	☐	☐
45. Centers the central ray perpendicularly at the level of the iliac crest.	☐	☐	☐	☐	☐	☐

Prone
The student:

	Procedure		Repeat		Competency	
	Yes	No	Yes	No	Yes	No
46. Places the patient in the prone position on the radiographic table, with arms at sides and without rotation.	☐	☐	☐	☐	☐	☐
47. Selects the appropriate receptor or places the cassette lengthwise. For conventional cassettes, the flash must be at the bottom and away from any anatomy.	☐	☐	☐	☐	☐	☐
48. Centers the central ray to the midsagittal plane of the body.	☐	☐	☐	☐	☐	☐
49. Directs the central ray perpendicularly at the level of the iliac crest.	☐	☐	☐	☐	☐	☐

Prevoid Bladder
The student:

	Procedure		Repeat		Competency	
	Yes	No	Yes	No	Yes	No
50. Places the patient in the supine position on the radiographic table, with arms at sides and without rotation.	☐	☐	☐	☐	☐	☐
51. Selects the appropriate receptor or places the cassette crosswise in the Bucky drawer.	☐	☐	☐	☐	☐	☐
52. Centers the central ray to the midsagittal plane of the body.	☐	☐	☐	☐	☐	☐
53. Directs the central ray perpendicularly, midway between the iliac crest and the symphysis pubis, with the top of the cassette/receptor at the top of the crest.	☐	☐	☐	☐	☐	☐

Supine Postvoid Bladder
The student:

	Procedure		Repeat		Competency	
	Yes	No	Yes	No	Yes	No
54. Places the patient in the supine position on the radiographic table, with arms at sides and without rotation.	☐	☐	☐	☐	☐	☐
55. Selects the appropriate receptor or places the cassette crosswise in the Bucky drawer.	☐	☐	☐	☐	☐	☐
56. Centers the central ray to the midsagittal plane of the body.	☐	☐	☐	☐	☐	☐
57. Directs the central ray perpendicularly, midway between the iliac crest and the symphysis pubis, with the top of the cassette/receptor at the top of the crest.	☐	☐	☐	☐	☐	☐

Erect or Supine Postvoid KUB
The student:

	Procedure		Repeat		Competency	
	Yes	No	Yes	No	Yes	No
58. Places the patient in the erect position at the upright Bucky/receptor or supine on the radiographic table, with arms at sides and without rotation.	☐	☐	☐	☐	☐	☐
59. Selects the appropriate receptor or places the cassette lengthwise in the Bucky drawer.	☐	☐	☐	☐	☐	☐
60. Centers the central ray to the midsagittal plane of the body.	☐	☐	☐	☐	☐	☐
61. Directs the central ray perpendicularly at the level of the iliac crest.	☐	☐	☐	☐	☐	☐

Compression
The student:

	Procedure		Repeat		Competency	
	Yes	No	Yes	No	Yes	No
62. Is able to apply and perform appropriate compression images as requested by the radiologist	☐	☐	☐	☐	☐	☐

Comments:

_____

_____

IMPORTANT DETAILS
The student:

	Procedure		Repeat		Competency	
	Yes	No	Yes	No	Yes	No
63. Instills confidence in the patient by exhibiting self-confidence throughout the examination.	☐	☐	☐	☐	☐	☐
64. Places a lead marker in the appropriate area of the cassette/receptor (top/bottom/anteriorly/laterally), where it will be visualized on the finished radiograph, on the proper anatomical side (right/left), and in the appropriate position (face up/face down), depending on the patient's position; also uses number markers for tomograms.	☐	☐	☐	☐	☐	☐
65. Provides radiation protection (shield) for the patient (when appropriate), self, and others (closes doors).	☐	☐	☐	☐	☐	☐
66. Applies proper collimation and makes adjustments as necessary.	☐	☐	☐	☐	☐	☐
67. Properly measures the patient along the course of the central ray and accurately sets the proper fulcrum levels.	☐	☐	☐	☐	☐	☐
68. Sets the proper technique (kVp, mA, time) *and all projections, including tomograms,* making adjustments in technique and fulcrum levels as necessary.	☐	☐	☐	☐	☐	☐

Conventional systems

• Sets the proper kVp, mA, and time and makes adjustments as necessary.

or

CR or DR systems
• Identifies the patient on the work-list (or manually types the patient information into the system).
• Selects appropriate body region, specific body part, and accurate view/projection.
• Double-checks preset parameters:
 —Adult vs. pediatric patients
  ○ Small, medium, or large
 —Bucky/receptor (upright vs. table) *or* non-Bucky
 —AEC vs. fixed
  ○ If AEC, checks ion chambers
  ○ Density setting
 —kVp and mA; adjusts if necessary
 —Focal spot/filament size

	Procedure		Repeat		Competency	
	Yes	No	Yes	No	Yes	No
69. Exposes the cassette/receptor after telling the patient to hold still and after giving him or her proper breathing instructions (expiration) *for each projection.*	☐	☐	☐	☐	☐	☐
70. Provides each radiograph with the proper identification (flash) and/or processes each cassette (image) without difficulty (regardless of technology—film, CR, or DR).	▦	▦	▦	▦	☐	☐
71. Properly completes the examination by filling out all necessary paperwork, entering the examination in the computer, having the images checked by the appropriate staff members, answering any last-minute questions, and informing the patient that he or she is finished. Provides proper post-exam instructions as required.	▦	▦	▦	▦	☐	☐

(continued)

	Procedure		Repeat		Competency	
	Yes	No	Yes	No	Yes	No
72. Exhibits the ability to adapt to new and difficult situations if and when necessary.	☑	☑	☑	☑	☐	☐
73. Accepts constructive criticism and uses it to his or her advantage.	☐	☐	☐	☐	☐	☐
74. Leaves the radiographic room neat and clean for the next examination.	☑	☑	☑	☑	☐	☐
75. Completes the examination within a reasonable time frame.	☐	☐	☐	☐	☐	☐

Comments:

_____

RADIOGRAPHIC IMAGE QUALITY

The student is able to critique his or her radiographs as to whether they demonstrate:

	Procedure		Repeat		Competency	
	Yes	No	Yes	No	Yes	No
76. Proper technique/optimal density	☑	☑	☑	☑	☐	☐
77. Enhanced detail, without evidence of motion and without any visible artifacts	☑	☑	☑	☑	☐	☐
78. Proper positioning (all anatomy included, evidence of proper centering/alignment, etc.)	☑	☑	☑	☑	☐	☐
79. Proper marker placement						
80. Evidence of proper collimation and radiation protection	☑	☑	☑	☑	☐	☐
81. Long vs. short scale of contrast	☑	☑	☑	☑	☐	☐
82. Image/projection identification and/or other identification	☑	☑	☑	☑	☐	☐

Comments:

_____

ABDOMEN ANATOMY

The student is able to identify:

	Procedure		Repeat		Competency	
	Yes	No	Yes	No	Yes	No
83. Kidneys	☑	☑	☑	☑	☐	☐
84. Ureter	☑	☑	☑	☑	☐	☐
85. Bladder	☑	☑	☑	☑	☐	☐
86. Diaphragm	☑	☑	☑	☑	☐	☐
87. Symphysis pubis	☑	☑	☑	☑	☐	☐
88. Iliac crest	☑	☑	☑	☑	☐	☐
89. Bowel gas	☑	☑	☑	☑	☐	☐
90. Renal pelvis	☑	☑	☑	☑	☐	☐
91. Major and minor calyces	☑	☑	☑	☑	☐	☐
92. Upper vs. lower poles of the kidney	☑	☑	☑	☑	☐	☐
93. Trigone	☑	☑	☑	☑	☐	☐
94. Location of adrenal glands	☑	☑	☑	☑	☐	☐
95. Obvious pathology	☑	☑	☑	☑	☐	☐

Comments:

_____

_____	_____	_____
Procedure Evaluator Signature	Repeat Evaluator Signature	Competency Evaluator Signature
_____	_____	_____
Date	Date	Date

END INTRAVENOUS UROGRAM (IVU) OR TOMOGRAPHIC INTRAVENOUS PYELOGRAM (IVP) EVALUATION

The objective of this evaluation is to determine the student's competency level when performing specific radiographic examinations.

Student Name:_____

Procedure Grade	Repeat Grade	Competency Grade

PATIENT INFORMATION OR SIMULATED PROCEDURE *(circle if simulated)*

	Procedure	Repeat	Competency
Age			
Medical Record No.			
Ability to Cooperate			
Condition/Pathology			
Technical Factors Used			
Exposure Index			

FACILITY PREPARATION
The student:

	Procedure Yes	No	Repeat Yes	No	Competency Yes	No
1. Examines the radiographic room and cleans/straightens it before escorting the patient in.	☐	☐	☐	☐	☐	☐
2. Has all equipment and supplies (markers, tape, cassettes, lead aprons, proper contrast material, etc.) readily available before escorting the patient in.	☐	☐	☐	☐	☐	☐

Additional supplies:

_____
_____
_____
_____

	Procedure Yes	No	Repeat Yes	No	Competency Yes	No
3. Selects and prepares the contrast material without difficulty.	▦	▦	▦	▦	☐	☐
4. Is able to manipulate all radiographic equipment with ease, and centers the central ray to the cassette/receptor *for all projections.*	☐	☐	☐	☐	☐	☐
5. Adjusts the tube to the proper SID *for each projection.*	☐	☐	☐	☐	☐	☐
6. Selects cassettes/receptor of the appropriate sizes *for all projections,* according to the patient's size and examination.	☐	☐	☐	☐	☐	☐

Comments:

_____

_____

PATIENT PREPARATION
The student:

	Procedure Yes	No	Repeat Yes	No	Competency Yes	No
7. Identifies the correct patient and examination according to the requisition.	☐	☐	☐	☐	☐	☐
8. Obtains and documents the patient's history before the examination, including whether the patient are before the examination and preparation instructions, and asks whether the patient has had a contrast study before.	▦	▦	▦	▦	☐	☐

(continued)

	Procedure		Repeat		Competency	
	Yes	No	Yes	No	Yes	No
9. Thoroughly explains the examination in terms the patient fully understands (how the study is performed) and properly communicates with the patient throughout the examination.	☐	☐	☐	☐	☐	☐
10. Asks female patients of childbearing age the date of their last menstrual period and documents this; inquires about the possibility of pregnancy and has them sign pregnancy consent forms.	☐	☐	☐	☐	☐	☐
11. Removes all obscuring objects (snaps, zippers, jewelry, belts, etc.) so as *not* to produce radiographic artifacts.	☐	☐	☐	☐	☐	☐
12. Respects the patient's modesty and provides ample comfort for the patient while positioning him or her to begin the examination.	☐	☐	☐	☐	☐	☐
13. Ensures that the patient's bladder is empty before performing the initial radiographs.	☐	☐	☐	☐	☐	☐
14. Performs a scout radiograph when indicated.	☐	☐	☐	☐	☐	☐

Comments:

_____

_____

TASKS DURING FLUOROSCOPY
The student:

	Procedure		Repeat		Competency	
	Yes	No	Yes	No	Yes	No
15. Relays the patient's history to the radiologist.	■	■	■	■	☐	☐
16. Assists staff members and the physician throughout the examination.	■	■	■	■	☐	☐
17. Monitors, communicates with, and assists the patient throughout the examination.	■	■	■	■	☐	☐
18. Takes charge of the examination when the radiologist departs.	■	■	■	■	☐	☐

Comments:

_____

_____

PATIENT POSITIONING FOR A RETROGRADE UROGRAM
AP Abdomen
The student:

	Procedure		Repeat		Competency	
	Yes	No	Yes	No	Yes	No
19. Assists in placing the patient in the supine position on the radiographic/ surgical table, ensuring that there is no rotation.	☐	☐	☐	☐	☐	☐
20. Selects the appropriate receptor or places the cassette lengthwise. For conventional cassettes, the flash must be at the bottom and away from any anatomy.	☐	☐	☐	☐	☐	☐
21. Centers the central ray to the midsagittal plane of the body.	☐	☐	☐	☐	☐	☐
22. Directs the central ray perpendicularly to the iliac crest, making sure the symphysis pubis is included on the cassette/receptor.	☐	☐	☐	☐	☐	☐

AP or Obliques During Injection
The student:

	Procedure		Repeat		Competency	
	Yes	No	Yes	No	Yes	No
23. Assists in placing the patient in the supine or semi-supine position on the table.	☐	☐	☐	☐	☐	☐
24. Selects the appropriate receptor or places the cassette lengthwise. For conventional cassettes, the flash must be at the bottom and away from any anatomy.	☐	☐	☐	☐	☐	☐
25. Centers the central ray midway between the lateral surfaces of the body.	☐	☐	☐	☐	☐	☐

	Procedure		Repeat		Competency	
	Yes	No	Yes	No	Yes	No
26. Directs the central ray perpendicularly to the iliac crest, making sure the symphysis pubis is included on the cassette/receptor.	☐	☐	☐	☐	☐	☐

Comments:

_____

_____

IMPORTANT DETAILS
The student:

	Procedure		Repeat		Competency	
	Yes	No	Yes	No	Yes	No
27. Instills confidence in the patient by exhibiting self-confidence throughout the examination.	☐	☐	☐	☐	☐	☐
28. Places a lead marker in the appropriate area of the cassette/receptor (top/bottom/anteriorly/laterally), where it will be visualized on the finished radiograph, on the proper anatomical side (right/left), and in the appropriate position (face up/face down), depending on the patient's position.	☐	☐	☐	☐	☐	☐
29. Provides radiation protection (shield) for the patient (when appropriate), self, and others (closes doors).	☐	☐	☐	☐	☐	☐
30. Applies proper collimation and makes adjustments as necessary.	☐	☐	☐	☐	☐	☐
31. Properly measures the patient along the course of the central ray *for each projection.*	☐	☐	☐	☐	☐	☐

32. Sets the proper technique *for fluoroscopy* (kVp, mA, time).

And all projections/spot images:

Conventional systems

* Sets the proper kVp, mA, and time and makes adjustments as necessary.

or

CR or DR systems
* Identifies the patient on the work-list (or manually types the patient information into the system).
* Selects appropriate body region, specific body part, and accurate view/projection.
* Double-checks preset parameters:
  —Adult vs. pediatric patients
    ○ Small, medium, or large
  —Bucky/receptor (upright vs. table) *or* non-Bucky
  —AEC vs. fixed
    ○ If AEC, checks ion chambers
    ○ Density setting
  —kVp and mA; adjusts if necessary
  —Focal spot/filament size

	Procedure		Repeat		Competency	
	Yes	No	Yes	No	Yes	No
33. Exposes the cassette/receptor while watching the patient (expiration) *for each projection.*	☐	☐	☐	☐	☐	☐
34. Provides each radiograph with the proper identification (flash) and/or processes each cassette (image) without difficulty (regardless of technology—film, CR, or DR).	▨	▨	▨	▨	☐	☐
35. Properly completes the examination by filling out all necessary paperwork, entering the examination in the computer, having the images checked by the appropriate staff members, answering any last-minute questions, and informing the patient that he or she is finished. Provides proper post-exam instructions as required.	▨	▨	▨	▨	☐	☐
36. Exhibits the ability to adapt to new and difficult situations if and when necessary.	▨	▨	▨	▨	☐	☐

(continued)

	Procedure		Repeat		Competency	
	Yes	No	Yes	No	Yes	No
37. Accepts constructive criticism and uses it to his or her advantage.	☐	☐	☐	☐	☐	☐
38. Completes the examination within a reasonable time frame.	☐	☐	☐	☐	☐	☐
39. Leaves the radiographic room neat and clean for the next examination.	■	■	■	■	☐	☐

Comments:

_____

_____

RADIOGRAPHIC IMAGE QUALITY
The student is able to critique his or her radiographs as to whether they demonstrate:

	Procedure		Repeat		Competency	
	Yes	No	Yes	No	Yes	No
40. Proper technique/optimal density	■	■	■	■	☐	☐
41. Enhanced detail, without evidence of motion and without any visible artifacts	■	■	■	■	☐	☐
42. Proper positioning (all anatomy included, evidence of proper centering/alignment, etc.)	■	■	■	■	☐	☐
43. Proper marker placement	■	■	■	■	☐	☐
44. Evidence of proper collimation and radiation protection	■	■	■	■	☐	☐
45. Long vs. short scale of contrast	■	■	■	■	☐	☐
46. Image/projection identification and/or other identification	■	■	■	■	☐	☐

Comments:

_____

_____

ABDOMEN ANATOMY
The student is able to identify:

	Procedure		Repeat		Competency	
	Yes	No	Yes	No	Yes	No
47. Kidneys	■	■	■	■	☐	☐
48. Ureter	■	■	■	■	☐	☐
49. Bladder	■	■	■	■	☐	☐
50. Urethra	■	■	■	■	☐	☐
51. Diaphragm	■	■	■	■	☐	☐
52. Iliac crest	■	■	■	■	☐	☐
53. Bowel gas	■	■	■	■	☐	☐
54. Renal pelvis	■	■	■	■	☐	☐
55. Major and minor calyces	■	■	■	■	☐	☐
56. Upper vs. lower poles of the kidney	■	■	■	■	☐	☐
57. Obvious pathology	■	■	■	■	☐	☐

Comments:

_____

_____

_____   _____   _____
Procedure Evaluator Signature   Repeat Evaluator Signature   Competency Evaluator Signature

_____   _____   _____
Date   Date   Date

END RETROGRADE UROGRAM OR RETROGRADE PYELOGRAPHY EVALUATION

Retrograde Urethrogram

The objective of this evaluation is to determine the student's competency level when performing specific radiographic examinations.

Student Name:_____

Procedure Grade	Repeat Grade	Competency Grade

PATIENT INFORMATION OR SIMULATED PROCEDURE *(circle if simulated)*

	Procedure	Repeat	Competency
Age			
Medical Record No.			
Ability to Cooperate			
Condition/Pathology			
Technical Factors Used			
Exposure Index			

FACILITY PREPARATION
The student:

	Procedure Yes	Procedure No	Repeat Yes	Repeat No	Competency Yes	Competency No
1. Examines the operating room and prepares the radiographic equipment for the procedure.	☐	☐	☐	☐	☐	☐
2. Has all equipment and supplies (markers, tape, cassettes, lead aprons, proper contrast material, etc.) readily available before escorting the patient in.	☐	☐	☐	☐	☐	☐

Additional supplies:

_____

_____

_____

_____

	Procedure Yes	Procedure No	Repeat Yes	Repeat No	Competency Yes	Competency No
3. Selects and prepares the contrast material without difficulty.	☒	☒	☒	☒	☐	☐
4. Is able to manipulate all radiographic equipment with ease, and centers the central ray to the cassette/receptor *for all projections.*	☐	☐	☐	☐	☐	☐
5. Adjusts the tube to the proper SID *for each projection.*	☐	☐	☐	☐	☐	☐
6. Selects cassettes/receptor of the appropriate sizes *for all projections,* according to the patient's size and examination.	☐	☐	☐	☐	☐	☐

Comments:

_____

_____

PATIENT PREPARATION
The student:

	Procedure Yes	Procedure No	Repeat Yes	Repeat No	Competency Yes	Competency No
7. Identifies the correct patient and examination according to the requisition.	☐	☐	☐	☐	☐	☐
8. Obtains and documents the patient's history before the examination, including whether the patient ate before the examination and preparation instructions, and asks if the patient has had a contrast study before.	☒	☒	☒	☒	☐	☐

(continued)

	Procedure		Repeat		Competency	
	Yes	No	Yes	No	Yes	No
9. Thoroughly explains the examination (how the study is performed) and properly communicates with the patient throughout the examination.	☐	☐	☐	☐	☐	☐
10. Asks female patients of childbearing age the date of their last menstrual period and documents this; inquires about the possibility of pregnancy and has them sign pregnancy consent forms.	☐	☐	☐	☐	☐	☐
11. Removes all obscuring objects (snaps, zippers, jewelry, belts, etc.) so as *not* to produce radiographic artifacts.	☐	☐	☐	☐	☐	☐
12. Respects the patient's modesty and provides ample comfort for the patient while positioning him or her to begin the examination.	☐	☐	☐	☐	☐	☐
13. Ensures that the patient's bladder is empty before performing the initial radiographs.	☐	☐	☐	☐	☐	☐
14. Performs a scout radiograph when indicated.	☐	☐	☐	☐	☐	☐

Comments:

_____

_____

TASKS DURING FLUOROSCOPY
The student:

	Procedure		Repeat		Competency	
	Yes	No	Yes	No	Yes	No
15. Relays the patient's history to the radiologist.	▦	▦	▦	▦	☐	☐
16. Assists staff members and the physician throughout the examination.	▦	▦	▦	▦	☐	☐
17. Monitors, communicates with, and assists the patient throughout the examination.	▦	▦	▦	▦	☐	☐
18. Takes charge of the examination when the radiologist departs.	▦	▦	▦	▦	☐	☐

Comments:

_____

_____

PATIENT POSITIONING FOR A RETROGRADE URETHROGRAM
AP Abdomen
The student:

	Procedure		Repeat		Competency	
	Yes	No	Yes	No	Yes	No
19. Assists in placing the patient in the supine position on the radiographic/ surgical table, without rotation.	☐	☐	☐	☐	☐	☐
20. Selects the appropriate receptor or places the cassette lengthwise. For conventional cassettes, the flash must be at the bottom and away from any anatomy.	☐	☐	☐	☐	☐	☐
21. Centers the central ray to the midsagittal plane of the body.	☐	☐	☐	☐	☐	☐
22. Directs the central ray perpendicularly to the iliac crest, making sure the symphysis pubis is included on the cassette/receptor.	☐	☐	☐	☐	☐	☐

Voiding AP or Obliques
The student:

	Procedure		Repeat		Competency	
	Yes	No	Yes	No	Yes	No
23. Assists in placing the patient in the supine or semi-supine position on the table.	☐	☐	☐	☐	☐	☐
24. Selects the appropriate receptor or places the cassette lengthwise. For conventional cassettes, the flash must be at the bottom and away from any anatomy.	☐	☐	☐	☐	☐	☐
25. Centers the central ray midway between the lateral surfaces of the body.	☐	☐	☐	☐	☐	☐

	Procedure		Repeat		Competency	
	Yes	No	Yes	No	Yes	No
26. Directs the central ray perpendicularly to the iliac crest, making sure the symphysis pubis included on the cassette/receptor.	☐	☐	☐	☐	☐	☐

Comments:

_____

_____

IMPORTANT DETAILS
The student:

	Procedure		Repeat		Competency	
	Yes	No	Yes	No	Yes	No
27. Instills confidence in the patient by exhibiting self-confidence throughout the examination.	☐	☐	☐	☐	☐	☐
28. Places a lead marker in the appropriate area of the cassette/receptor (top/bottom/anteriorly/laterally), where it will be visualized on the finished radiograph, on the proper anatomical side (right/left), and in the appropriate position (face up/face down), depending on the patient's position.	☐	☐	☐	☐	☐	☐
29. Provides radiation protection (shield) for the patient (when appropriate), self, and others (closes doors).	☐	☐	☐	☐	☐	☐
30. Applies proper collimation and makes adjustments as necessary.	☐	☐	☐	☐	☐	☐
31. Properly measures the patient along the course of the central ray *for each projection.*	☐	☐	☐	☐	☐	☐

32. Sets the proper technique *for fluoroscopy* (kVp, mA, time).

And all projections/spot images:

Conventional systems

- Sets the proper kVp, mA, and time and makes adjustments as necessary.

or

CR or DR systems

- Identifies the patient on the work-list (or manually types the patient information into the system).
- Selects appropriate body region, specific body part, and accurate view/projection.
- Double-checks preset parameters:
  —Adult vs. pediatric patients
    ◦ Small, medium, or large
  —Bucky/receptor (upright vs. table) *or* non-Bucky
  —AEC vs. fixed
    ◦ If AEC, checks ion chambers
    ◦ Density setting
  —kVp and mA; adjusts if necessary
  —Focal spot/filament size

	Procedure		Repeat		Competency	
33. Exposes the cassette/receptor while watching the patient (expiration) *for each projection.*	☐	☐	☐	☐	☐	☐
34. Provides each radiograph with the proper identification (flash) and/or processes each cassette (image) without difficulty (regardless of technology—film, CR, or DR).	▦	▦	▦	▦	☐	☐
35. Properly completes the examination by filling out all necessary paperwork, entering the examination in the computer, having the images checked by the appropriate staff members, answering any last-minute questions, and informing the patient that he or she is finished. Provides proper post-exam instructions as required.	▦	▦	▦	▦	☐	☐
36. Exhibits the ability to adapt to new and difficult situations if and when necessary.	▦	▦	▦	▦	☐	☐

(continued)

	Procedure		Repeat		Competency	
	Yes	No	Yes	No	Yes	No
37. Accepts constructive criticism and uses it to his or her advantage.	☐	☐	☐	☐	☐	☐
38. Completes the examination within a reasonable time frame.	☐	☐	☐	☐	☐	☐
39. Leaves the radiographic room neat and clean for the next examination.	▣	▣	▣	▣	☐	☐

Comments:

_____

_____

RADIOGRAPHIC IMAGE QUALITY
The student is able to critique his or her radiographs as to whether they demonstrate:

	Procedure		Repeat		Competency	
	Yes	No	Yes	No	Yes	No
40. Proper technique/optimal density	▣	▣	▣	▣	☐	☐
41. Enhanced detail, without evidence of motion and without any visible artifacts	▣	▣	▣	▣	☐	☐
42. Proper positioning (all anatomy included, evidence of proper centering/alignment, etc.)	▣	▣	▣	▣	☐	☐
43. Proper marker placement	▣	▣	▣	▣	☐	☐
44. Evidence of proper collimation and radiation protection	▣	▣	▣	▣	☐	☐
45. Long vs. short scale of contrast	▣	▣	▣	▣	☐	☐
46. Image/projection identification and/or other identification	▣	▣	▣	▣	☐	☐

Comments:

_____

_____

ABDOMEN ANATOMY
The student is able to identify:

	Procedure		Repeat		Competency	
	Yes	No	Yes	No	Yes	No
47. Bladder	▣	▣	▣	▣	☐	☐
48. Urethra	▣	▣	▣	▣	☐	☐
49. Symphysis pubis	▣	▣	▣	▣	☐	☐
50. Iliac crest	▣	▣	▣	▣	☐	☐
51. Bowel gas	▣	▣	▣	▣	☐	☐
52. Obvious pathology	▣	▣	▣	▣	☐	☐

Comments:

_____

_____

_____   _____   _____
Procedure Evaluator Signature   Repeat Evaluator Signature   Competency Evaluator Signature

_____   _____   _____
Date   Date   Date

END RETROGRADE URETHROGRAM EVALUATION

Student Name:_____

<table>
<tr><td>Procedure Grade</td><td>Repeat Grade</td><td>Competency Grade</td></tr>
<tr><td></td><td></td><td></td></tr>
</table>

PATIENT INFORMATION OR SIMULATED PROCEDURE *(circle if simulated)*

	Procedure	Repeat	Competency
Age			
Medical Record No.			
Ability to Cooperate			
Condition/Pathology			
Technical Factors Used			
Exposure Index			

FACILITY PREPARATION
The student:

	Procedure Yes	No	Repeat Yes	No	Competency Yes	No
1. Examines the radiographic room and cleans/straightens it before escorting the patient in.	☐	☐	☐	☐	☐	☐
2. Has all equipment and supplies (markers, tape, cassettes, lead aprons, proper contrast material, etc.) readily available before escorting the patient in.	☐	☐	☐	☐	☐	☐

Additional supplies:

_____

_____

_____

_____

	Procedure Yes	No	Repeat Yes	No	Competency Yes	No
3. Selects and prepares the contrast material without difficulty.	■	■	■	■	☐	☐
4. Is able to manipulate all radiographic equipment with ease, and centers the central ray to the cassette/receptor *for all projections.*	☐	☐	☐	☐	☐	☐
5. Adjusts the tube to the proper SID *for each projection.*	☐	☐	☐	☐	☐	☐
6. Selects cassettes/receptor of the appropriate sizes *for all projections,* according to the patient's size and examination.	☐	☐	☐	☐	☐	☐

Comments:

_____

_____

PATIENT PREPARATION
The student:

	Procedure Yes	No	Repeat Yes	No	Competency Yes	No
7. Identifies the correct patient and examination according to the requisition while establishing a good rapport with him or her.	☐	☐	☐	☐	☐	☐

(continued)

	Procedure		Repeat		Competency	
	Yes	No	Yes	No	Yes	No
8. Obtains and documents the patient's history before the examination, including whether the patient ate before the examination and preparation instructions, and asks if the patient has had a contrast study before.	▣	▣	▣	▣	☐	☐
9. Thoroughly explains the examination (how the study is performed) and properly communicates with the patient throughout the examination.	☐	☐	☐	☐	☐	☐
10. Asks female patients of childbearing age the date of their last menstrual period and documents this; inquires about the possibility of pregnancy and has them sign pregnancy consent forms.	☐	☐	☐	☐	☐	☐
11. Removes all obscuring objects (snaps, zippers, jewelry, belts, etc.) so as *not* to produce radiographic artifacts.	☐	☐	☐	☐	☐	☐
12. Respects the patient's modesty and provides ample comfort for the patient while positioning him or her to begin the examination.	☐	☐	☐	☐	☐	☐
13. Ensures that the patient's bladder is empty before performing the initial radiographs.	☐	☐	☐	☐	☐	☐
14. Performs a scout radiograph when indicated.	☐	☐	☐	☐	☐	☐

Comments:

_____

_____

TASKS DURING FLUOROSCOPY
The student:

	Procedure		Repeat		Competency	
	Yes	No	Yes	No	Yes	No
15. Relays the patient's history to the radiologist.	▣	▣	▣	▣	☐	☐
16. Assists staff members and the physician throughout the examination.	▣	▣	▣	▣	☐	☐
17. Monitors, communicates with, and assists the patient throughout the examination.	▣	▣	▣	▣	☐	☐
18. Takes charge of the examination after the radiologist departs.	▣	▣	▣	▣	☐	☐

Comments:

_____

_____

PATIENT POSITIONING FOR A CYSTOGRAM
AP Bladder
The student:

	Procedure		Repeat		Competency	
	Yes	No	Yes	No	Yes	No
19. Places the patient in the supine position on the radiographic table, without rotation.	☐	☐	☐	☐	☐	☐
20. Selects the appropriate receptor or places the cassette lengthwise. For conventional cassettes, the flash must be at the bottom and away from any anatomy.	▣	▣	▣	▣	☐	☐
21. Centers the central ray to the midsagittal plane of the body.	▣	▣	▣	▣	☐	☐
22. Directs the central ray perpendicularly at the level of the soft tissue depression just above the greater trochanter.	▣	▣	▣	▣	☐	☐

AP or Obliques During Contrast Administration (or During Voiding)
The student:

	Procedure		Repeat		Competency	
	Yes	No	Yes	No	Yes	No
23. Places the patient in the supine or semisupine position on the radiographic table.	▣	▣	▣	▣	☐	☐

	Procedure		Repeat		Competency	
	Yes	No	Yes	No	Yes	No
24. Selects the appropriate receptor or places the cassette lengthwise. For conventional cassettes, the flash must be at the bottom and away from any anatomy.	☐	☐	☐	☐	☐	☐
25. Centers the central ray midway between the lateral surfaces of the body.	☐	☐	☐	☐	☐	☐
26. Directs the central ray perpendicularly at the level of the soft tissue depression just above the greater trochanter.	☐	☐	☐	☐	☐	☐

Comments:

_____

_____

IMPORTANT DETAILS
The student:

	Procedure		Repeat		Competency	
	Yes	No	Yes	No	Yes	No
27. Instills confidence in the patient by exhibiting self-confidence throughout the examination.	☐	☐	☐	☐	☐	☐
28. Places a lead marker in the appropriate area of the cassette/receptor (top/bottom/anteriorly/laterally), where it will be visualized on the finished radiograph, on the proper anatomical side (right/left), and in the appropriate position (face up/face down), depending on the patient's position.	☐	☐	☐	☐	☐	☐
29. Provides radiation protection (shield) for the patient (when appropriate), self, and others (closes doors).	☐	☐	☐	☐	☐	☐
30. Applies proper collimation and makes adjustments as necessary.	☐	☐	☐	☐	☐	☐
31. Properly measures the patient along the course of the central ray *for each projection.*	☐	☐	☐	☐	☐	☐

32. Sets the proper technique *for fluoroscopy* (kVp, mA, time).

And all projections/spot images:

Conventional systems

- Sets the proper kVp, mA, and time and makes adjustments as necessary.

or

CR or DR systems
- Identifies the patient on the work-list (or manually types the patient information into the system).
- Selects appropriate body region, specific body part, and accurate view/projection.
- Double-checks preset parameters:
  —Adult vs. pediatric patients
  ○ Small, medium, or large
  —Bucky/receptor (upright vs. table) *or* non-Bucky
  —AEC vs. fixed
  ○ If AEC, checks ion chambers
  ○ Density setting
  —kVp and mA; adjusts if necessary
  —Focal spot/filament size

	Procedure		Repeat		Competency	
33. Exposes the cassette/receptor after telling the patient to hold still and after giving him or her proper breathing instructions (expiration) *for each projection.*	☐	☐	☐	☐	☐	☐
34. Provides each radiograph with the proper identification (flash) and/or processes each cassette (image) without difficulty (regardless of technology—film, CR, or DR).	☐	☐	☐	☐	☐	☐

(continued)

	Procedure		Repeat		Competency	
	Yes	No	Yes	No	Yes	No
35. Properly completes the examination by filling out all necessary paperwork, entering the examination in the computer, having the images checked by the appropriate staff members, answering any last-minute questions, and informing the patient that he or she is finished. Provides proper post-exam instructions as required.	☐	☐	☐	☐	☐	☐
36. Exhibits the ability to adapt to new and difficult situations if and when necessary.	☐	☐	☐	☐	☐	☐
37. Accepts constructive criticism and uses it to his or her advantage.	☐	☐	☐	☐	☐	☐
38. Leaves the radiographic room neat and clean for the next examination.	☐	☐	☐	☐	☐	☐
39. Completes the examination within a reasonable time frame.	☐	☐	☐	☐	☐	☐

Comments:

_____

_____

RADIOGRAPHIC IMAGE QUALITY
The student is able to critique his or her radiographs as to whether they demonstrate:

	Procedure		Repeat		Competency	
	Yes	No	Yes	No	Yes	No
40. Proper technique/optimal density	☐	☐	☐	☐	☐	☐
41. Enhanced detail, without evidence of motion and without any visible artifacts	☐	☐	☐	☐	☐	☐
42. Proper positioning (all anatomy included, evidence of proper centering/alignment, etc.)	☐	☐	☐	☐	☐	☐
43. Proper marker placement	☐	☐	☐	☐	☐	☐
44. Evidence of proper collimation and radiation protection	☐	☐	☐	☐	☐	☐
45. Long vs. short scale of contrast	☐	☐	☐	☐	☐	☐
46. Image/projection identification and/or other identification	☐	☐	☐	☐	☐	☐

Comments:

_____

_____

ABDOMEN ANATOMY
The student is able to identify:

	Procedure		Repeat		Competency	
	Yes	No	Yes	No	Yes	No
47. Bladder	☐	☐	☐	☐	☐	☐
48. Urethra	☐	☐	☐	☐	☐	☐
49. Symphysis pubis	☐	☐	☐	☐	☐	☐
50. Iliac crest	☐	☐	☐	☐	☐	☐
51. Bowel gas	☐	☐	☐	☐	☐	☐
52. Obvious pathology	☐	☐	☐	☐	☐	☐

Comments:

_____

_____

_____

Procedure Evaluator Signature	Repeat Evaluator Signature	Competency Evaluator Signature
Date	Date	Date

END CYSTOGRAM EVALUATION

Student Name:_____

Procedure Grade	Repeat Grade	Competency Grade

PATIENT INFORMATION OR SIMULATED PROCEDURE *(circle if simulated)*

	Procedure	Repeat	Competency
Age			
Medical Record No.			
Ability to Cooperate			
Condition/Pathology			
Technical Factors Used			
Exposure Index			

FACILITY PREPARATION
The student:

	Procedure Yes	No	Repeat Yes	No	Competency Yes	No
1. Examines the radiographic room and cleans/straightens it before escorting the patient in.	☐	☐	☐	☐	☐	☐
2. Has all equipment and supplies (markers, tape, cassettes, lead aprons, urinal/female voiding device, including a catheterization kit if necessary, proper contrast material, etc.) readily available before escorting the patient in.	☐	☐	☐	☐	☐	☐

Additional supplies:

_____
_____
_____
_____

	Procedure Yes	No	Repeat Yes	No	Competency Yes	No
3. Selects and prepares the contrast material without difficulty.	▨	▨	▨	▨	☐	☐
4. Is able to manipulate all radiographic equipment with ease, and centers the central ray to the cassette/receptor *for all projections.*	☐	☐	☐	☐	☐	☐
5. Adjusts the tube to the proper SID *for each projection.*	☐	☐	☐	☐	☐	☐
6. Selects cassettes/receptor of the appropriate sizes *for each projection,* according to the patient's size and examination.	☐	☐	☐	☐	☐	☐

Comments:

_____

_____

PATIENT PREPARATION
The student:

	Procedure Yes	No	Repeat Yes	No	Competency Yes	No
7. Identifies the correct patient and examination according to the requisition while establishing a good rapport with him or her.	☐	☐	☐	☐	☐	☐

(continued)

	Procedure		Repeat		Competency	
	Yes	No	Yes	No	Yes	No
8. Obtains and documents the patient's history before the examination, including whether the patient ate before the examination and preparation instructions, and asks if the patient has had a contrast study before.	▩	▩	▩	▩	☐	☐
9. Thoroughly explains the examination (how the examination is performed), *emphasizing the voiding procedure,* and properly communicates with the patient throughout the examination.	☐	☐	☐	☐	☐	☐
10. Asks female patients of childbearing age the date of their last menstrual period and documents this; inquires about the possibility of pregnancy and has them sign pregnancy consent forms.	☐	☐	☐	☐	☐	☐
11. Removes all obscuring objects (snaps, zippers, jewelry, belts, etc.) so as *not* to produce radiographic artifacts.	☐	☐	☐	☐	☐	☐
12. Respects the patient's modesty and provides ample comfort for the patient while positioning him or her to begin the examination.	☐	☐	☐	☐	☐	☐
13. Ensures that the patient's bladder is empty before performing the initial radiographs.	☐	☐	☐	☐	☐	☐
14. Performs a scout radiograph when indicated.	☐	☐	☐	☐	☐	☐

Comments:

_____

_____

TASKS DURING FLUOROSCOPY
The student:

	Procedure		Repeat		Competency	
	Yes	No	Yes	No	Yes	No
15. Relays the patient's history to the radiologist.	▩	▩	▩	▩	☐	☐
16. Assists staff and the physician throughout the examination.	▩	▩	▩	▩	☐	☐
17. Monitors, communicates with, and assists the patient throughout the examination.	▩	▩	▩	▩	☐	☐
18. Takes charge of the examination after the radiologist departs.	▩	▩	▩	▩	☐	☐

Comments:

_____

_____

PATIENT POSITIONING FOR A VOIDING CYSTOURETHROGRAM
AP Abdomen
The student:

	Procedure		Repeat		Competency	
	Yes	No	Yes	No	Yes	No
19. Places the patient in the supine position on the radiographic table, without rotation.	☐	☐	☐	☐	☐	☐
20. Selects the appropriate receptor or places the cassette lengthwise. For conventional cassettes, the flash must be at the bottom and away from any anatomy.	☐	☐	☐	☐	☐	☐
21. Centers the central ray to the midsagittal plane of the body.	☐	☐	☐	☐	☐	☐
22. Directs the central ray perpendicularly to a point 2 inches above the symphysis pubis.	☐	☐	☐	☐	☐	☐

AP or Obliques During Injection
The student:

	Procedure		Repeat		Competency	
	Yes	No	Yes	No	Yes	No
23. Places the patient in the supine or 35–40° oblique/semi-supine position on the radiographic table.	☐	☐	☐	☐	☐	☐
24. Selects the appropriate receptor or places the cassette lengthwise. For conventional cassettes, the flash must be at the bottom and away from any anatomy.	☐	☐	☐	☐	☐	☐
25. Centers the central ray to the midsagittal plane of the body.	☐	☐	☐	☐	☐	☐
26. Directs the central ray perpendicularly to a point 2 inches above the symphysis pubis.	☐	☐	☐	☐	☐	☐

Voiding AP
The student:

	Procedure		Repeat		Competency	
	Yes	No	Yes	No	Yes	No
27. Places the patient in the supine position on the radiographic table, without rotation.	☐	☐	☐	☐	☐	☐
28. Selects the appropriate receptor or places the cassette lengthwise. For conventional cassettes, the flash must be at the bottom and away from any anatomy.	☐	☐	☐	☐	☐	☐
29. Centers the central ray to the midway between the lateral surfaces of the body.	☐	☐	☐	☐	☐	☐
30. Directs the central ray 5–15° caudad to a point 2 inches above the pubic symphysis, making sure the cassette/receptor extends 3 inches below the symphysis pubis so that the urethra is included on the cassette/receptor.	☐	☐	☐	☐	☐	☐

Voiding Obliques
The student:

	Procedure		Repeat		Competency	
	Yes	No	Yes	No	Yes	No
31. Places the patient in the oblique position, angled 35–40°, on the radiographic table.	☐	☐	☐	☐	☐	☐
32. Selects the appropriate receptor or places the cassette lengthwise. For conventional cassettes, the flash must be at the bottom and away from any anatomy.	☐	☐	☐	☐	☐	☐
33. Centers the central ray midway between the lateral surfaces of the body.	☐	☐	☐	☐	☐	☐
34. Directs the central ray perpendicularly to a point 2 inches above the pubic symphysis, making sure the cassette/receptor extends 3 inches below the symphysis pubis so that the urethra is included on the cassette/receptor.	☐	☐	☐	☐	☐	☐

Postvoid AP
The student:

	Procedure		Repeat		Competency	
	Yes	No	Yes	No	Yes	No
35. Places the patient in the supine position on the radiographic table, without rotation.	☐	☐	☐	☐	☐	☐
36. Selects the appropriate receptor or places the cassette lengthwise. For conventional cassettes, the flash must be at the bottom and away from any anatomy.	☐	☐	☐	☐	☐	☐
37. Centers the central ray to the midsagittal plane of the body.	☐	☐	☐	☐	☐	☐
38. Directs the central ray perpendicularly to a point 2 inches above the symphysis pubis.	☐	☐	☐	☐	☐	☐

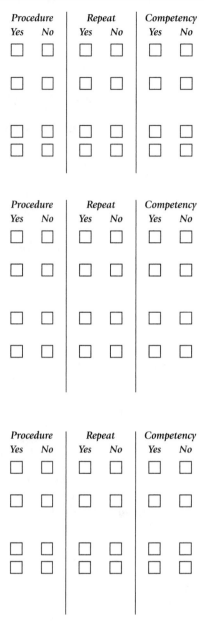

Comments:

_____

_____

(continued)

IMPORTANT DETAILS
The student:

	Procedure		Repeat		Competency	
	Yes	No	Yes	No	Yes	No
39. Instills confidence in the patient by exhibiting self-confidence throughout the examination.	☐	☐	☐	☐	☐	☐
40. Places a lead marker in the appropriate area of the cassette/receptor (top/bottom/anteriorly/laterally), where it will be visualized on the finished radiograph, on the proper anatomical side (right/left), and in the appropriate position (face up/face down), depending on the patient's position.	☐	☐	☐	☐	☐	☐
41. Provides radiation protection (shield) for the patient (when appropriate), self, and others (closes doors).	☐	☐	☐	☐	☐	☐
42. Applies proper collimation and makes adjustments as necessary.	☐	☐	☐	☐	☐	☐
43. Properly measures the patient along the course of the central ray *for each projection.*	☐	☐	☐	☐	☐	☐

44. Sets the proper technique *for fluoroscopy* (kVp, mA, time).

   And all projections/spot images:

   Conventional systems

   • Sets the proper kVp, mA, and time and makes adjustments as necessary.

   or

   CR or DR systems

   • Identifies the patient on the work-list (or manually types the patient information into the system).
   • Selects appropriate body region, specific body part, and accurate view/projection.
   • Double-checks preset parameters:
   　—Adult vs. pediatric patients
   　　○ Small, medium, or large
   　—Bucky/receptor (upright vs. table) *or* non-Bucky
   　—AEC vs. fixed
   　　○ If AEC, checks ion chambers
   　　○ Density setting
   　—kVp and mA; adjusts if necessary
   　—Focal spot/filament size

	Procedure		Repeat		Competency	
	Yes	No	Yes	No	Yes	No
45. Exposes the cassette/receptor after telling the patient to hold still and after giving him or her proper breathing instructions (expiration) *for each projection.*	☐	☐	☐	☐	☐	☐
46. Provides each radiograph with the proper identification (flash) and/or processes each cassette (image) without difficulty (regardless of technology—film, CR, or DR).	▣	▣	▣	▣	☐	☐
47. Properly completes the examination by filling out all necessary paperwork, entering the examination in the computer, having the images checked by the appropriate staff members, answering any last-minute questions, and informing the patient that he or she is finished. Provides proper post-exam instructions as required.	▣	▣	▣	▣	☐	☐
48. Exhibits the ability to adapt to new and difficult situations if and when necessary.	▣	▣	▣	▣	☐	☐
49. Accepts constructive criticism and uses it to his or her advantage.	☐	☐	☐	☐	☐	☐
50. Leaves the radiographic room neat and clean for the next examination.	▣	▣	▣	▣	☐	☐
51. Completes the examination within a reasonable time frame.	☐	☐	☐	☐	☐	☐

Comments:

_____

_____

RADIOGRAPHIC IMAGE QUALITY
The student is able to critique his or her radiographs as to whether they demonstrate:

	Procedure Yes	No	Repeat Yes	No	Competency Yes	No
52. Proper technique/optimal density	☐	☐	☐	☐	☐	☐
53. Enhanced detail, without evidence of motion and without any visible artifacts	☐	☐	☐	☐	☐	☐
54. Proper positioning (all anatomy included, evidence of proper centering/alignment, etc.)	☐	☐	☐	☐	☐	☐
55. Proper marker placement	☐	☐	☐	☐	☐	☐
56. Evidence of proper collimation and radiation protection	☐	☐	☐	☐	☐	☐
57. Long vs. short scale of contrast	☐	☐	☐	☐	☐	☐
58. Image/projection identification and/or other identification	☐	☐	☐	☐	☐	☐

Comments:

_____

_____

ABDOMEN ANATOMY
The student is able to identify:

	Procedure Yes	No	Repeat Yes	No	Competency Yes	No
59. Bladder	☐	☐	☐	☐	☐	☐
60. Urethra	☐	☐	☐	☐	☐	☐
61. Symphysis pubis	☐	☐	☐	☐	☐	☐
62. Iliac crest	☐	☐	☐	☐	☐	☐
63. Obvious pathology	☐	☐	☐	☐	☐	☐

Comments:

_____

_____

_____	_____	_____
Procedure Evaluator Signature	Repeat Evaluator Signature	Competency Evaluator Signature
_____	_____	_____
Date	Date	Date

END VOIDING CYSTOURETHROGRAM EVALUATION

Cholecystogram

The objective of this evaluation is to determine the student's competency level when performing specific radiographic examinations.

Student Name:_____

	Procedure Grade	Repeat Grade	Competency Grade

PATIENT INFORMATION OR SIMULATED PROCEDURE *(circle if simulated)*

	Procedure	Repeat	Competency
Age			
Medical Record No.			
Ability to Cooperate			
Condition/Pathology			
Technical Factors Used			
Exposure Index			

FACILITY PREPARATION
The student:

	Procedure Yes No	Repeat Yes No	Competency Yes No
1. Examines the radiographic room and cleans/straightens it before escorting the patient in.	☐ ☐	☐ ☐	☐ ☐
2. Has all equipment and supplies (patient gown, shield, markers, tape, cassettes, lead aprons, blockers, hemostats, compression paddle, lubricant, proper contrast material, etc.) readily available before escorting the patient in, the Bucky drawer in the proper position, the monitor by the table, and the fluoro on.	☐ ☐	☐ ☐	☐ ☐

Additional supplies:

_____
_____
_____
_____

	Procedure Yes No	Repeat Yes No	Competency Yes No
3. Selects and prepares the contrast material without difficulty.	▨ ▨	▨ ▨	☐ ☐
4. Is able to manipulate all radiographic equipment with ease, and centers the central ray to the cassette/receptor *for all projections.*	☐ ☐	☐ ☐	☐ ☐
5. Adjusts the tube to the proper SID *for each projection.*	☐ ☐	☐ ☐	☐ ☐
6. Selects cassettes/receptor of the appropriate sizes *for all projections,* according to the patient's size and examination.	☐ ☐	☐ ☐	☐ ☐

Comments:

_____

_____

PATIENT PREPARATION
The student:

	Procedure Yes No	Repeat Yes No	Competency Yes No
7. Identifies the correct patient and examination according to the requisition while establishing a good rapport with him or her.	☐ ☐	☐ ☐	☐ ☐

(continued)

	Procedure		Repeat		Competency	
	Yes	No	Yes	No	Yes	No
8. Obtains and documents the patient's history before the examination, including whether the patient ate before the examination and preparation instructions	▪	▪	▪	▪	☐	☐
9. Thoroughly explains the examination in terms the patient fully understands and properly communicates with the patient throughout the examination.	☐	☐	☐	☐	☐	☐
10. Asks female patients of childbearing age the date of their last menstrual period and documents this; inquires about the possibility of pregnancy and has them sign pregnancy consent forms.	☐	☐	☐	☐	☐	☐
11. Removes all obscuring objects (snaps, zippers, jewelry, belts, etc.) so as *not* to produce radiographic artifacts.	☐	☐	☐	☐	☐	☐
12. Respects the patient's modesty and provides ample comfort for the patient while positioning him or her to begin the examination.	☐	☐	☐	☐	☐	☐
13. Performs a scout radiograph when indicated.	☐	☐	☐	☐	☐	☐

Comments:

_____

_____

TASKS DURING FLUOROSCOPY
The student:

	Procedure		Repeat		Competency	
	Yes	No	Yes	No	Yes	No
14. Relays the patient's history to the radiologist.	▪	▪	▪	▪	☐	☐
15. Assists staff and the physician throughout the examination.	▪	▪	▪	▪	☐	☐
16. Monitors, communicates with, and assists the patient throughout the examination.	▪	▪	▪	▪	☐	☐
17. Takes charge of the examination after the radiologist departs.	▪	▪	▪	▪	☐	☐

Comments:

_____

_____

PATIENT POSITIONING FOR A CHOLECYSTOGRAM
Posteroanterior
The student:

	Procedure		Repeat		Competency	
	Yes	No	Yes	No	Yes	No
18. Places the patient in the prone position on the radiographic table, without rotation.	☐	☐	☐	☐	☐	☐
19. Selects the appropriate receptor or places the cassette lengthwise. For conventional cassettes, the flash must be at the bottom and away from any anatomy.	☐	☐	☐	☐	☐	☐
20. Centers the central ray on the *right side,* midway between the midsagittal plane and the right lateral margin of the body.	☐	☐	☐	☐	☐	☐
21. Directs the central ray perpendicularly 2–3 inches above the subcostal plane.	☐	☐	☐	☐	☐	☐

Left Anterior Oblique
The student:

	Procedure		Repeat		Competency	
	Yes	No	Yes	No	Yes	No
22. Places the patient semiprone at an angle of 15–30° on the radiographic table.	☐	☐	☐	☐	☐	☐
23. Selects the appropriate receptor or places the cassette lengthwise. For conventional cassettes, the flash must be at the bottom and away from any anatomy.	☐	☐	☐	☐	☐	☐

	Procedure		Repeat		Competency	
	Yes	No	Yes	No	Yes	No
24. Centers the central ray midway between the midsagittal plane and the lateral margin of the body, over the *right side*/up side.	☐	☐	☐	☐	☐	☐

Right Lateral Decubitus
The student:

	Procedure		Repeat		Competency	
	Yes	No	Yes	No	Yes	No
25. Places the patient in the right lateral recumbent position, with the patient built up to adequately demonstrate the right side.	☐	☐	☐	☐	☐	☐
26. Selects the appropriate receptor or places the grid/cassette lengthwise lengthwise, as close to the patient as possible. For conventional cassettes, the flash must be at the bottom and away from any anatomy.	☐	☐	☐	☐	☐	☐
27. Instructs the patient to raise his or her arms above the area of interest and adjusts the thorax to a true lateral position, making sure there is no rotation.	☐	☐	☐	☐	☐	☐
28. Centers the central ray to midway between the midsagittal plane and the right lateral margin of the body.	☐	☐	☐	☐	☐	☐
29. Using a horizontal beam, directs the central ray perpendicularly 2–3 inches above the subcostal plane.	☐	☐	☐	☐	☐	☐

Comments:

_____

_____

IMPORTANT DETAILS
The student:

	Procedure		Repeat		Competency	
	Yes	No	Yes	No	Yes	No
30. Instills confidence in the patient by exhibiting self-confidence throughout the examination.	☐	☐	☐	☐	☐	☐
31. Places a lead marker in the appropriate area of the cassette/receptor (top/bottom/anteriorly/laterally), where it will be visualized on the finished radiograph, on the proper anatomical side (right/left), and in the appropriate position (face up/face down), depending on the patient's position.	☐	☐	☐	☐	☐	☐
32. Provides radiation protection (shield) for the patient (when appropriate), self, and others (closes doors).	☐	☐	☐	☐	☐	☐
33. Applies proper collimation and makes adjustments as necessary.	☐	☐	☐	☐	☐	☐
34. Properly measures the patient along the course of the central ray *for each projection.*	☐	☐	☐	☐	☐	☐
35. Sets the proper technique *for fluoroscopy* (kVp, mA, time).	☐	☐	☐	☐	☐	☐

And all projections/spot images:

Conventional systems

- Sets the proper kVp, mA, and time and makes adjustments as necessary.

or

CR or DR systems
- Identifies the patient on the work-list (or manually types the patient information into the system).
- Selects appropriate body region, specific body part, and accurate view/projection.
- Double-checks preset parameters:
  —Adult vs. pediatric patients
    ○ Small, medium, or large
  —Bucky/receptor (upright vs. table) *or* non-Bucky

(continued)

	Procedure		Repeat		Competency	
	Yes	No	Yes	No	Yes	No

—AEC vs. fixed
    ◦ If AEC, checks ion chambers
    ◦ Density setting
—kVp and mA; adjusts if necessary
—Focal spot/filament size

	Procedure		Repeat		Competency	
36. Exposes the cassette/receptor after telling the patient to hold still and after giving him or her proper breathing instructions (expiration) *for each projection.*	☐	☐	☐	☐	☐	☐
37. Provides each radiograph with the proper identification (flash) and/or processes each cassette (image) without difficulty (regardless of technology—film, CR, or DR).	▨	▨	▨	▨	☐	☐
38. Properly completes the examination by filling out all necessary paperwork, entering the examination in the computer, having the images checked by the appropriate staff members, answering any last-minute questions, and informing the patient that he or she is finished. Provides proper post-exam instructions as required.	▨	▨	▨	▨	☐	☐
39. Exhibits the ability to adapt to new and difficult situations if and when necessary.	▨	▨	▨	▨	☐	☐
40. Accepts constructive criticism and uses it to his or her advantage.	☐	☐	☐	☐	☐	☐
41. Leaves the radiographic room neat and clean for the next examination.	▨	▨	▨	▨	☐	☐
42. Completes the examination within a reasonable time frame.	☐	☐	☐	☐	☐	☐

Comments:

_____

_____

RADIOGRAPHIC IMAGE QUALITY
The student is able to critique his or her radiographs as to whether they demonstrate:

	Procedure		Repeat		Competency	
	Yes	No	Yes	No	Yes	No
43. Proper technique/optimal density	▨	▨	▨	▨	☐	☐
44. Enhanced detail, without evidence of motion and without any visible artifacts	▨	▨	▨	▨	☐	☐
45. Proper positioning (all anatomy included, evidence of proper centering/alignment, etc.)	▨	▨	▨	▨	☐	☐
46. Proper marker placement	▨	▨	▨	▨	☐	☐
47. Evidence of proper collimation and radiation protection	▨	▨	▨	▨	☐	☐
48. Long vs. short scale of contrast	▨	▨	▨	▨	☐	☐
49. Image/projection identification and/or other identification	▨	▨	▨	▨	☐	☐

Comments:

_____

_____

ABDOMEN ANATOMY
The student is able to identify:

	Procedure		Repeat		Competency	
	Yes	No	Yes	No	Yes	No
50. Gallbladder	▨	▨	▨	▨	☐	☐
51. Stones in the gallbladder	▨	▨	▨	▨	☐	☐
52. Biliary ducts	▨	▨	▨	▨	☐	☐
53. Bowel gas	▨	▨	▨	▨	☐	☐
54. Diaphragm	▨	▨	▨	▨	☐	☐
55. Kidney	▨	▨	▨	▨	☐	☐

	Procedure		Repeat		Competency	
	Yes	No	Yes	No	Yes	No
56. Rib cage	☐	☐	☐	☐	☐	☐
57. Obvious pathology	☐	☐	☐	☐	☐	☐

Comments:

_____

_____

_____	_____	_____
Procedure Evaluator Signature	Repeat Evaluator Signature	Competency Evaluator Signature
_____	_____	_____
Date	Date	Date

END CHOLECYSTOGRAM EVALUATION

Three-Textured Barium Swallow

The objective of this evaluation is to determine the student's competency level when performing specific radiographic examinations.

Student Name:_____

Procedure Grade	Repeat Grade	Competency Grade

PATIENT INFORMATION OR SIMULATED PROCEDURE *(circle if simulated)*

	Procedure	Repeat	Competency
Age			
Medical Record No.			
Ability to Cooperate			
Condition/Pathology			
Technical Factors Used			
Exposure Index			

FACILITY PREPARATION
The student:

	Procedure Yes	No	Repeat Yes	No	Competency Yes	No
1. Examines the radiographic room and cleans/straightens it before escorting the patient in.	☐	☐	☐	☐	☐	☐
2. Has all equipment and supplies (patient gown, shield, markers, tape, cassettes, lead aprons, blockers, hemostats, compression paddle, proper contrast material, etc.) readily available before escorting the patient in, the Bucky drawer in the proper position, the tower lead drape removed, the fluoro on, the foot board removed, and the letters properly placed on machine.	☐	☐	☐	☐	☐	☐

Additional supplies:

_____
_____
_____
_____

	Procedure Yes	No	Repeat Yes	No	Competency Yes	No
3. Selects and prepares the contrast material without difficulty.	■	■	■	■	☐	☐
4. Is able to manipulate all radiographic equipment with ease, and centers the central ray to the cassette/receptor *for all projections.*	☐	☐	☐	☐	☐	☐
5. Adjusts the tube to the proper SID *for each projection.*	☐	☐	☐	☐	☐	☐
6. Selects cassettes/receptor of the appropriate sizes *for all projections,* according to the patient's size and examination.	☐	☐	☐	☐	☐	☐

Comments:

_____

_____

PATIENT PREPARATION
The student:

	Procedure Yes	No	Repeat Yes	No	Competency Yes	No
7. Identifies the correct patient and examination according to the requisition while establishing a good rapport with him or her.	☐	☐	☐	☐	☐	☐

(continued)

	Procedure		Repeat		Competency	
	Yes	No	Yes	No	Yes	No
8. Obtains and documents the patient's history before the examination, including whether the patient ate before the examination and preparation instructions	▩	▩	▩	▩	☐	☐
9. Thoroughly explains the examination in terms the patient fully understands and properly communicates with the patient throughout the examination.	☐	☐	☐	☐	☐	☐
10. Asks female patients of childbearing age the date of their last menstrual period and documents this; inquires about the possibility of pregnancy and has them sign pregnancy consent forms.	☐	☐	☐	☐	☐	☐
11. Removes all obscuring objects (snaps, zippers, jewelry, belts, etc.) so as *not* to produce radiographic artifacts.	☐	☐	☐	☐	☐	☐
12. Respects the patient's modesty and provides ample comfort for the patient while positioning him or her to begin the examination.	☐	☐	☐	☐	☐	☐
13. Performs a scout radiograph when indicated.	☐	☐	☐	☐	☐	☐

Comments:

_____

_____

TASKS DURING FLUOROSCOPY
The student:

	Procedure		Repeat		Competency	
	Yes	No	Yes	No	Yes	No
14. Relays the patient's history to the radiologist.	▩	▩	▩	▩	☐	☐
15. Assists the radiologist throughout the examination.	▩	▩	▩	▩	☐	☐
16. Monitors, communicates with, and assists the patient throughout the examination.	▩	▩	▩	▩	☐	☐
17. Takes charge of the examination after the radiologist departs.	▩	▩	▩	▩	☐	☐

Comments:

_____

_____

PATIENT POSITIONING FOR A THREE-TEXTURED BARIUM SWALLOW
Anteroposterior
The student:

	Procedure		Repeat		Competency	
	Yes	No	Yes	No	Yes	No
18. Places the patient in the erect AP position, without rotation.	☐	☐	☐	☐	☐	☐
19. Selects the appropriate receptor or places the cassette lengthwise. For conventional cassettes, the flash must be at the bottom and away from any anatomy.	☐	☐	☐	☐	☐	☐
20. Centers the central ray to the midsagittal plane of the body.	☐	☐	☐	☐	☐	☐
21. Directs the central ray perpendicularly.	☐	☐	☐	☐	☐	☐

Lateral
The student:

	Procedure		Repeat		Competency	
	Yes	No	Yes	No	Yes	No
22. Places the patient in the lateral position, without rotation.	☐	☐	☐	☐	☐	☐
23. Selects the appropriate receptor or places the cassette lengthwise. For conventional cassettes, the flash must be at the bottom and away from any anatomy.	☐	☐	☐	☐	☐	☐
24. Centers the central ray to the midcoronal plane of the body.	☐	☐	☐	☐	☐	☐
25. Directs the central ray perpendicularly.	☐	☐	☐	☐	☐	☐

Comments:

_____

_____

IMPORTANT DETAILS
The student:

	Procedure		Repeat		Competency	
	Yes	No	Yes	No	Yes	No
26. Instills confidence in the patient by exhibiting self-confidence throughout the examination.	☐	☐	☐	☐	☐	☐
27. Places a lead marker in the appropriate area of the cassette/receptor (top/bottom/anteriorly/laterally), where it will be visualized on the finished radiograph, on the proper anatomical side (right/left), and in the appropriate position (face up/face down), depending on the patient's position.	☐	☐	☐	☐	☐	☐
28. Provides radiation protection (shield) for the patient (when appropriate), self, and others (closes doors).	☐	☐	☐	☐	☐	☐
29. Applies proper collimation and makes adjustments as necessary.	☐	☐	☐	☐	☐	☐
30. Properly measures the patient along the course of the central ray *for each projection.*	☐	☐	☐	☐	☐	☐
31. Sets the proper technique *for fluoroscopy* (kVp, mA, time).	☐	☐	☐	☐	☐	☐

And all projections/spot images:

Conventional systems

• Sets the proper kVp, mA, and time and makes adjustments as necessary.

or

CR or DR systems

• Identifies the patient on the work-list (or manually types the patient information into the system).
• Selects appropriate body region, specific body part, and accurate view/projection.
• Double-checks preset parameters:
  —Adult vs. pediatric patients
    ○ Small, medium, or large
  —Bucky/receptor (upright vs. table) *or* non-Bucky
  —AEC vs. fixed
    ○ If AEC, checks ion chambers
    ○ Density setting
  —kVp and mA; adjusts if necessary
  —Focal spot/filament size

	Procedure		Repeat		Competency	
32. If additional images are required, exposes the cassette/receptor after telling the patient to hold still and after giving him or her proper breathing instructions (expiration) *for each projection.*	☐	☐	☐	☐	☐	☐
33. Provides each radiograph with the proper identification (flash) and/or processes each cassette (image) without difficulty (regardless of technology—film, CR, or DR).	▨	▨	▨	▨	☐	☐
34. Properly completes the examination by filling out all necessary paperwork, entering the examination in the computer, having the images checked by the appropriate staff members, answering any last-minute questions, and informing the patient that he or she is finished. Provides proper post-exam instructions as required.	▨	▨	▨	▨	☐	☐
35. Exhibits the ability to adapt to new and difficult situations if and when necessary.	▨	▨	▨	▨	☐	☐
36. Accepts constructive criticism and uses it to his or her advantage.	☐	☐	☐	☐	☐	☐
37. Leaves the radiographic room neat and clean for the next examination.	▨	▨	▨	▨	☐	☐
38. Completes the examination within a reasonable time frame.	☐	☐	☐	☐	☐	☐

(continued)

Comments:

_____

_____

RADIOGRAPHIC IMAGE QUALITY
The student is able to critique his or her radiographs as to whether they demonstrate:

	Procedure Yes	No	Repeat Yes	No	Competency Yes	No
39. Proper technique/optimal density	▪	▪	▪	▪	☐	☐
40. Enhanced detail, without evidence of motion and without any visible artifacts	▪	▪	▪	▪	☐	☐
41. Proper positioning (all anatomy included, evidence of proper centering/alignment, etc.)	▪	▪	▪	▪	☐	☐
42. Proper marker placement	▪	▪	▪	▪	☐	☐
43. Evidence of proper collimation and radiation protection	▪	▪	▪	▪	☐	☐
44. Long vs. short scale of contrast	▪	▪	▪	▪	☐	☐
45. Image/projection identification and/or other identification	▪	▪	▪	▪	☐	☐

Comments:

_____

_____

ANATOMY
The student is able to identify:

	Procedure Yes	No	Repeat Yes	No	Competency Yes	No
46. Cervical spine	▪	▪	▪	▪	☐	☐
47. Esophagus	▪	▪	▪	▪	☐	☐
48. Nasopharynx	▪	▪	▪	▪	☐	☐
49. Trachea	▪	▪	▪	▪	☐	☐
50. Hyoid bone	▪	▪	▪	▪	☐	☐
51. Obvious pathology	▪	▪	▪	▪	☐	☐

Comments:

_____

_____

_____ _____ _____
Procedure Evaluator Signature   Repeat Evaluator Signature   Competency Evaluator Signature

_____ _____ _____
Date   Date   Date

END THREE-TEXTURED BARIUM SWALLOW EVALUATION

Student Name:_____

	Procedure Grade	Repeat Grade	Competency Grade

PATIENT INFORMATION OR SIMULATED PROCEDURE *(circle if simulated)*

	Procedure	Repeat	Competency
Age			
Medical Record No.			
Ability to Cooperate			
Condition/Pathology			
Technical Factors Used			
Exposure Index			

FACILITY PREPARATION
The student:

	Procedure Yes	No	Repeat Yes	No	Competency Yes	No
1. Examines the radiographic room and cleans/straightens it before escorting the patient in.	☐	☐	☐	☐	☐	☐
2. Has all equipment and supplies (patient gown, shield, markers, lead aprons, blockers, tape, cassettes, etc.) readily available before escorting the patient in, and has the Bucky drawer in the proper position, the monitor by the table, the fluoro on, and the image on the equipment so that it is reversed.	☐	☐	☐	☐	☐	☐

Additional supplies:

_____
_____
_____
_____

	Procedure Yes	No	Repeat Yes	No	Competency Yes	No
3. Is able to manipulate all radiographic equipment with ease, and centers the central ray to the cassette/receptor *for all projections.*	☐	☐	☐	☐	☐	☐
4. Adjusts the tube to the proper SID *for each projection.*	☐	☐	☐	☐	☐	☐
5. Selects cassettes/receptor of the appropriate sizes *for all projections,* according to the patient's size and examination.	☐	☐	☐	☐	☐	☐

Comments:

_____
_____

PATIENT PREPARATION
The student:

	Procedure Yes	No	Repeat Yes	No	Competency Yes	No
6. Identifies the correct patient and examination according to the requisition while establishing a good rapport with him or her.	☐	☐	☐	☐	☐	☐
7. Obtains and documents the patient's history before the examination, including whether the patient ate before the examination and preparation instructions	▦	▦	▦	▦	☐	☐

(continued)

	Procedure		Repeat		Competency	
	Yes	No	Yes	No	Yes	No
8. Thoroughly explains the examination in terms the patient fully understands and properly communicates with the patient throughout the examination.	☐	☐	☐	☐	☐	☐
9. Asks female patients of childbearing age the date of their last menstrual period and documents this; inquires about the possibility of pregnancy and has them sign pregnancy consent forms.	☐	☐	☐	☐	☐	☐
10. Removes all obscuring objects (snaps, zippers, jewelry, belts, etc.) so as *not* to produce radiographic artifacts.	☐	☐	☐	☐	☐	☐
11. Respects the patient's modesty and provides ample comfort for the patient while positioning him or her to begin the examination (RAO).	☐	☐	☐	☐	☐	☐
12. Performs a scout radiograph when indicated.	☐	☐	☐	☐	☐	☐

Comments:

_____

_____

TASKS DURING FLUOROSCOPY
The student:

	Procedure		Repeat		Competency	
	Yes	No	Yes	No	Yes	No
13. Ensures proper image orientation on the monitor relative to patient position and equipment ("flips" the image as required).	■	■	■	■	☐	☐
14. Relays the patient's history to the radiologist.	■	■	■	■	☐	☐
15. Assists the radiologist throughout the examination.	■	■	■	■	☐	☐
16. Monitors, communicates with, and assists the patient throughout the examination.	■	■	■	■	☐	☐
17. Takes charge of the examination after the radiologist departs.	■	■	■	■	☐	☐

Comments:

_____

_____

IMPORTANT DETAILS
The student:

	Procedure		Repeat		Competency	
	Yes	No	Yes	No	Yes	No
18. Instills confidence in the patient by exhibiting self-confidence throughout the examination.	☐	☐	☐	☐	☐	☐
19. Places a lead marker in the appropriate area of the cassette/receptor (top/bottom/anteriorly/laterally), where it will be visualized on the finished radiograph, on the proper anatomical side (right/left), and in the appropriate position (face up/face down), depending on the patient's position.	☐	☐	☐	☐	☐	☐
20. Provides radiation protection (shield) for the patient (when appropriate), self, and others (closes doors).	☐	☐	☐	☐	☐	☐
21. Applies proper collimation and makes adjustments as necessary.	☐	☐	☐	☐	☐	☐
22. Properly measures the patient along the course of the central ray *for each projection.*	☐	☐	☐	☐	☐	☐
23. Sets the proper technique *for fluoroscopy* (kVp, mA, time).	☐	☐	☐	☐	☐	☐

And all projections/spot images:

Conventional systems

• Sets the proper kVp, mA, and time and makes adjustments as necessary.

or

	Procedure		Repeat		Competency	
	Yes	No	Yes	No	Yes	No

CR or DR systems
- Identifies the patient on the work-list (or manually types the patient information into the system).
- Selects appropriate body region, specific body part, and accurate view/projection.
- Double-checks preset parameters:
  - —Adult vs. pediatric patients
    - ○ Small, medium, or large
  - —Bucky/receptor (upright vs. table) *or* non-Bucky
  - —AEC vs. fixed
    - ○ If AEC, checks ion chambers
    - ○ Density setting
  - —kVp and mA; adjusts if necessary
  - —Focal spot/filament size

	Procedure		Repeat		Competency	
	Yes	No	Yes	No	Yes	No
24. Exposes the cassette/receptor after telling the patient to hold still and after giving him or her proper breathing instructions (expiration) *for each projection.*	☐	☐	☐	☐	☐	☐
25. Provides each radiograph with the proper identification (flash) and/or processes each cassette (image) without difficulty (regardless of technology—film, CR, or DR).	▣	▣	▣	▣	☐	☐
26. Properly completes the examination by filling out all necessary paperwork, entering the examination in the computer, having the images checked by the appropriate staff members, answering any last-minute questions, and informing the patient that he or she is finished. Provides proper post-exam instructions as required.	▣	▣	▣	▣	☐	☐
27. Exhibits the ability to adapt to new and difficult situations if and when necessary.	▣	▣	▣	▣	☐	☐
28. Accepts constructive criticism and uses it to his or her advantage.	☐	☐	☐	☐	☐	☐
29. Leaves the radiographic room neat and clean for the next examination.	▣	▣	▣	▣	☐	☐
30. Completes the examination within a reasonable time frame.	☐	☐	☐	☐	☐	☐

Comments:

_____

_____

RADIOGRAPHIC IMAGE QUALITY
The student is able to critique his or her radiographs as to whether they demonstrate:

	Procedure		Repeat		Competency	
	Yes	No	Yes	No	Yes	No
31. Proper technique/optimal density	▣	▣	▣	▣	☐	☐
32. Enhanced detail, without evidence of motion and without any visible artifacts	▣	▣	▣	▣	☐	☐
33. Proper positioning (all anatomy included, evidence of proper centering/alignment, etc.)	▣	▣	▣	▣	☐	☐
34. Proper marker placement	▣	▣	▣	▣	☐	☐
35. Evidence of proper collimation and radiation protection	▣	▣	▣	▣	☐	☐
36. Long vs. short scale of contrast	▣	▣	▣	▣	☐	☐
37. Image/projection identification and/or other identification	▣	▣	▣	▣	☐	☐

Comments:

_____

_____

(continued)

ANATOMY
The student is able to identify:

	Procedure		Repeat		Competency	
	Yes	No	Yes	No	Yes	No
38. Endoscope	☐	☐	☐	☐	☐	☐
39. Common bile duct	☐	☐	☐	☐	☐	☐
40. Pancreatic duct	☐	☐	☐	☐	☐	☐
41. Duodenum	☐	☐	☐	☐	☐	☐
42. Obvious pathology or stone	☐	☐	☐	☐	☐	☐

Comments:

_____

_____

Procedure Evaluator Signature	Repeat Evaluator Signature	Competency Evaluator Signature

Date	Date	Date

END ENDOSCOPIC RETROGRADE CHOLANGIOGRAPHIC PANCREATOGRAPHY EVALUATION

Student Name:_____

<table>
<tr><td>Procedure Grade</td><td>Repeat Grade</td><td>Competency Grade</td></tr>
<tr><td></td><td></td><td></td></tr>
</table>

PATIENT INFORMATION OR SIMULATED PROCEDURE *(circle if simulated)*

	Procedure	Repeat	Competency
Age			
Medical Record No.			
Ability to Cooperate			
Condition/Pathology			
Technical Factors Used			
Exposure Index			

FACILITY PREPARATION
The student:

	Procedure Yes	No	Repeat Yes	No	Competency Yes	No
1. While wearing operative attire, identifies the appropriate OR suite to perform the procedure.	☐	☐	☐	☐	☐	☐
2. Has all equipment and supplies (markers, tape, cassettes, lead aprons, etc.) readily available before the case begins.	☐	☐	☐	☐	☐	☐

Additional supplies:

_____
_____
_____
_____

	Procedure Yes	No	Repeat Yes	No	Competency Yes	No
3. Is able to manipulate all radiographic equipment with ease (C-arm or portable unit, and/or centers the central ray to the appropriate-size cassette/receptor) *for all projections.*	☐	☐	☐	☐	☐	☐
4. Adjusts the tube to the proper SID *for each projection.*	☐	☐	☐	☐	☐	☐
5. Observes and does not interfere with the sterile field.	☐	☐	☐	☐	☐	☐

Comments:

_____

_____

PATIENT PREPARATION
The student:

	Procedure Yes	No	Repeat Yes	No	Competency Yes	No
6. Ensures that all obscuring objects (snaps, zippers, jewelry, belts, etc.) are removed so as *not* to produce radiographic artifacts.	☐	☐	☐	☐	☐	☐

Comments:

_____

_____

(continued)

TASKS DURING THE PROCEDURE
The student:

	Procedure Yes	No	Repeat Yes	No	Competency Yes	No
7. Assists the staff members throughout the examination.	☑	☑	☑	☑	☐	☐
8. Monitors the patient and communicates with the staff members throughout the examination.	☑	☑	☑	☑	☐	☐
9. Informs the surgical staff when exposures are about to be taken and takes the exposures only as directed by the physician.	☑	☑	☑	☑	☐	☐

Comments:

_____

_____

PATIENT POSITIONING FOR AN OPERATIVE CHOLANGIOGRAM
Anteroposterior
The student:

	Procedure Yes	No	Repeat Yes	No	Competency Yes	No
10. Selects the appropriate receptor or places the cassette under the patient appropriately.	☐	☐	☐	☐	☐	☐
11. Centers the central ray 3 inches above the iliac crest, or as per the surgeon's directions.	☐	☐	☐	☐	☐	☐
12. Instructs the anesthesiologist to suspend the patient's respiration.	☐	☐	☐	☐	☐	☐
13. Processes the radiograph, and then returns to the surgical suite and hangs it for the surgeon's evaluation.	☐	☐	☐	☐	☐	☐
14. Follows instructions for additional radiographs.	☐	☐	☐	☐	☐	☐

Comments:

_____

_____

IMPORTANT DETAILS
The student:

	Procedure Yes	No	Repeat Yes	No	Competency Yes	No
15. Instills confidence in the patient by exhibiting self-confidence throughout the examination.	☐	☐	☐	☐	☐	☐
16. Places a lead marker in the appropriate area of the cassette/receptor (top/bottom/anteriorly/laterally), where it will be visualized on the finished radiograph, on the proper anatomical side (right/left), and in the appropriate position (face up/face down), depending on the patient's position.	☐	☐	☐	☐	☐	☐
17. Provides radiation protection (shield) for the patient (when appropriate), self, and others (closes doors).	☐	☐	☐	☐	☐	☐
18. Applies proper collimation and makes adjustments as necessary.	☐	☐	☐	☐	☐	☐
19. Sets the proper technique *for fluoroscopy* (kVp, mA, time).	☐	☐	☐	☐	☐	☐

and all projections/spot images:

Conventional systems

• Sets the proper kVp, mA, and time and makes adjustments as necessary.

or

CR or DR systems
• Identifies the patient on the work-list (or manually types the patient information into the system).
• Selects appropriate body region, specific body part, and accurate view/projection.
• Double-checks preset parameters:
  —Adult vs. pediatric patients
    ○ Small, medium, or large
  —Bucky/receptor (upright vs. table) *or* non-Bucky

	Procedure Yes	Procedure No	Repeat Yes	Repeat No	Competency Yes	Competency No

—AEC vs. fixed
    ○ If AEC, checks ion chambers
    ○ Density setting
—kVp and mA; adjusts if necessary
—Focal spot/filament size

	Procedure Yes	Procedure No	Repeat Yes	Repeat No	Competency Yes	Competency No
20. Provides each radiograph with the proper identification (flash) and/or processes each cassette (image) without difficulty (regardless of technology—film, CR, or DR).	☐	☐	☐	☐	☐	☐
21. Properly completes the examination by filling out all necessary paperwork.	☐	☐	☐	☐	☐	☐
22. Exhibits the ability to adapt to new and difficult situations if and when necessary.	☐	☐	☐	☐	☐	☐
23. Accepts constructive criticism and uses it to his or her advantage.	☐	☐	☐	☐	☐	☐
24. Completes the examination within a reasonable time frame.	☐	☐	☐	☐	☐	☐

Comments:

_____

_____

RADIOGRAPHIC IMAGE QUALITY
The student is able to critique his or her radiographs as to whether they demonstrate:

	Procedure Yes	Procedure No	Repeat Yes	Repeat No	Competency Yes	Competency No
25. Proper technique/optimal density	☐	☐	☐	☐	☐	☐
26. Enhanced detail, without evidence of motion and without any visible artifacts	☐	☐	☐	☐	☐	☐
27. Proper positioning (all anatomy included, evidence of proper centering/alignment, etc.)	☐	☐	☐	☐	☐	☐
28. Proper marker placement	☐	☐	☐	☐	☐	☐
29. Evidence of proper collimation and radiation protection	☐	☐	☐	☐	☐	☐
30. Long vs. short scale of contrast	☐	☐	☐	☐	☐	☐
31. Image/projection identification and/or other identification	☐	☐	☐	☐	☐	☐

Comments:

_____

_____

ANATOMY
The student is able to identify:

	Procedure Yes	Procedure No	Repeat Yes	Repeat No	Competency Yes	Competency No
32. Common bile duct	☐	☐	☐	☐	☐	☐
33. Hepatic duct	☐	☐	☐	☐	☐	☐
34. Duodenum	☐	☐	☐	☐	☐	☐
35. Obvious pathology or stone	☐	☐	☐	☐	☐	☐

Comments:

_____

_____

_____ | _____ | _____
Procedure Evaluator Signature   Repeat Evaluator Signature   Competency Evaluator Signature

_____ | _____ | _____
Date   Date   Date

END SURGICAL/OPERATIVE CHOLANGIOGRAM EVALUATION

Student Name:_____

Procedure Grade	Repeat Grade	Competency Grade

PATIENT INFORMATION OR SIMULATED PROCEDURE *(circle if simulated)*

	Procedure	Repeat	Competency
Age			
Medical Record No.			
Ability to Cooperate			
Condition/Pathology			
Technical Factors Used			
Exposure Index			

FACILITY PREPARATION
The student:

	Procedure Yes	Procedure No	Repeat Yes	Repeat No	Competency Yes	Competency No
1. Examines the radiographic room and cleans/straightens it before escorting the patient in.	☐	☐	☐	☐	☐	☐
2. Has all equipment and supplies (patient gown, shield, markers, tape, cassettes, lead aprons, blockers, hemostats, proper contrast material, etc.) readily available before escorting the patient in, the Bucky drawer in the proper position, the monitor by the table, and the fluoro on.	☐	☐	☐	☐	☐	☐

Additional supplies:

_____

_____

_____

_____

	Procedure Yes	Procedure No	Repeat Yes	Repeat No	Competency Yes	Competency No
3. Selects and prepares the contrast material without difficulty.	▣	▣	▣	▣	☐	☐
4. Is able to manipulate all radiographic equipment with ease, and centers the central ray to the cassette/receptor *for all projections.*	☐	☐	☐	☐	☐	☐
5. Adjusts the tube to the proper SID *for each projection.*	☐	☐	☐	☐	☐	☐
6. Selects cassettes/receptor of the appropriate sizes *for all projections,* according to the patient's size and examination.	☐	☐	☐	☐	☐	☐

Comments:

_____

_____

PATIENT PREPARATION
The student:

	Procedure Yes	Procedure No	Repeat Yes	Repeat No	Competency Yes	Competency No
7. Identifies the correct patient and examination according to the requisition while establishing a good rapport with him or her.	☐	☐	☐	☐	☐	☐

(continued)

453

	Procedure		Repeat		Competency	
	Yes	No	Yes	No	Yes	No
8. Obtains and documents the patient's history before the examination, including whether the patient ate before the examination and preparation instructions.	☒	☒	☒	☒	☐	☐
9. If necessary, thoroughly explains the examination in terms the patient fully understands and properly communicates with the patient throughout the examination.	☐	☐	☐	☐	☐	☐
10. Asks female patients of childbearing age the date of their last menstrual period and documents this; inquires about the possibility of pregnancy and has them sign pregnancy consent forms.	☐	☐	☐	☐	☐	☐
11. Removes all obscuring objects (snaps, zippers, jewelry, belts, etc.) so as *not* to produce radiographic artifacts.	☐	☐	☐	☐	☐	☐
12. Respects the patient's modesty and provides ample comfort for the patient while positioning him or her to begin the examination (RPO: 25–30°).	☐	☐	☐	☐	☐	☐
13. Performs a scout radiograph when indicated.	☐	☐	☐	☐	☐	☐

Comments:

_____

_____

TASKS DURING FLUOROSCOPY
The student:

	Procedure		Repeat		Competency	
	Yes	No	Yes	No	Yes	No
14. Relays the patient's history to the radiologist.	☒	☒	☒	☒	☐	☐
15. Assists the radiologist throughout the examination.	☒	☒	☒	☒	☐	☐
16. Monitors, communicates with, and assists the patient throughout the examination.	☒	☒	☒	☒	☐	☐
17. Takes charge of the examination after the radiologist departs.	☒	☒	☒	☒	☐	☐

Comments:

_____

_____

PATIENT POSITIONING FOR FOR A T-TUBE CHOLANGIOGRAM
Right Posterior Oblique
The student:

	Procedure		Repeat		Competency	
	Yes	No	Yes	No	Yes	No
18. Places the patient in the oblique position on the radiographic table, adjusting his or her angle to 25–30°.	☐	☐	☐	☐	☐	☐
19. Selects the appropriate receptor or places the cassette lengthwise. For conventional cassettes, the flash must be at the bottom and away from any anatomy.	☐	☐	☐	☐	☐	☐
20. Centers the central ray midway between the midsagittal plane and the lateral rib margin.	☐	☐	☐	☐	☐	☐
21. Directs the central ray perpendicularly to a level 2 inches above the subcostal plane.	☐	☐	☐	☐	☐	☐

Comments:

_____

_____

IMPORTANT DETAILS
The student:

	Procedure		Repeat		Competency	
	Yes	No	Yes	No	Yes	No
22. Instills confidence in the patient by exhibiting self-confidence throughout the examination.	☐	☐	☐	☐	☐	☐
23. Places a lead marker in the appropriate area of the cassette/receptor (top/bottom/anteriorly/laterally), where it will be visualized on the finished radiograph, on the proper anatomical side (right/left), and in the appropriate position (face up/face down), depending on the patient's position.	☐	☐	☐	☐	☐	☐
24. Provides radiation protection (shield) for the patient (when appropriate), self, and others (closes doors).	☐	☐	☐	☐	☐	☐
25. Applies proper collimation and makes adjustments as necessary.	☐	☐	☐	☐	☐	☐
26. Properly measures the patient along the course of the central ray *for each projection.*	☐	☐	☐	☐	☐	☐
27. Sets the proper technique *for fluoroscopy* (kVp, mA, time).	☐	☐	☐	☐	☐	☐

And all projections/spot images:

Conventional systems

- Sets the proper kVp, mA, and time and makes adjustments as necessary.

or

CR or DR systems

- Identifies the patient on the work-list (or manually types the patient information into the system).
- Selects appropriate body region, specific body part, and accurate view/projection.
- Double-checks preset parameters:
  —Adult vs. pediatric patients
   ○ Small, medium, or large
  —Bucky/receptor (upright vs. table) *or* non-Bucky
  —AEC vs. fixed
   ○ If AEC, checks ion chambers
   ○ Density setting
  —kVp and mA; adjusts if necessary
  —Focal spot/filament size

	Procedure		Repeat		Competency	
28. Exposes the cassette/receptor after telling the patient to hold still and after giving him or her proper breathing instructions (expiration) *for each projection.*	☐	☐	☐	☐	☐	☐
29. Provides each radiograph with the proper identification (flash) and/or processes each cassette (image) without difficulty (regardless of technology—film, CR, or DR).	■	■	■	■	☐	☐
30. Properly completes the examination by filling out all necessary paperwork, entering the examination in the computer, having the images checked by the appropriate staff members, answering any last-minute questions, and informing the patient that he or she is finished. Provides proper post-exam instructions as required.	■	■	■	■	☐	☐
31. Exhibits the ability to adapt to new and difficult situations if and when necessary.	■	■	■	■	☐	☐
32. Accepts constructive criticism and uses it to his or her advantage.	☐	☐	☐	☐	☐	☐
33. Leaves the radiographic room neat and clean for the next examination.	■	■	■	■	☐	☐
34. Completes the examination within a reasonable time frame.	☐	☐	☐	☐	☐	☐

Comments:

_____

_____

(continued)

RADIOGRAPHIC IMAGE QUALITY
The student is able to critique his or her radiographs as to whether they demonstrate:

	Procedure Yes	Procedure No	Repeat Yes	Repeat No	Competency Yes	Competency No
35. Proper technique/optimal density	☐	☐	☐	☐	☐	☐
36. Enhanced detail, without evidence of motion and without any visible artifacts	☐	☐	☐	☐	☐	☐
37. Proper positioning (all anatomy included, evidence of proper centering/alignment, etc.)	☐	☐	☐	☐	☐	☐
38. Proper marker placement	☐	☐	☐	☐	☐	☐
39. Evidence of proper collimation and radiation protection	☐	☐	☐	☐	☐	☐
40. Long vs. short scale of contrast	☐	☐	☐	☐	☐	☐
41. Image/projection identification and/or other identification	☐	☐	☐	☐	☐	☐

Comments:

_____

ANATOMY
The student is able to identify:

	Procedure Yes	Procedure No	Repeat Yes	Repeat No	Competency Yes	Competency No
42. Common bile duct	☐	☐	☐	☐	☐	☐
43. Hepatic duct	☐	☐	☐	☐	☐	☐
44. Obvious pathology or stone	☐	☐	☐	☐	☐	☐

Comments:

_____

_____   _____   _____
Procedure Evaluator Signature   Repeat Evaluator Signature   Competency Evaluator Signature

_____   _____   _____
Date   Date   Date

END T-TUBE CHOLANGIOGRAM EVALUATION

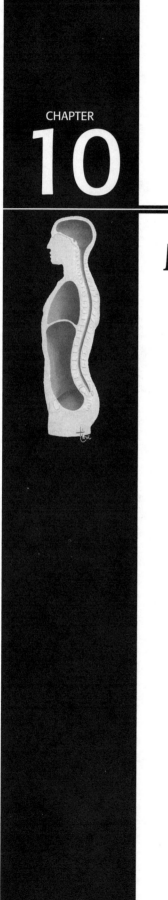

Miscellaneous

Hysterosalpingogram

The objective of this evaluation is to determine the student's competency level when performing specific radiographic examinations.

Student Name:_____

Procedure Grade	Repeat Grade	Competency Grade

PATIENT INFORMATION OR SIMULATED PROCEDURE *(circle if simulated)*

	Procedure	Repeat	Competency
Age			
Medical Record No.			
Ability to Cooperate			
Condition/Pathology			
Technical Factors Used			
Exposure Index			

FACILITY PREPARATION
The student:

	Procedure Yes	Procedure No	Repeat Yes	Repeat No	Competency Yes	Competency No
1. Examines the radiographic room and cleans/straightens it before escorting the patient in.	☐	☐	☐	☐	☐	☐
2. Has all equipment and supplies readily available before escorting the patient in, including patient gown, shield, markers, tape, cassettes, Bucky drawer in proper position, monitor by table, fluoro on, lead aprons and blockers, compression paddle, hemostats, lubricant, and proper contrast material.	☐	☐	☐	☐	☐	☐

Additional supplies:

_____
_____
_____
_____

	Procedure Yes	Procedure No	Repeat Yes	Repeat No	Competency Yes	Competency No
3. Selects and prepares the contrast material without difficulty.	▨	▨	▨	▨	☐	☐
4. Selects and prepares the appropriate sterile tray (maintains the sterile environment).	▨	▨	▨	▨	☐	☐
5. Is able to manipulate all radiographic equipment with ease, and centers the central ray to the cassette/receptor *for all projections.*	☐	☐	☐	☐	☐	☐
6. Adjusts the tube to the proper SID *for each projection.*	☐	☐	☐	☐	☐	☐
7. Selects the appropriate receptor or cassettes of the appropriate size *for all projections,* according to the patient's size and examination.	☐	☐	☐	☐	☐	☐

Comments:

_____
_____

(continued)

PATIENT PREPARATION
The student:

	Procedure		Repeat		Competency	
	Yes	No	Yes	No	Yes	No
8. Identifies the correct patient and examination according to the requisition while establishing a good rapport with him or her.	☐	☐	☐	☐	☐	☐
9. Obtains and documents the patient's history before the examination, including preparation instructions.	▣	▣	▣	▣	☐	☐
10. Asks patients of childbearing age the date of their last menstrual period and documents this; inquires about the possibility of pregnancy and has them sign pregnancy consent forms	☐	☐	☐	☐	☐	☐
11. Ensures that the patient's bladder is empty.	☐	☐	☐	☐	☐	☐
12. Explains the examination in terms the patient fully understands, and properly communicates with the patient throughout the examination.	☐	☐	☐	☐	☐	☐
13. Removes all obscuring objects (snaps, zippers, jewelry, etc.) so as *not* to produce radiographic artifacts.	☐	☐	☐	☐	☐	☐
14. Respects the patient's modesty and provides ample comfort for her while positioning her to begin the examination.	☐	☐	☐	☐	☐	☐
15. Performs a scout radiograph when indicated.	☐	☐	☐	☐	☐	☐

Comments:

_____

_____

TASKS DURING FLUOROSCOPY
The student:

	Procedure		Repeat		Competency	
	Yes	No	Yes	No	Yes	No
16. Relays the patient's history to the radiologist.	▣	▣	▣	▣	☐	☐
17. Assists the radiologist throughout the examination (aseptic conditions).	▣	▣	▣	▣	☐	☐
18. Monitors, communicates with, and assists the patient throughout the examination.	▣	▣	▣	▣	☐	☐
19. Takes charge of the examination after the radiologist departs.	▣	▣	▣	▣	☐	☐

Comments:

_____

_____

PATIENT POSITIONING FOR A HYSTEROSALPINGOGRAM (WITH OVERHEADS, IF INDICATED)
AP Cystoscopic Position
The student:

	Procedure		Repeat		Competency	
	Yes	No	Yes	No	Yes	No
20. Places the patient in the supine position on the radiographic table, with her arms at her sides, without rotation, and with the knees flexed.	☐	☐	☐	☐	☐	☐
21. Selects the appropriate receptor or places the cassette lengthwise. For conventional cassettes, the flash must be away from any anatomy.	☐	☐	☐	☐	☐	☐
22. Centers the central ray to the midsagittal plane of the body.	☐	☐	☐	☐	☐	☐
23. Directs the central ray perpendicularly at a level 2 inches proximal to the pubic symphysis.	☐	☐	☐	☐	☐	☐

As indicated or requested:
AP Axial
Left Posterior Oblique (LPO)
Right Posterior Oblique (RPO)
Lateral

Comments:

_____

_____

IMPORTANT DETAILS
The student:

	Procedure		Repeat		Competency	
	Yes	No	Yes	No	Yes	No
24. Instills confidence in the patient by exhibiting self-confidence throughout the examination.	☐	☐	☐	☐	☐	☐
25. Places a lead marker in the appropriate area of the cassette/receptor (top/bottom/anteriorly/laterally), where it will be visualized on the finished radiograph, on the proper anatomical side (right/left), and in the appropriate position (face up/face down), depending on the patient's position.	☐	☐	☐	☐	☐	☐
26. Provides radiation protection (shield) for the patient (when appropriate), self, and others (closes doors).	☐	☐	☐	☐	☐	☐
27. Applies proper collimation and makes adjustments as necessary.	☐	☐	☐	☐	☐	☐
28. Properly measures the patient along the course of the central ray *for each projection.*	☐	☐	☐	☐	☐	☐
29. Sets the proper technique *for fluoroscopy* (kVp, mA, time).	☐	☐	☐	☐	☐	☐

And all projections/spot images:

Conventional systems

- Sets the proper kVp, mA, and time and makes adjustments as necessary.

or

CR or DR systems
- Identifies the patient on the work-list (or manually types the patient information into the system).
- Selects appropriate body region, specific body part, and accurate view/projection.
- Double-checks preset parameters:
  —Adult vs. pediatric patients
  ○ Small, medium, or large
  —Bucky/receptor (upright vs. table) or non-Bucky
  —AEC vs. fixed
  ○ If AEC, checks ion chambers
  ○ Density setting
  —kVp and mA; adjusts if necessary
  —Focal spot/filament size

	Procedure		Repeat		Competency	
30. Exposes the cassette/receptor after telling the patient to hold still and after giving him or her proper breathing instructions (expiration) *for each projection.*	☐	☐	☐	☐	☐	☐
31. Provides each radiograph with the proper identification (flash) and/or processes each cassette (image) without difficulty (regardless of technology—film, CR, or DR).	▨	▨	▨	▨	☐	☐
32. Properly completes the examination by filling out all necessary paperwork, entering the examination in the computer, having the images checked by the appropriate staff members, answering any last-minute questions, and informing the patient that he or she is finished. Provides proper post-exam instructions as required.	▨	▨	▨	▨	☐	☐
33. Exhibits the ability to adapt to new and difficult situations if and when necessary.	▨	▨	▨	▨	☐	☐
34. Accepts constructive criticism and uses it to his or her advantage.	☐	☐	☐	☐	☐	☐
35. Leaves the radiographic room neat and clean for the next examination.	▨	▨	▨	▨	☐	☐
36. Completes the examination within a reasonable time frame.	☐	☐	☐	☐	☐	☐

Comments:

_____

_____

(continued)

RADIOGRAPHIC IMAGE QUALITY
The student is able to critique his or her radiographs as to whether they demonstrate:

	Procedure		Repeat		Competency	
	Yes	No	Yes	No	Yes	No
37. Proper technique/optimal density	☐	☐	☐	☐	☐	☐
38. Enhanced detail, without evidence of motion and without any visible artifacts	☐	☐	☐	☐	☐	☐
39. Proper positioning (all anatomy included, evidence of proper centering/alignment, etc.)	☐	☐	☐	☐	☐	☐
40. Proper marker placement						
41. Evidence of proper collimation and radiation protection	☐	☐	☐	☐	☐	☐
42. Long vs. short scale of contrast	☐	☐	☐	☐	☐	☐

Comments:

_____

_____

ANATOMY
The student is able to identify:

	Procedure		Repeat		Competency	
	Yes	No	Yes	No	Yes	No
43. Fallopian tubes	☐	☐	☐	☐	☐	☐
44. Uterus	☐	☐	☐	☐	☐	☐
45. "Spill" into the peritoneal cavity	☐	☐	☐	☐	☐	☐
46. Cervical canal	☐	☐	☐	☐	☐	☐
47. Obvious pathology	☐	☐	☐	☐	☐	☐

Comments:

_____

_____

Procedure Evaluator Signature	Repeat Evaluator Signature	Competency Evaluator Signature
Date	Date	Date

END HYSTEROSALPINGOGRAM EVALUATION

specific radiographic examinations.

Student Name:_____

Procedure Grade	Repeat Grade	Competency Grade

PATIENT INFORMATION OR SIMULATED PROCEDURE *(circle if simulated)*

	Procedure	Repeat	Competency
Age			
Medical Record No.			
Ability to Cooperate			
Condition/Pathology			
Technical Factors Used			
Exposure Index			

FACILITY PREPARATION
The student:

	Procedure Yes No	Repeat Yes No	Competency Yes No
1. Examines the radiographic room and cleans/straightens it before escorting the patient in.	☐ ☐	☐ ☐	☐ ☐
2. Has all equipment and supplies readily available before escorting the patient in, including patient gown, shield, markers, tape, cassettes, Bucky drawer in proper position, monitor by table, fluoro on, lead aprons and blockers, compression paddle, hemostats, sheets, chucks, appropriate myelogram tray, and portable Mayo stand. Additional supplies: _____ _____ _____ _____	☐ ☐	☐ ☐	☐ ☐
3. Selects and prepares the contrast material without difficulty.	▣ ▣	▣ ▣	☐ ☐
4. Selects and prepares the appropriate sterile tray (maintains the sterile environment).	▣ ▣	▣ ▣	☐ ☐
5. Is able to manipulate all radiographic equipment with ease, and centers the central ray to the cassette/receptor *for all projections.*	☐ ☐	☐ ☐	☐ ☐
6. Adjusts the tube to the proper SID *for each projection.*	☐ ☐	☐ ☐	☐ ☐
7. Selects the appropriate receptor or cassettes of the appropriate sizes *for all projections,* according to the patient's size and examination.	☐ ☐	☐ ☐	☐ ☐

Comments:

_____

_____

(continued)

PATIENT PREPARATION
The student:

	Procedure		Repeat		Competency	
	Yes	No	Yes	No	Yes	No
8. Identifies the correct patient and examination according to the requisition while establishing a good rapport with him or her.	☐	☐	☐	☐	☐	☐
9. Obtains and documents the patient's history before the examination, including preparation instructions.	▨	▨	▨	▨	☐	☐
10. Explains the examination in terms the patient fully understands, and properly communicates with the patient throughout the examination.	☐	☐	☐	☐	☐	☐
11. Asks female patients of childbearing age the date of their last menstrual period and documents this; inquires about the possibility of pregnancy and has them sign pregnancy consent forms	☐	☐	☐	☐	☐	☐
12. Ensures that the proper consent forms are signed.	☐	☐	☐	☐	☐	☐
13. Removes all obscuring objects (snaps, zippers, jewelry, etc.) so as *not* to produce radiographic artifacts.	☐	☐	☐	☐	☐	☐
14. Respects the patient's modesty and provides ample comfort for him or her while positioning him or her to begin the examination.	☐	☐	☐	☐	☐	☐
15. Performs a scout radiograph when indicated.	☐	☐	☐	☐	☐	☐

Comments:

_____

_____

TASKS DURING FLUOROSCOPY
The student:

	Procedure		Repeat		Competency	
	Yes	No	Yes	No	Yes	No
16. Relays the patient's history to the radiologist.	▨	▨	▨	▨	☐	☐
17. Assists the radiologist throughout the examination (aseptic conditions).	▨	▨	▨	▨	☐	☐
18. Monitors, communicates with, and assists the patient throughout the examination.	▨	▨	▨	▨	☐	☐
19. Takes charge of the examination after the radiologist departs.	▨	▨	▨	▨	☐	☐

Comments:

_____

_____

PATIENT POSITIONING FOR A MYELOGRAM/IMMEDIATE CROSS-TABLE LATERAL
The student:

	Procedure		Repeat		Competency	
	Yes	No	Yes	No	Yes	No
20. Places the patient in the prone position on the radiographic table.	☐	☐	☐	☐	☐	☐
21. Selects the appropriate receptor or places the grid/cassette lengthwise, as close to the patient as possible. For conventional cassettes, the flash must be away from any anatomy.	☐	☐	☐	☐	☐	☐
22. Places the patient's arms so that they do not interfere with the area of interest.	☐	☐	☐	☐	☐	☐
23. Horizontally directs the central ray, perpendicularly centered to the area of interest.	☐	☐	☐	☐	☐	☐

Comments:

_____

_____

PATIENT POSITIONING FOR ADDITIONAL IMAGES AS REQUESTED BY THE RADIOLOGIST
The student:

	Procedure		Repeat		Competency	
	Yes	No	Yes	No	Yes	No
24. Places the patient in the _____ position on the radiographic table.	☐	☐	☐	☐	☐	☐
25. Selects the appropriate receptor. For conventional cassettes, the flash must be at the bottom and away from any anatomy.	☐	☐	☐	☐	☐	☐
26. Places the patient's arms so that they do not interfere with the area of interest.	☐	☐	☐	☐	☐	☐
27. Directs the central ray appropriately, centered to the area of interest.	☐	☐	☐	☐	☐	☐

Comments:

_____

_____

IMPORTANT DETAILS
The student:

	Procedure		Repeat		Competency	
	Yes	No	Yes	No	Yes	No
28. Instills confidence in the patient by exhibiting self-confidence throughout the examination.	☐	☐	☐	☐	☐	☐
29. Places a lead marker in the appropriate area of the cassette/receptor (top/bottom/anteriorly/laterally), where it will be visualized on the finished radiograph, on the proper anatomical side (right/left), and in the appropriate position (face up/face down), depending on the patient's position.	☐	☐	☐	☐	☐	☐
30. Provides radiation protection (shield) for the patient (when appropriate), self, and others (closes doors).	☐	☐	☐	☐	☐	☐
31. Applies proper collimation and makes adjustments as necessary.	☐	☐	☐	☐	☐	☐
32. Properly measures the patient along the course of the central ray *for each projection.*	☐	☐	☐	☐	☐	☐
33. Sets the proper technique *for fluoroscopy* (kVp, mA, time).	☐	☐	☐	☐	☐	☐

And all projections/spot images:

Conventional systems

- Sets the proper kVp, mA, and time and makes adjustments as necessary.

or

CR or DR systems
- Identifies the patient on the work-list (or manually types the patient information into the system).
- Selects appropriate body region, specific body part, and accurate view/projection.
- Double-checks preset parameters:
  —Adult vs. pediatric patients
    ○ Small, medium, or large
  —Bucky/receptor (upright vs. table) or non-Bucky
  —AEC vs. fixed
    ○ If AEC, checks ion chambers
    ○ Density setting
  —kVp and mA; adjusts if necessary
  —Focal spot/filament size

	Procedure		Repeat		Competency	
34. Exposes the cassette/receptor after telling the patient to hold still and after giving him or her proper breathing instructions (expiration) *for each projection.*	☐	☐	☐	☐	☐	☐
35. Provides each radiograph with the proper identification (flash) and/or processes each cassette (image) without difficulty (regardless of technology—film, CR, or DR).	▨	▨	▨	▨	☐	☐

(continued)

	Procedure		Repeat		Competency	
	Yes	No	Yes	No	Yes	No
36. Properly completes the examination by filling out all necessary paperwork, entering the examination in the computer, having the images checked by the appropriate staff members, answering any last-minute questions, and informing the patient that he or she is finished. Provides proper post-exam instructions as required.	▢	▢	▢	▢	☐	☐
37. Exhibits the ability to adapt to new and difficult situations if and when necessary.	▢	▢	▢	▢	☐	☐
38. Accepts constructive criticism and uses it to his or her advantage.	☐	☐	☐	☐	☐	☐
39. Leaves the radiographic room neat and clean for the next examination.	▢	▢	▢	▢	☐	☐
40. Completes the examination within a reasonable time frame.	☐	☐	☐	☐	☐	☐

Comments:

_____

_____

RADIOGRAPHIC IMAGE QUALITY
The student is able to critique his or her radiographs as to whether they demonstrate:

	Procedure		Repeat		Competency	
	Yes	No	Yes	No	Yes	No
41. Proper technique/optimal density	▢	▢	▢	▢	☐	☐
42. Enhanced detail, without evidence of motion and without any visible artifacts	▢	▢	▢	▢	☐	☐
43. Proper positioning (all anatomy included, evidence of proper centering/alignment, etc.)	▢	▢	▢	▢	☐	☐
44. Proper marker placement						
45. Evidence of proper collimation and radiation protection	▢	▢	▢	▢	☐	☐
46. Long vs. short scale of contrast	▢	▢	▢	▢	☐	☐

Comments:

_____

_____

ANATOMY
The student is able to identify:

	Procedure		Repeat		Competency	
	Yes	No	Yes	No	Yes	No
47. Nerve roots	▢	▢	▢	▢	☐	☐
48. Axillary pouches	▢	▢	▢	▢	☐	☐
49. Contrast in spinal canal	▢	▢	▢	▢	☐	☐
50. Vertebrae	▢	▢	▢	▢	☐	☐
51. Obvious pathology	▢	▢	▢	▢	☐	☐

Comments:

_____

_____

Procedure Evaluator Signature	Repeat Evaluator Signature	Competency Evaluator Signature
Date	Date	Date

END MYELOGRAM EVALUATION

Student Name:_____

Procedure Grade	Repeat Grade	Competency Grade

PATIENT INFORMATION OR SIMULATED PROCEDURE *(circle if simulated)*

	Procedure	Repeat	Competency
Age			
Medical Record No.			
Ability to Cooperate			
Condition/Pathology			
Technical Factors Used			
Exposure Index			

FACILITY PREPARATION
The student:

	Procedure Yes / No	Repeat Yes / No	Competency Yes / No
1. Examines the radiographic room and cleans/straightens it before escorting the patient in.	☐ ☐	☐ ☐	☐ ☐
2. Has all equipment and supplies readily available before escorting the patient in, including patient gown, shield, markers, tape, cassettes, Bucky drawer in proper position, monitor by table, fluoro on, lead aprons and blockers, hemostats, Betadine, and sterile markers; supplies the requested contrast material as per the physician's preference; and prepares the appropriate arthrogram tray according to the examination and protocol.	☐ ☐	☐ ☐	☐ ☐

Additional supplies:

_____
_____
_____
_____

	Procedure Yes / No	Repeat Yes / No	Competency Yes / No
3. Selects and prepares the contrast material without difficulty.	■ ■	■ ■	☐ ☐
4. Selects and prepares the appropriate sterile tray (maintains the sterile environment).	■ ■	■ ■	☐ ☐
5. Is able to manipulate all radiographic equipment with ease, and centers the central ray to the cassette/receptor *for all projections.*	☐ ☐	☐ ☐	☐ ☐
6. Adjusts the tube to the proper SID *for each projection.*	☐ ☐	☐ ☐	☐ ☐
7. Selects the appropriate receptor or cassettes of the appropriate sizes *for all projections,* according to the patient's size and examination.	☐ ☐	☐ ☐	☐ ☐

Comments:

_____

_____

(continued)

PATIENT PREPARATION
The student:

	Procedure		Repeat		Competency	
	Yes	No	Yes	No	Yes	No
8. Identifies the correct patient and examination according to the requisition while establishing a good rapport with him or her.	☐	☐	☐	☐	☐	☐
9. Obtains and documents the patient's history before the examination.	▨	▨	▨	▨	☐	☐
10. Explains the examination in terms the patient fully understands, and properly communicates with the patient throughout the examination.	☐	☐	☐	☐	☐	☐
11. Asks female patients of childbearing age the date of their last menstrual period and documents this; inquires about the possibility of pregnancy and has them sign pregnancy consent forms	☐	☐	☐	☐	☐	☐
12. Ensures that the proper consent forms are signed.	☐	☐	☐	☐	☐	☐
13. Removes all obscuring objects (snaps, zippers, jewelry, etc.) so as *not* to produce radiographic artifacts.	☐	☐	☐	☐	☐	☐
14. Respects the patient's modesty and provides ample comfort for the patient while positioning him or her to begin the examination.	☐	☐	☐	☐	☐	☐
15. Retrieves previous images for reproduction.	☐	☐	☐	☐	☐	☐
16. Performs a scout radiograph when indicated.	☐	☐	☐	☐	☐	☐

Comments:

_____

_____

TASKS DURING FLUOROSCOPY
The student:

	Procedure		Repeat		Competency	
	Yes	No	Yes	No	Yes	No
17. Relays the patient's history to the radiologist.	▨	▨	▨	▨	☐	☐
18. Assists the radiologist throughout the examination (aseptic conditions).	▨	▨	▨	▨	☐	☐
19. Monitors, communicates with, and assists the patient throughout the examination.	▨	▨	▨	▨	☐	☐
20. Takes charge of the examination after the radiologist departs.	▨	▨	▨	▨	☐	☐

Comments:

_____

_____

PATIENT POSITIONING FOR AN ARTHROGRAM (UNLESS OTHERWISE DIRECTED BY THE PHYSICIAN)
AP or PA
The student:

	Procedure		Repeat		Competency	
	Yes	No	Yes	No	Yes	No
21. Places the patient in the supine or prone position on the radiographic table, without rotation.	☐	☐	☐	☐	☐	☐
22. Selects the appropriate receptor. For conventional cassettes, the flash must be at the bottom and away from any anatomy.	☐	☐	☐	☐	☐	☐
23. Centers the central ray midway between the lateral borders of the area of interest.	☐	☐	☐	☐	☐	☐
24. Directs the central ray appropriately (angles if necessary), centered to the area of interest.	☐	☐	☐	☐	☐	☐

Lateral
The student:

	Procedure		Repeat		Competency	
	Yes	No	Yes	No	Yes	No
25. Places the patient in the lateral position, without rotation.	☐	☐	☐	☐	☐	☐
26. Selects the appropriate receptor. For conventional cassettes, the flash must be at the bottom and away from any anatomy.	☐	☐	☐	☐	☐	☐
27. Centers the central ray midway between the anterior and posterior borders of the area of interest.	☐	☐	☐	☐	☐	☐
28. Directs the central ray appropriately (angles if necessary), centered to the area of interest.	☐	☐	☐	☐	☐	☐

Comments:

_____

_____

IMPORTANT DETAILS
The student:

	Procedure		Repeat		Competency	
	Yes	No	Yes	No	Yes	No
29. Instills confidence in the patient by exhibiting self-confidence throughout the examination.	☐	☐	☐	☐	☐	☐
30. Places a lead marker in the appropriate area of the cassette/receptor (top/bottom/anteriorly/laterally), where hey will be visualized, on the proper anatomical side (right/left), and in the appropriate position (face up/face down), depending on the patient's position.	☐	☐	☐	☐	☐	☐
31. Provides radiation protection (shield) for the patient (when appropriate), self, and others (closes doors).	☐	☐	☐	☐	☐	☐
32. Applies proper collimation and makes adjustments as necessary.	☐	☐	☐	☐	☐	☐
33. Properly measures the patient along the course of the central ray *for each projection.*	☐	☐	☐	☐	☐	☐
34. Sets the proper technique *for fluoroscopy* (kVp, mA, time).	☐	☐	☐	☐	☐	☐

And all projections/spot images:

Conventional systems

• Sets the proper kVp, mA, and time and makes adjustments as necessary.

or

CR or DR systems
• Identifies the patient on the work-list (or manually types the patient information into the system).
• Selects appropriate body region, specific body part, and accurate view/projection.
• Double-checks preset parameters:
—Adult vs. pediatric patients
   ○ Small, medium, or large
—Bucky/receptor (upright vs. table) or non-Bucky
—AEC vs. fixed
   ○ If AEC, checks ion chambers
   ○ Density setting
—kVp and mA; adjusts if necessary
—Focal spot/filament size

	Procedure		Repeat		Competency	
35. Exposes the cassette/receptor after telling the patient to hold still and after giving him or her proper breathing instructions (if necessary) *for each projection.*	☐	☐	☐	☐	☐	☐
36. Provides each radiograph with the proper identification (flash) and/or processes each cassette (image) without difficulty (regardless of technology—film, CR, or DR).	▨	▨	▨	▨	☐	☐

(continued)

	Procedure		Repeat		Competency	
	Yes	No	Yes	No	Yes	No
37. Properly completes the examination by filling out all necessary paperwork, entering the examination in the computer, having the images checked by the appropriate staff members, answering any last-minute questions, and informing the patient that he or she is finished. Provides proper post-exam instructions as required.	☐	☐	☐	☐	☐	☐
38. Exhibits the ability to adapt to new and difficult situations if and when necessary.	☐	☐	☐	☐	☐	☐
39. Accepts constructive criticism and uses it to his or her advantage.	☐	☐	☐	☐	☐	☐
40. Leaves the radiographic room neat and clean for the next examination.	☐	☐	☐	☐	☐	☐
41. Completes the examination within a reasonable time frame.	☐	☐	☐	☐	☐	☐

Comments:

_____

_____

RADIOGRAPHIC IMAGE QUALITY
The student is able to critique his or her radiographs as to whether they demonstrate:

	Procedure		Repeat		Competency	
	Yes	No	Yes	No	Yes	No
42. Proper technique/optimal density	☐	☐	☐	☐	☐	☐
43. Enhanced detail, without evidence of motion and without any visible artifacts	☐	☐	☐	☐	☐	☐
44. Proper positioning (all anatomy included, evidence of proper centering/alignment, etc.)	☐	☐	☐	☐	☐	☐
45. Proper marker placement						
46. Evidence of proper collimation and radiation protection	☐	☐	☐	☐	☐	☐
47. Long vs. short scale of contrast	☐	☐	☐	☐	☐	☐

Comments:

_____

_____

ANATOMY
Shoulder Arthrogram
The student is able to identify:

	Procedure		Repeat		Competency	
	Yes	No	Yes	No	Yes	No
48. Clavicle	☐	☐	☐	☐	☐	☐
49. Humeral head	☐	☐	☐	☐	☐	☐
50. Glenoid cavity	☐	☐	☐	☐	☐	☐
51. Coracoid vs. acromion	☐	☐	☐	☐	☐	☐
52. Obvious pathology	☐	☐	☐	☐	☐	☐

Wrist Arthrogram
The student is able to identify:

	Procedure		Repeat		Competency	
	Yes	No	Yes	No	Yes	No
53. Radius vs. ulna	☐	☐	☐	☐	☐	☐
54. Distal radioulnar joint	☐	☐	☐	☐	☐	☐
55. Intercarpal articulations	☐	☐	☐	☐	☐	☐
56. Carpometacarpal articulations	☐	☐	☐	☐	☐	☐
57. Obvious pathology	☐	☐	☐	☐	☐	☐

Hip Arthrogram
The student is able to identify:

	Procedure Yes	Procedure No	Repeat Yes	Repeat No	Competency Yes	Competency No
58. Acetabulum	☐	☐	☐	☐	☐	☐
59. Femoral head and neck	☐	☐	☐	☐	☐	☐
60. Greater vs. lesser trochanters	☐	☐	☐	☐	☐	☐
61. Ischium	☐	☐	☐	☐	☐	☐
62. Ilium	☐	☐	☐	☐	☐	☐
63. Obvious pathology	☐	☐	☐	☐	☐	☐

Knee Arthrogram
The student is able to identify:

	Procedure Yes	Procedure No	Repeat Yes	Repeat No	Competency Yes	Competency No
64. Medial vs. lateral meniscus	☐	☐	☐	☐	☐	☐
65. Medial vs. lateral femoral condyles	☐	☐	☐	☐	☐	☐
66. Tibial spine	☐	☐	☐	☐	☐	☐
67. Tibial plateau	☐	☐	☐	☐	☐	☐
68. Obvious pathology	☐	☐	☐	☐	☐	☐

Ankle Arthrogram
The student is able to identify:

	Procedure Yes	Procedure No	Repeat Yes	Repeat No	Competency Yes	Competency No
69. Talotibial joint	☐	☐	☐	☐	☐	☐
70. Medial vs. lateral malleolus	☐	☐	☐	☐	☐	☐
71. Talus	☐	☐	☐	☐	☐	☐
72. Tibia vs. fibula	☐	☐	☐	☐	☐	☐
73. Obvious pathology	☐	☐	☐	☐	☐	☐

Comments:

_____

_____

_____ _____ _____
Procedure Evaluator Signature   Repeat Evaluator Signature   Competency Evaluator Signature

_____ _____ _____
Date   Date   Date

END ARTHROGRAM EVALUATION

The objective of this evaluation is to determine the student's competency level when performing specific radiographic examinations.

Student Name:_____

Procedure Grade	Repeat Grade	Competency Grade

PATIENT INFORMATION OR SIMULATED PROCEDURE *(circle if simulated)*

	Procedure	Repeat	Competency
Age			
Medical Record No.			
Ability to Cooperate			
Condition/Pathology			
Technical Factors Used			
Exposure Index			

FACILITY PREPARATION
The student:

	Procedure Yes	Procedure No	Repeat Yes	Repeat No	Competency Yes	Competency No
1. Examines the radiographic room and cleans/straightens it before escorting the patient in.	☐	☐	☐	☐	☐	☐
2. Has all equipment and supplies readily available before escorting the patient in, including patient gown, shield, markers, tape, cassettes, monitor by table, fluoro on, lead aprons and blockers, hemostats, support box for patient to stand on, and portable Mayo stand; supplies the requested contrast material as per the physician's preference; and prepares the appropriate venogram tray according to the examination and protocol.	☐	☐	☐	☐	☐	☐

Additional supplies:

_____
_____
_____
_____

	Procedure Yes	Procedure No	Repeat Yes	Repeat No	Competency Yes	Competency No
3. Selects and prepares the contrast material without difficulty.	▓	▓	▓	▓	☐	☐
4. Is able to manipulate all radiographic equipment with ease, and centers the central ray to the cassette/receptor *for all projections.*	☐	☐	☐	☐	☐	☐
5. Adjusts the tube to the proper SID *for each projection.*	☐	☐	☐	☐	☐	☐
6. Selects the appropriate receptor or cassettes of the appropriate sizes *for all projections,* according to the patient's size and examination.	☐	☐	☐	☐	☐	☐

Comments:

_____
_____

(continued)

PATIENT PREPARATION
The student:

	Procedure		Repeat		Competency	
	Yes	No	Yes	No	Yes	No
7. Identifies the correct patient and examination according to the requisition while establishing a good rapport with him or her.	☐	☐	☐	☐	☐	☐
8. Obtains and documents the patient's history before the examination, including preparation instructions.	▨	▨	▨	▨	☐	☐
9. Explains the examination in terms the patient fully understands, and properly communicates with the patient throughout the examination.	☐	☐	☐	☐	☐	☐
10. Asks female patients of childbearing age the date of their last menstrual period and documents this; inquires about the possibility of pregnancy and has them sign pregnancy consent forms	☐	☐	☐	☐	☐	☐
11. Ensures that the physician had the proper consent forms signed.	☐	☐	☐	☐	☐	☐
12. Removes all obscuring objects (snaps, zippers, jewelry, etc.) so as *not* to produce radiographic artifacts.	☐	☐	☐	☐	☐	☐
13. Respects the patient's modesty and provides ample comfort for the patient while positioning him or her to begin the examination by placing the unaffected leg on the support box.	☐	☐	☐	☐	☐	☐
14. Performs a scout radiograph when indicated.	☐	☐	☐	☐	☐	☐

Comments:

_____

_____

TASKS DURING FLUOROSCOPY
The student:

	Procedure		Repeat		Competency	
	Yes	No	Yes	No	Yes	No
15. Relays the patient's history to the radiologist.	▨	▨	▨	▨	☐	☐
16. Assists the radiologist throughout the examination.	▨	▨	▨	▨	☐	☐
17. Monitors, communicates with, and assists the patient throughout the examination.	▨	▨	▨	▨	☐	☐
18. Takes charge of the examination after the radiologist departs.	▨	▨	▨	▨	☐	☐
19. Allows approximately 100 cc of NaCl to flush the intravenous (IV) line.	▨	▨	▨	▨	☐	☐
20. Removes the IV line.	▨	▨	▨	▨	☐	☐

Comments:

_____

_____

PATIENT POSITIONING FOR A VENOGRAM
Immediate APs
(Tibia/Fibula and Ankle, Knee, Thigh and Right/Left Iliac/Pelvis)
The student:

	Procedure		Repeat		Competency	
	Yes	No	Yes	No	Yes	No
21. Places the patient in the supine position on the radiographic table	☐	☐	☐	☐	☐	☐
22. Selects the appropriate receptor. For conventional cassettes, the flash must be at the bottom and away from any anatomy.	☐	☐	☐	☐	☐	☐
23. Places the patient's arms so that they do not interfere with the area of interest.	☐	☐	☐	☐	☐	☐
24. Centers midway between the lateral aspects of the area of interest.	☐	☐	☐	☐	☐	☐
25. Directs the central ray perpendicularly, centered midway between the superior and inferior regions of the area of interest.	☐	☐	☐	☐	☐	☐

Comments:

_____

_____

Immediate Lateral
(True Lateral or Cross-Table; Tibia/Fibula and Ankle, Knee, Thigh)
The student:

	Procedure		Repeat		Competency	
	Yes	No	Yes	No	Yes	No
26. Places the patient's leg in the lateral position on the radiographic table, without rotation.	☐	☐	☐	☐	☐	☐
27. Selects the appropriate receptor. For conventional cassettes, the flash must be at the bottom and away from any anatomy.	☐	☐	☐	☐	☐	☐
28. Places the patient's arms so that they do not interfere with the area of interest.	☐	☐	☐	☐	☐	☐
29. Centers midway between the anterior and posterior aspects of the area of interest.	☐	☐	☐	☐	☐	☐
30. Directs the central ray perpendicularly, centered midway between the superior and inferior regions of the area of interest.	☐	☐	☐	☐	☐	☐

Comments:

_____

_____

IMPORTANT DETAILS
The student:

	Procedure		Repeat		Competency	
	Yes	No	Yes	No	Yes	No
31. Instills confidence in the patient by exhibiting self-confidence throughout the examination.	☐	☐	☐	☐	☐	☐
32. Places a lead marker in the appropriate area of the cassette/receptor (top/bottom/anteriorly/laterally), where hey will be visualized, on the proper anatomical side (right/left), and in the appropriate position (face up/face down), depending on the patient's position.	☐	☐	☐	☐	☐	☐
33. Provides radiation protection (shield) for the patient (when appropriate), self, and others (closes doors).	☐	☐	☐	☐	☐	☐
34. Applies proper collimation and makes adjustments as necessary.	☐	☐	☐	☐	☐	☐
35. Properly measures the patient along the course of the central ray *for each projection.*	☐	☐	☐	☐	☐	☐
36. Sets the proper technique *for fluoroscopy* (kVp, mA, time).	☐	☐	☐	☐	☐	☐

And all projections/spot images:

Conventional systems

- Sets the proper kVp, mA, and time and makes adjustments as necessary.

or

CR or DR systems
- Identifies the patient on the work-list (or manually types the patient information into the system).
- Selects appropriate body region, specific body part, and accurate view/projection.
- Double-checks preset parameters:
  —Adult vs. pediatric patients
    ○ Small, medium, or large
  —Bucky/receptor (upright vs. table) or non-Bucky
  —AEC vs. fixed
    ○ If AEC, checks ion chambers
    ○ Density setting
  —kVp and mA; adjusts if necessary
  —Focal spot/filament size

	Procedure		Repeat		Competency	
37. Exposes the cassette/receptor after telling the patient to hold still and after giving him or her proper breathing instructions (if necessary) *for each projection.*	☐	☐	☐	☐	☐	☐

(continued)

	Procedure		Repeat		Competency	
	Yes	No	Yes	No	Yes	No
38. Provides each radiograph with the proper identification (flash) and/or processes each cassette (image) without difficulty (regardless of technology—film, CR, or DR).	☑	☑	☑	☑	☐	☐
39. Properly completes the examination by filling out all necessary paperwork, entering the examination in the computer, having the images checked by the appropriate staff members, answering any last-minute questions, and informing the patient that he or she is finished. Provides proper post-exam instructions as required.	☑	☑	☑	☑	☐	☐
40. Exhibits the ability to adapt to new and difficult situations if and when necessary.	☑	☑	☑	☑	☐	☐
41. Accepts constructive criticism and uses it to his or her advantage.	☐	☐	☐	☐	☐	☐
42. Leaves the radiographic room neat and clean for the next examination.	☑	☑	☑	☑	☐	☐
43. Completes the examination within a reasonable time frame.	☐	☐	☐	☐	☐	☐

Comments:

_____

_____

RADIOGRAPHIC IMAGE QUALITY
The student is able to critique his or her radiographs as to whether they demonstrate:

	Procedure		Repeat		Competency	
	Yes	No	Yes	No	Yes	No
44. Proper technique/optimal density	☑	☑	☑	☑	☐	☐
45. Enhanced detail, without evidence of motion and without any visible artifacts	☑	☑	☑	☑	☐	☐
46. Proper positioning (all anatomy included, evidence of proper centering/alignment, etc.)	☑	☑	☑	☑	☐	☐
47. Proper marker placement						
48. Evidence of proper collimation and radiation protection	☑	☑	☑	☑	☐	☐
49. Long vs. short scale of contrast	☑	☑	☑	☑	☐	☐

Comments:

_____

_____

ANATOMY
The student is able to identify:

	Procedure		Repeat		Competency	
	Yes	No	Yes	No	Yes	No
50. Inferior vena cava	☑	☑	☑	☑	☐	☐
51. Common vs. external iliac vein	☑	☑	☑	☑	☐	☐
52. Popliteal vein	☑	☑	☑	☑	☐	☐
53. Femoral vein	☑	☑	☑	☑	☐	☐
54. Corresponding bony landmarks and joints	☑	☑	☑	☑	☐	☐
55. Obvious pathology	☑	☑	☑	☑	☐	☐

Comments:

_____

_____

Procedure Evaluator Signature	Repeat Evaluator Signature	Competency Evaluator Signature

Date	Date	Date

END VENOGRAM EVALUATION

Student Name:_____

Procedure Grade	Repeat Grade	Competency Grade

PATIENT INFORMATION OR SIMULATED PROCEDURE *(circle if simulated)*

	Procedure	Repeat	Competency
Age			
Medical Record No.			
Ability to Cooperate			
Condition/Pathology			
Technical Factors Used			
Exposure Index			

FACILITY PREPARATION
The student:

	Procedure Yes No	Repeat Yes No	Competency Yes No
1. Examines the radiographic room and cleans/straightens it before escorting the patient in.	☐ ☐	☐ ☐	☐ ☐
2. Has all equipment (image receptor, compression paddle) set up and supplies (patient gown, shield, markers, tape, cassettes) readily available before escorting the patient in. Additional supplies: _____ _____ _____ _____	☐ ☐	☐ ☐	☐ ☐
3. Is able to manipulate all radiographic equipment with ease and able to load cassette with the proper side toward the patient *for all projections.*	☐ ☐	☐ ☐	☐ ☐
4. Selects the appropriate receptor or cassettes of the appropriate size *for all projections,* according to the patient's size.	☐ ☐	☐ ☐	☐ ☐
5. Enters the patient's information into the computer.	☐ ☐	☐ ☐	☐ ☐

Comments:

_____

_____

PATIENT PREPARATION
The student:

	Procedure Yes No	Repeat Yes No	Competency Yes No
6. Identifies the correct patient and examination according to the requisition while establishing a good rapport with him or her.	☐ ☐	☐ ☐	☐ ☐
7. Obtains and documents the patient's history before the examination and records it on the appropriate form.	■ ■	■ ■	☐ ☐

(continued)

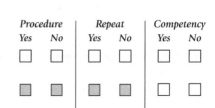

	Procedure		Repeat		Competency	
	Yes	No	Yes	No	Yes	No
8. Explains the examination in terms the patient fully understands, and properly communicates with the patient throughout the examination.	☐	☐	☐	☐	☐	☐
9. Asks female patients of childbearing age the date of their last menstrual period and documents this; inquires about the possibility of pregnancy and has them sign pregnancy consent forms.	☐	☐	☐	☐	☐	☐
10. Ensures that the patient does not have powder and/or deodorant on; if he or she does, politely instructs the patient to wash it off.	☐	☐	☐	☐	☐	☐
11. Removes all obscuring objects (snaps, zippers, jewelry, etc.) so as *not* to produce radiographic artifacts.	☐	☐	☐	☐	☐	☐
12. Respects the patient's modesty and provides ample comfort for the patient while positioning him or her to begin the examination.	☐	☐	☐	☐	☐	☐

Comments:

_____

_____

TASKS DURING A MAMMOGRAM
The student:

	Procedure		Repeat		Competency	
	Yes	No	Yes	No	Yes	No
13. Relays the patient's history to the radiologist.	■	■	■	■	☐	☐
14. Monitors, communicates with, and assists the patient throughout the examination.	■	■	■	■	☐	☐

Comments:

_____

_____

PATIENT POSITIONING FOR A MAMMOGRAM
Craniocaudal
The student gently:

	Procedure		Repeat		Competency	
	Yes	No	Yes	No	Yes	No
15. Selects the appropriate receptor. For conventional cassettes, the flash must be at the bottom and away from any anatomy.	☐	☐	☐	☐	☐	☐
16. Places the patient so that he or she is facing the mammographic equipment.	☐	☐	☐	☐	☐	☐
17. Raises the inframammary fold to its maximum height and places the patient's breast on the radiographic Bucky/receptor.	☐	☐	☐	☐	☐	☐
18. Adjusts the height of the Bucky/receptor to an appropriate height.	☐	☐	☐	☐	☐	☐
19. Using both hands, pulls the breast forward onto the image receptor, centering the breast over the appropriate photocell.	☐	☐	☐	☐	☐	☐
20. Rotates the patient's head away from the area being examined, and instructs him or her to relax the shoulder.	☐	☐	☐	☐	☐	☐
21. Checks that the nipple is in profile (does not sacrifice tissue to do so).	☐	☐	☐	☐	☐	☐
22. Drapes the opposite breast over the corner of the Bucky/receptor so that the medial tissue of the affected breast will be well demonstrated on the finished radiograph.	☐	☐	☐	☐	☐	☐
23. Pulls the lateral tissue onto the Bucky/receptor (without losing the medial tissue).	☐	☐	☐	☐	☐	☐
24. Applies appropriate compression while anchoring the breast with one hand.	☐	☐	☐	☐	☐	☐
25. Releases compression immediately following the exposure.	☐	☐	☐	☐	☐	☐

Mediolateral Oblique
The student gently:

	Procedure		Repeat		Competency	
	Yes	No	Yes	No	Yes	No
26. Rotates the mammographic equipment so that it is perpendicular to the pectoral muscle.	☐	☐	☐	☐	☐	☐
27. Selects the appropriate receptor. For conventional cassettes, the flash must be at the bottom and away from any anatomy.	☐	☐	☐	☐	☐	☐
28. Places the patient in the lateral position.	☐	☐	☐	☐	☐	☐
29. Adjusts the height of the Bucky/receptor so that the top is level with the axilla.	☐	☐	☐	☐	☐	☐
30. Lifts the arm of the side being examined up over the corner of the Bucky/receptor.	☐	☐	☐	☐	☐	☐
31. Helps adjust the patient so that his or her arm is draped over the machine, with the elbow flexed and shoulder relaxed.	☐	☐	☐	☐	☐	☐
32. Lifts and pulls the breast and pectoral muscle anteriorly and medially.	☐	☐	☐	☐	☐	☐
33. Turns the patient toward the machine (feet facing machine), and places the breast tissue against the Bucky/receptor.	☐	☐	☐	☐	☐	☐
34. Holding the breast up and out, applies appropriate compression.	☐	☐	☐	☐	☐	☐
35. Pulls the abdominal tissue down to open the inframammary fold.	☐	☐	☐	☐	☐	☐
36. Checks that the nipple is in profile before making the exposure.	☐	☐	☐	☐	☐	☐
37. Releases compression immediately following the exposure.	☐	☐	☐	☐	☐	☐

Comments:

_____

_____

IMPORTANT DETAILS
The student:

	Procedure		Repeat		Competency	
	Yes	No	Yes	No	Yes	No
38. Instills confidence in the patient by exhibiting self-confidence throughout the examination.	☐	☐	☐	☐	☐	☐
39. Provides radiation protection (shield) for the patient (when appropriate), self, and others (closes doors).	☐	☐	☐	☐	☐	☐
40. Applies proper collimation and makes adjustments as necessary.	☐	☐	☐	☐	☐	☐
41. Places lead markers in the appropriate area of the Bucky/receptor, where they will be visualized, on the proper anatomical side (near right/left; craniocaudal [CC]—lateral) *each projection.*	☐	☐	☐	☐	☐	☐
42. Sets the proper technique:	☐	☐	☐	☐	☐	☐

Conventional systems
- Sets the proper kVp, mA, and time and makes adjustments as necessary.

or

CR or DR systems
- Identifies the patient on the work-list (or manually types the patient information into the system).
- Selects appropriate body region, specific body part, and accurate view/projection.
- Double-checks preset parameters:
  —Adult vs. pediatric patients
  ○ Small, medium, or large
  —Bucky/receptor (upright vs. table) or non-Bucky
  —AEC vs. fixed
  ○ If AEC, checks ion chambers
  ○ Density setting

(continued)

	Procedure		Repeat		Competency	
	Yes	No	Yes	No	Yes	No

 —kVp and mA; adjusts if necessary
 —Focal spot/filament size

	Procedure		Repeat		Competency	
	Yes	No	Yes	No	Yes	No
43. Exposes the cassette/receptor after telling the patient to hold still and after giving him or her proper breathing instructions (suspended) for each projection.	☐	☐	☐	☐	☐	☐
44. Provides each radiograph with the proper identification (flash) and/or processes each cassette (image) without difficulty (regardless of technology—film, CR, or DR).	■	■	■	■	☐	☐
45. Properly completes the examination by filling out all necessary paperwork, entering the examination in the computer, having images checked by the appropriate staff members, providing postprocedural instructions and answering last-minute questions, and informing the patient that he or she is finished. Provides proper post-exam instructions as required.	■	■	■	■	☐	☐
46. Exhibits the ability to adapt to new and difficult situations if and when necessary.	■	■	■	■	☐	☐
47. Accepts constructive criticism and uses it to his or her advantage.	☐	☐	☐	☐	☐	☐
48. Leaves the radiographic room neat and clean for the next examination.	■	■	■	■	☐	☐
49. Completes the examination within a reasonable time frame.	☐	☐	☐	☐	☐	☐

Comments:

_____

_____

RADIOGRAPHIC IMAGE QUALITY
The student is able to critique his or her radiographs as to whether they demonstrate:

	Procedure		Repeat		Competency	
	Yes	No	Yes	No	Yes	No
50. Proper technique/optimal density	■	■	■	■	☐	☐
51. Enhanced detail, without evidence of motion and without any visible artifacts	■	■	■	■	☐	☐
52. Proper positioning (all anatomy included, evidence of proper centering/alignment, etc.)	■	■	■	■	☐	☐
53. Proper marker placement						
54. Evidence of proper collimation and radiation protection	■	■	■	■	☐	☐
55. Long vs. short scale of contrast	■	■	■	■	☐	☐

Comments:

_____

_____

ANATOMY
The student is able to identify:

	Procedure		Repeat		Competency	
	Yes	No	Yes	No	Yes	No
56. Fat tissue	■	■	■	■	☐	☐
57. Nipple	■	■	■	■	☐	☐
58. Lactiferous tubules (if visible)	■	■	■	■	☐	☐
59. Pectoralis muscle	■	■	■	■	☐	☐
60. Axillary border	■	■	■	■	☐	☐
61. Obvious pathology	■	■	■	■	☐	☐

Comments:

_____

_____

_____

Procedure Evaluator Signature	Repeat Evaluator Signature	Competency Evaluator Signature

Date	Date	Date

Specific radiographic examinations.

Student Name:_____	Procedure Grade	Repeat Grade	Competency Grade

PATIENT INFORMATION OR SIMULATED PROCEDURE *(circle if simulated)*

	Procedure	Repeat	Competency
Age			
Medical Record No.			
Ability to Cooperate			
Condition/Pathology			
Technical Factors Used			
Exposure Index			

FACILITY PREPARATION
The student:

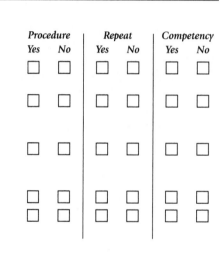

	Procedure Yes No	Repeat Yes No	Competency Yes No
1. Examines the radiographic room and cleans/straightens it before escorting the patient in.	☐ ☐	☐ ☐	☐ ☐
2. Has all equipment and supplies (patient gown, shield, markers, number markers, tape, cassettes, etc.) readily available before escorting the patient in.	☐ ☐	☐ ☐	☐ ☐
3. Is able to manipulate all radiographic and tomographic equipment with ease, and centers the central ray to the cassette/receptor *for all projections.*	☐ ☐	☐ ☐	☐ ☐
4. Adjusts the tube to the proper SID *for each projection.*	☐ ☐	☐ ☐	☐ ☐
5. Selects the appropriate receptor or cassettes of the appropriate size *for all projections,* according to the patient's size and examination.	☐ ☐	☐ ☐	☐ ☐

Comments:

_____

_____

PATIENT PREPARATION
The student:

	Procedure Yes No	Repeat Yes No	Competency Yes No
6. Identifies the correct patient and examination according to the requisition while establishing a good rapport with him or her.	☐ ☐	☐ ☐	☐ ☐
7. Obtains and documents the patient's history before the examination.	▨ ▨	▨ ▨	☐ ☐
8. Explains the examination in terms the patient fully understands, *emphasizing movement of equipment,* and properly communicates with the patient throughout the examination.	☐ ☐	☐ ☐	☐ ☐
9. Asks female patients of childbearing age the date of their last menstrual period and documents this; inquires about the possibility of pregnancy and has them sign pregnancy consent forms.	☐ ☐	☐ ☐	☐ ☐

(continued)

483

	Procedure		Repeat		Competency	
	Yes	No	Yes	No	Yes	No
10. Removes all obscuring objects (snaps, zippers, jewelry, etc.) so as *not* to produce radiographic artifacts.	☐	☐	☐	☐	☐	☐
11. Respects the patient's modesty and provides ample comfort for the patient while positioning him or her to begin the examination.	☐	☐	☐	☐	☐	☐

Comments:

_____

_____

TASKS DURING A CONVENTIONAL TOMOGRAM
The student:

	Procedure		Repeat		Competency	
	Yes	No	Yes	No	Yes	No
12. Relays the patient's history to the radiologist.	☐	☐	☐	☐	☐	☐
13. Monitors, communicates with, and assists the patient throughout the examination.	☐	☐	☐	☐	☐	☐
14. Communicates with the radiologist throughout the examination.	☐	☐	☐	☐	☐	☐

Comments:

_____

_____

PATIENT POSITIONING FOR A TOMOGRAM
Anteroposterior/Posteroanterior
The student:

	Procedure		Repeat		Competency	
	Yes	No	Yes	No	Yes	No
15. Places the patient in the supine or prone position on the radiographic table, without rotation.	☐	☐	☐	☐	☐	☐
16. Selects the appropriate receptor. For conventional cassettes, the flash must be at the bottom and away from any anatomy.	☐	☐	☐	☐	☐	☐
17. Centers the central ray midway between the lateral borders of the area of interest.	☐	☐	☐	☐	☐	☐
18. Directs the central ray appropriately, centered to the area of interest.	☐	☐	☐	☐	☐	☐

Lateral
The student:

	Procedure		Repeat		Competency	
	Yes	No	Yes	No	Yes	No
19. Places the patient in the lateral position, without rotation.	☐	☐	☐	☐	☐	☐
20. Selects the appropriate receptor. For conventional cassettes, the flash must be at the bottom and away from any anatomy.	☐	☐	☐	☐	☐	☐
21. Centers the central ray midway between the anterior and posterior borders of the area of interest.	☐	☐	☐	☐	☐	☐
22. Directs the central ray appropriately, centered to the area of interest.	☐	☐	☐	☐	☐	☐

Comments:

_____

_____

IMPORTANT DETAILS
The student:

	Procedure		Repeat		Competency	
	Yes	No	Yes	No	Yes	No
23. Instills confidence in the patient by exhibiting self-confidence throughout the examination.	☐	☐	☐	☐	☐	☐

	Procedure		Repeat		Competency	
	Yes	No	Yes	No	Yes	No
24. Places lead markers in the appropriate area of the cassette/receptor (top/bottom/anteriorly/laterally), where they will be visualized, on the proper anatomical side (right/left), and in the appropriate position (face up/face down), depending on the patient's position.	☐	☐	☐	☐	☐	☐
25. Provides radiation protection (shield) for the patient (when appropriate), self, and others (closes doors).	☐	☐	☐	☐	☐	☐
26. Applies proper collimation and makes adjustments as necessary.	☐	☐	☐	☐	☐	☐
27. Properly measures the patient along the course of the central ray and accurately sets fulcrum levels.	☐	☐	☐	☐	☐	☐
28. Sets the proper technique (kVp, mA, time) *and all projections, including tomograms,* making adjustments in technique and fulcrum levels as necessary.	☐	☐	☐	☐	☐	☐

28. (continued)

Conventional systems
- Sets the proper kVp, mA, and time and makes adjustments as necessary.

or

CR or DR systems
- Identifies the patient on the work-list (or manually types the patient information into the system).
- Selects appropriate body region, specific body part, and accurate view/projection.
- Double-checks preset parameters:
  —Adult vs. pediatric patients
    ○ Small, medium, or large
  —Bucky/receptor (upright vs. table) or non-Bucky
  —AEC vs. fixed
    ○ If AEC, checks ion chambers
    ○ Density setting
  —kVp and mA; adjusts if necessary
  —Focal spot/filament size

	Procedure		Repeat		Competency	
29. Exposes the cassette/receptor after telling the patient to hold still and after giving him or her proper breathing instructions (if necessary) *for each projection.*	☐	☐	☐	☐	☐	☐
30. Provides each radiograph with the proper identification (flash) and/or processes each cassette (image) without difficulty (regardless of technology—film, CR, or DR).	▨	▨	▨	▨	☐	☐
31. Properly completes the examination by filling out all necessary paperwork, entering the examination in the computer, having images checked by the appropriate staff members, providing postprocedural instructions and answering last-minute questions, and informing the patient that he or she is finished. Provides proper post-exam instructions as required.	▨	▨	▨	▨	☐	☐
32. Exhibits the ability to adapt to new and difficult situations if and when necessary.	▨	▨	▨	▨	☐	☐
33. Accepts constructive criticism and uses it to his or her advantage.	☐	☐	☐	☐	☐	☐
34. Leaves the radiographic room neat and clean for the next examination.	▨	▨	▨	▨	☐	☐
35. Completes the examination within a reasonable time frame.	☐	☐	☐	☐	☐	☐

Comments:

_____

_____

(continued)

RADIOGRAPHIC IMAGE QUALITY
The student is able to critique his or her radiographs as to whether they demonstrate:

	Procedure		Repeat		Competency	
	Yes	No	Yes	No	Yes	No
36. Proper technique/optimal density	☐	☐	☐	☐	☐	☐
37. Enhanced detail, without any visible artifacts and with evidence of proper motion/blur	☐	☐	☐	☐	☐	☐
38. Proper positioning (all anatomy included, evidence of proper centering/alignment, etc.)	☐	☐	☐	☐	☐	☐
39. Proper marker placement	☐	☐	☐	☐	☐	☐
40. Evidence of proper collimation and radiation protection	☐	☐	☐	☐	☐	☐
41. Long vs. short scale of contrast	☐	☐	☐	☐	☐	☐

Comments:

_____

_____

ANATOMY
The student is able to identify:

	Procedure		Repeat		Competency	
	Yes	No	Yes	No	Yes	No
42. _____	☐	☐	☐	☐	☐	☐
43. _____	☐	☐	☐	☐	☐	☐
44. _____	☐	☐	☐	☐	☐	☐
45. _____	☐	☐	☐	☐	☐	☐
46. _____	☐	☐	☐	☐	☐	☐
47. _____	☐	☐	☐	☐	☐	☐
48. _____	☐	☐	☐	☐	☐	☐
49. Obvious pathology	☐	☐	☐	☐	☐	☐

Comments:

_____

_____

Procedure Evaluator Signature	Repeat Evaluator Signature	Competency Evaluator Signature
Date	Date	Date

END CONVENTIONAL TOMOGRAM EVALUATION

Student Name:_____

Procedure Grade	Repeat Grade	Competency Grade

PATIENT INFORMATION OR SIMULATED PROCEDURE *(circle if simulated)*

	Procedure	Repeat	Competency
Age			
Medical Record No.			
Ability to Cooperate			
Condition/Pathology			
Technical Factors Used			
Exposure Index			

FACILITY PREPARATION
The student:

	Procedure Yes No	Repeat Yes No	Competency Yes No
1. Examines the radiographic room and cleans/straightens it before escorting the patient in.	☐ ☐	☐ ☐	☐ ☐
2. Has all equipment and supplies (patient gown, shield, markers, tape, cassettes, etc.) readily available before escorting the patient in.	☐ ☐	☐ ☐	☐ ☐
3. Is able to manipulate all radiographic equipment with ease, and centers the central ray to the cassette/receptor *for all projections.*	☐ ☐	☐ ☐	☐ ☐
4. Adjusts the tube to the proper SID *for each projection.*	☐ ☐	☐ ☐	☐ ☐
5. Selects the appropriate receptor or cassettes of the appropriate sizes *for all projections,* according to the patient's size and examination.	☐ ☐	☐ ☐	☐ ☐

Comments:

_____

_____

PATIENT PREPARATION
The student:

	Procedure Yes No	Repeat Yes No	Competency Yes No
6. Identifies the correct patient and examination according to the requisition while establishing a good rapport with him or her.	☐ ☐	☐ ☐	☐ ☐
7. Obtains and documents the patient's history before the examination.	☐ ☐	☐ ☐	☐ ☐
8. Explains the examination in terms the patient fully understands, and properly communicates with the patient throughout the examination.	☐ ☐	☐ ☐	☐ ☐
9. Asks female patients of childbearing age the date of their last menstrual period and documents this; inquires about the possibility of pregnancy and has them sign pregnancy consent forms	☐ ☐	☐ ☐	☐ ☐
10. Removes all obscuring objects (snaps, zippers, jewelry, etc.) so as *not* to produce radiographic artifacts.	☐ ☐	☐ ☐	☐ ☐

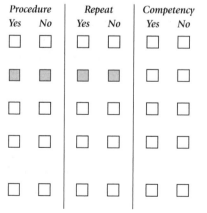

(continued)

	Procedure		Repeat		Competency	
	Yes	No	Yes	No	Yes	No
11. Respects the patient's modesty and provides ample comfort for the patient while positioning him or her to begin the examination.	☐	☐	☐	☐	☐	☐

Comments:

_____

_____

PATIENT POSITIONING FOR A SOFT TISSUE EXTREMITY
AP or PA
The student:

	Procedure		Repeat		Competency	
	Yes	No	Yes	No	Yes	No
12. Places the patient in the supine or prone position at the upright Bucky/receptor or on the radiographic table, without rotation.	☐	☐	☐	☐	☐	☐
13. Selects the appropriate receptor or places the cassette appropriately. For conventional cassettes, the flash must be at the bottom and away from any anatomy.	☐	☐	☐	☐	☐	☐
14. Centers the central ray to the midline (between the lateral surfaces) of the affected extremity.	☐	☐	☐	☐	☐	☐
15. Directs the central ray perpendicularly or with the appropriate angle relative to the part being radiographed.	☐	☐	☐	☐	☐	☐

Lateral
The student:

	Procedure		Repeat		Competency	
	Yes	No	Yes	No	Yes	No
16. Places the patient in the left lateral position, without rotation.	☐	☐	☐	☐	☐	☐
17. Selects the appropriate receptor or places the cassette appropriately. For conventional cassettes, the flash must be at the bottom and away from any anatomy.	☐	☐	☐	☐	☐	☐
18. Centers the central ray midway between the anterior and posterior surfaces of the affected extremity.	☐	☐	☐	☐	☐	☐
19. Directs the central ray perpendicularly.	☐	☐	☐	☐	☐	☐

Comments:

_____

_____

IMPORTANT DETAILS
The student:

	Procedure		Repeat		Competency	
	Yes	No	Yes	No	Yes	No
20. Instills confidence in the patient by exhibiting self-confidence throughout the examination.	☐	☐	☐	☐	☐	☐
21. Places a lead marker in the appropriate area of the cassette/receptor (top/bottom/anteriorly/laterally), where they will be visualized, on the proper anatomical side (right/left), and in the appropriate position (face up/face down), depending on the patient's position, and marks the image to indicate the affected area.	☐	☐	☐	☐	☐	☐
22. Provides radiation protection (shield) for the patient (when appropriate), self, and others (closes doors).	☐	☐	☐	☐	☐	☐
23. Applies proper collimation and makes adjustments as necessary.	☐	☐	☐	☐	☐	☐
24. Properly measures the patient along the course of the central ray.	☐	☐	☐	☐	☐	☐
25. Sets the proper exposure technique:	☐	☐	☐	☐	☐	☐

Conventional systems
- Sets the proper kVp, mA, and time and makes adjustments as necessary.

or

CR or DR systems
- Identifies the patient on the work-list (or manually types the patient information into the system).
- Selects appropriate body region, specific body part, and accurate view/projection.
- Double-checks preset parameters:
  —Adult vs. pediatric patients
   ◦ Small, medium, or large
  —Bucky/receptor (upright vs. table) or non-Bucky
  —AEC vs. fixed
   ◦ If AEC, checks ion chambers
   ◦ Density setting
  —kVp and mA; adjusts if necessary
  —Focal spot/filament size

	Procedure		Repeat		Competency	
	Yes	No	Yes	No	Yes	No
26. Exposes the cassette/receptor after telling the patient to hold still and after giving him or her proper breathing instructions (if necessary) *for each projection.*	☐	☐	☐	☐	☐	☐
27. Provides each radiograph with the proper identification (flash) and/or processes each cassette (image) without difficulty (regardless of technology—film, CR, or DR).	▦	▦	▦	▦	☐	☐
28. Properly completes the examination by filling out all necessary paperwork, entering the examination in the computer, having images checked by the appropriate staff members, providing postprocedural instructions and answering last-minute questions, and informing the patient that he or she is finished. Provides proper post-exam instructions as required.	▦	▦	▦	▦	☐	☐
29. Exhibits the ability to adapt to new and difficult situations if and when necessary.	▦	▦	▦	▦	☐	☐
30. Accepts constructive criticism and uses it to his or her advantage.	☐	☐	☐	☐	☐	☐
31. Leaves the radiographic room neat and clean for the next examination.	▦	▦	▦	▦	☐	☐
32. Completes the examination within a reasonable time frame.	☐	☐	☐	☐	☐	☐

Comments:

_____

_____

RADIOGRAPHIC IMAGE QUALITY
The student is able to critique his or her radiographs as to whether they demonstrate:

	Procedure		Repeat		Competency	
	Yes	No	Yes	No	Yes	No
33. Proper technique/optimal density	▦	▦	▦	▦	☐	☐
34. Enhanced detail, without evidence of motion and without any visible artifacts	▦	▦	▦	▦	☐	☐
35. Proper positioning (all anatomy included, evidence of proper centering/alignment, etc.)	▦	▦	▦	▦	☐	☐
36. Proper marker placement						
37. Evidence of proper collimation and radiation protection	▦	▦	▦	▦	☐	☐
38. Long vs. short scale of contrast	▦	▦	▦	▦	☐	☐

Comments:

_____

_____

(continued)

SOFT TISSUE EXTREMITY ANATOMY
The student is able to identify:

| | Procedure | | Repeat | | Competency | |
	Yes	No	Yes	No	Yes	No
39. _____	☐	☐	☐	☐	☐	☐
40. _____	☐	☐	☐	☐	☐	☐
41. _____	☐	☐	☐	☐	☐	☐
42. _____	☐	☐	☐	☐	☐	☐
43. _____	☐	☐	☐	☐	☐	☐
44. _____	☐	☐	☐	☐	☐	☐
45. _____	☐	☐	☐	☐	☐	☐
46. Obvious pathology	☐	☐	☐	☐	☐	☐

Comments:

_____

_____

_____   _____   _____
Procedure Evaluator Signature   Repeat Evaluator Signature   Competency Evaluator Signature

_____   _____   _____
Date   Date   Date

END SOFT TISSUE EXTREMITIES EVALUATION

Student Name:_____

Procedure Grade	Repeat Grade	Competency Grade

PATIENT INFORMATION OR SIMULATED PROCEDURE *(circle if simulated)*

	Procedure	Repeat	Competency
Age			
Medical Record No.			
Ability to Cooperate			
Condition/Pathology			
Technical Factors Used			
Exposure Index			

FACILITY PREPARATION
The student:

	Procedure Yes No	Repeat Yes No	Competency Yes No
1. Examines the radiographic room and cleans/straightens it before escorting the patient in.	☐ ☐	☐ ☐	☐ ☐
2. Has all equipment and supplies (patient gown, shield, markers, tape, cassettes, etc.) readily available before escorting the patient in.	☐ ☐	☐ ☐	☐ ☐
3. Is able to manipulate all radiographic equipment with ease, and centers the central ray to the cassette/receptor *for all projections.*	☐ ☐	☐ ☐	☐ ☐
4. Adjusts the tube to the proper SID *for each projection.*	☐ ☐	☐ ☐	☐ ☐
5. Selects the appropriate receptor or cassettes of the appropriate sizes *for all projections,* according to the patient's size and examination.	☐ ☐	☐ ☐	☐ ☐

Comments:

_____

_____

PATIENT PREPARATION
The student:

	Procedure Yes No	Repeat Yes No	Competency Yes No
6. Identifies the correct patient and examination according to the requisition while establishing a good rapport with him or her.	☐ ☐	☐ ☐	☐ ☐
7. Obtains and documents the patient's history before the examination.	▨ ▨	▨ ▨	☐ ☐
8. Explains the examination in terms the patient fully understands, and properly communicates with the patient throughout the examination.	☐ ☐	☐ ☐	☐ ☐
9. Asks female patients of childbearing age the date of their last menstrual period and documents this; inquires about the possibility of pregnancy and has them sign pregnancy consent forms	☐ ☐	☐ ☐	☐ ☐
10. Removes all obscuring objects (snaps, zippers, jewelry, etc.) so as *not* to produce radiographic artifacts.	☐ ☐	☐ ☐	☐ ☐

(continued)

	Procedure		Repeat		Competency	
	Yes	No	Yes	No	Yes	No
11. Respects the patient's modesty and provides ample comfort for the patient while positioning him or her to begin the examination.	☐	☐	☐	☐	☐	☐

Comments:

_____

_____

PATIENT POSITIONING FOR A CASTED EXTREMITY
Anteroposterior/Posteroanterior
The student:

	Procedure		Repeat		Competency	
	Yes	No	Yes	No	Yes	No
12. Places the patient in the supine or prone position at the upright Bucky/receptor or on the radiographic table, without rotation.	☐	☐	☐	☐	☐	☐
13. Selects the appropriate receptor or places the cassette appropriately. For conventional cassettes, the flash must be at the bottom and away from any anatomy.	☐	☐	☐	☐	☐	☐
14. Centers the central ray to the midline (between the lateral surfaces) of the affected extremity.	☐	☐	☐	☐	☐	☐
15. Directs the central ray perpendicularly or with the appropriate angle relative to the part being radiographed.	☐	☐	☐	☐	☐	☐

Lateral
The student:

	Procedure		Repeat		Competency	
	Yes	No	Yes	No	Yes	No
16. Places the patient in the true lateral position, without rotation.	☐	☐	☐	☐	☐	☐
17. Selects the appropriate receptor or places the cassette appropriately. For conventional cassettes, the flash must be at the bottom and away from any anatomy.	☐	☐	☐	☐	☐	☐
18. Centers the central ray midway between the anterior and posterior surfaces of the affected extremity.	☐	☐	☐	☐	☐	☐
19. Directs the central ray perpendicularly.	☐	☐	☐	☐	☐	☐

Comments:

_____

_____

IMPORTANT DETAILS
The student:

	Procedure		Repeat		Competency	
	Yes	No	Yes	No	Yes	No
20. Instills confidence in the patient by exhibiting self-confidence throughout the examination.	☐	☐	☐	☐	☐	☐
21. Places a lead marker in the appropriate area of the cassette/receptor (top/bottom/anteriorly/laterally), where they will be visualized, on the proper anatomical side (right/left), and in the appropriate position (face up/face down), depending on the patient's position.	☐	☐	☐	☐	☐	☐
22. Provides radiation protection (shield) for the patient (when appropriate), self, and others (closes doors).	☐	☐	☐	☐	☐	☐
23. Applies proper collimation and makes adjustments as necessary.	☐	☐	☐	☐	☐	☐
24. Properly measures the patient along the course of the central ray.	☐	☐	☐	☐	☐	☐
25. Sets the proper exposure technique:	☐	☐	☐	☐	☐	☐

Conventional systems
- Sets the proper kVp, mA, and time and makes adjustments as necessary.

or

	Procedure		Repeat		Competency	
	Yes	No	Yes	No	Yes	No

CR or DR systems
- Identifies the patient on the work-list (or manually types the patient information into the system).
- Selects appropriate body region, specific body part, and accurate view/projection.
- Double-checks preset parameters:
  —Adult vs. pediatric patients
  ○ Small, medium, or large
  —Bucky/receptor (upright vs. table) or non-Bucky
  —AEC vs. fixed
  ○ If AEC, checks ion chambers
  ○ Density setting
  —kVp and mA; adjusts if necessary
  —Focal spot/filament size

	Procedure		Repeat		Competency	
	Yes	No	Yes	No	Yes	No
26. Exposes the cassette/receptor after telling the patient to hold still and after giving him or her proper breathing instructions (if necessary) *for each projection.*	☐	☐	☐	☐	☐	☐
27. Provides each radiograph with the proper identification (flash) and/or processes each cassette (image) without difficulty (regardless of technology—film, CR, or DR).	☑	☑	☑	☑	☐	☐
28. Properly completes the examination by filling out all necessary paperwork, entering the examination in the computer, having images checked by the appropriate staff members, providing postprocedural instructions and answering last-minute questions, and informing the patient that he or she is finished. Provides proper post-exam instructions as required.	☑	☑	☑	☑	☐	☐
29. Exhibits the ability to adapt to new and difficult situations if and when necessary.	☑	☑	☑	☑	☐	☐
30. Accepts constructive criticism and uses it to his or her advantage.	☐	☐	☐	☐	☐	☐
31. Leaves the radiographic room neat and clean for the next examination.	☑	☑	☑	☑	☐	☐
32. Completes the examination within a reasonable time frame.	☐	☐	☐	☐	☐	☐

Comments:

_____

_____

RADIOGRAPHIC IMAGE QUALITY
The student is able to critique his or her radiographs as to whether they demonstrate:

	Procedure		Repeat		Competency	
	Yes	No	Yes	No	Yes	No
33. Proper technique/optimal density	☑	☑	☑	☑	☐	☐
34. Enhanced detail, without evidence of motion and without any visible artifacts	☑	☑	☑	☑	☐	☐
35. Proper positioning (all anatomy included, evidence of proper centering/alignment, etc.)	☑	☑	☑	☑	☐	☐
36. Proper marker placement						
37. Evidence of proper collimation and radiation protection	☑	☑	☑	☑	☐	☐
38. Long vs. short scale of contrast	☑	☑	☑	☑	☐	☐

Comments:

_____

_____

(continued)

CASTED EXTREMITY ANATOMY
The student is able to identify:

	Procedure		Repeat		Competency	
	Yes	No	Yes	No	Yes	No
39. _____	☐	☐	☐	☐	☐	☐
40. _____	☐	☐	☐	☐	☐	☐
41. _____	☐	☐	☐	☐	☐	☐
42. _____	☐	☐	☐	☐	☐	☐
43. _____	☐	☐	☐	☐	☐	☐
44. _____	☐	☐	☐	☐	☐	☐
45. _____	☐	☐	☐	☐	☐	☐
46. Obvious pathology	☐	☐	☐	☐	☐	☐

Comments:

_____

_____

_____   _____   _____
Procedure Evaluator Signature   Repeat Evaluator Signature   Competency Evaluator Signature

_____   _____   _____
Date   Date   Date

END CASTED EXTREMITIES EVALUATION

spcific radiographic examinations.

Student Name:_____

Procedure Grade	Repeat Grade	Competency Grade

PATIENT INFORMATION OR SIMULATED PROCEDURE *(circle if simulated)*

	Procedure	Repeat	Competency
Age			
Medical Record No.			
Ability to Cooperate			
Condition/Pathology			
Technical Factors Used			
Exposure Index			

FACILITY PREPARATION
The student:

	Procedure Yes No	Repeat Yes No	Competency Yes No
1. Examines the radiographic room and cleans/straightens it before escorting the patient in.	☐ ☐	☐ ☐	☐ ☐
2. Has all equipment and supplies (patient gown, shield, markers, tape, cassettes, etc.) readily available before escorting the patient in.	☐ ☐	☐ ☐	☐ ☐
3. Is able to manipulate all radiographic equipment with ease, and centers the central ray to the cassette/receptor *for all projections.*	☐ ☐	☐ ☐	☐ ☐
4. Adjusts the tube to the proper SID *for each projection.*	☐ ☐	☐ ☐	☐ ☐
5. Selects the appropriate receptor or cassettes of the appropriate sizes *for all projections,* according to the patient's size and examination.	☐ ☐	☐ ☐	☐ ☐

Comments:

_____

_____

PATIENT PREPARATION
The student:

	Procedure Yes No	Repeat Yes No	Competency Yes No
6. Identifies the correct patient and examination according to the requisition while establishing a good rapport with him or her.	☐ ☐	☐ ☐	☐ ☐
7. Obtains and documents the patient's history before the examination.	▦ ▦	▦ ▦	☐ ☐
8. Explains the examination in terms the patient fully understands, and properly communicates with the patient throughout the examination.	☐ ☐	☐ ☐	☐ ☐
9. Asks female patients of childbearing age the date of their last menstrual period and documents this; inquires about the possibility of pregnancy and has them sign pregnancy consent forms	☐ ☐	☐ ☐	☐ ☐
10. Removes all obscuring objects (snaps, zippers, jewelry, etc.) so as *not* to produce radiographic artifacts.	☐ ☐	☐ ☐	☐ ☐

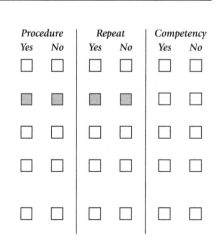

(continued)

	Procedure		Repeat		Competency	
	Yes	No	Yes	No	Yes	No
11. Respects the patient's modesty and provides ample comfort for the patient while positioning him or her to begin the examination.	☐	☐	☐	☐	☐	☐

Comments:

_____

_____

PATIENT POSITIONING FOR A SKELETAL/BONE SURVEY (FOR METASTASIS)
Skull
PA Caldwell
The student:

	Procedure		Repeat		Competency	
	Yes	No	Yes	No	Yes	No
12. Places the anterior surface of the patient's face against the Bucky/receptor.	☐	☐	☐	☐	☐	☐
13. Selects the appropriate receptor or places the cassette so that the upper border of the cassette/receptor is 2 inches above the vertex. For conventional cassettes, the flash must be away from any anatomy.	☐	☐	☐	☐	☐	☐
14. Places the patient's nose and forehead in contact with the Bucky/receptor.	☐	☐	☐	☐	☐	☐
15. Checks that the orbitomeatal line is perpendicular to the cassette/receptor.	☐	☐	☐	☐	☐	☐
16. Checks that the midsagittal line is perpendicular to the cassette/receptor.	☐	☐	☐	☐	☐	☐
17. Double-checks that the head is not tilted or rotated.	☐	☐	☐	☐	☐	☐
18. Centers the central ray to the midsagittal plane.	☐	☐	☐	☐	☐	☐
19. Directs the central ray at an angle of 15° caudad to the nasion.	☐	☐	☐	☐	☐	☐

Left Lateral
The student:

	Procedure		Repeat		Competency	
	Yes	No	Yes	No	Yes	No
20. Places the patient in the semiprone position.	☐	☐	☐	☐	☐	☐
21. Selects the appropriate receptor or places the cassette so that the upper border of the cassette/receptor is 2 inches above the vertex. For conventional cassettes, the flash must be away from any anatomy.	☐	☐	☐	☐	☐	☐
22. Places the patient's left side against the Bucky/receptor.	☐	☐	☐	☐	☐	☐
23. Checks that the infra-orbitomeatal line is parallel to the transverse axis of the cassette/receptor.	☐	☐	☐	☐	☐	☐
24. Checks that the head is not tilted (interpupillary line is perpendicular and midsagittal line is parallel to the cassette/receptor).	☐	☐	☐	☐	☐	☐
25. Centers the central ray 1–2 inches above the top of the ear attachment (EAM), and if the sella turcica is the primary interest, centers the central ray 3/4 inch superior and anterior to the EAM.	☐	☐	☐	☐	☐	☐
26. Directs the central ray perpendicularly.	☐	☐	☐	☐	☐	☐

Cervical Spine
Anteroposterior
The student:

	Procedure		Repeat		Competency	
	Yes	No	Yes	No	Yes	No
27. Places the patient's back against the upright Bucky/receptor (or supine on the radiographic table), without rotation.	☐	☐	☐	☐	☐	☐
28. Selects the appropriate receptor or places the cassette lengthwise. For conventional cassettes, the flash must be at the bottom and away from any anatomy.	☐	☐	☐	☐	☐	☐
29. Extends the head enough to place the occlusal plane and the mastoid tips in the same transverse plane, perpendicular to the cassette/receptor.	☐	☐	☐	☐	☐	☐
30. Centers the central ray to the midsagittal plane of the body.	☐	☐	☐	☐	☐	☐

	Procedure		Repeat		Competency	
	Yes	No	Yes	No	Yes	No
31. Directs the central ray at an angle of 15° cephalad to the thyroid cartilage/C4.	☐	☐	☐	☐	☐	☐

Lateral
The student:

	Procedure		Repeat		Competency	
	Yes	No	Yes	No	Yes	No
32. Places the patient in the left lateral position against the upright Bucky/receptor, without rotation.	☐	☐	☐	☐	☐	☐
33. Selects the appropriate receptor or places the cassette lengthwise, with the top of the cassette/receptor at the level of the EAM.	☐	☐	☐	☐	☐	☐
34. Elevates the patient's jaw/chin slightly forward.	☐	☐	☐	☐	☐	☐
35. Requests the patient to drop his or her shoulders and arms to the sides, reaching for the floor.	☐	☐	☐	☐	☐	☐
36. Directs the central ray to the center of the spine.	☐	☐	☐	☐	☐	☐
37. Centers the central ray perpendicularly to the thyroid cartilage/C4.	☐	☐	☐	☐	☐	☐

Thoracic Spine

Anteroposterior
The student:

	Procedure		Repeat		Competency	
	Yes	No	Yes	No	Yes	No
38. Places the patient in the supine position on the radiographic table, without rotation.	☐	☐	☐	☐	☐	☐
39. Selects the appropriate receptor or places the cassette lengthwise so that the upper edge of the cassette/receptor is approximately 1–2 inches above the patient's shoulders. For conventional cassettes, the flash must be at the bottom and away from any anatomy.	☐	☐	☐	☐	☐	☐
40. If possible, utilizes the anode heel effect and instructs the patient to flex his or her hips and knees slightly.	☐	☐	☐	☐	☐	☐
41. Centers the central ray to the midsagittal plane of the body.	☐	☐	☐	☐	☐	☐
42. Directs the central ray perpendicularly at the level to T6 (or 3–4 inches below the manubrial notch).	☐	☐	☐	☐	☐	☐

Lateral
The student:

	Procedure		Repeat		Competency	
	Yes	No	Yes	No	Yes	No
43. Places the patient in the left lateral position on the table, without rotation.	☐	☐	☐	☐	☐	☐
44. Selects the appropriate receptor or places the cassette lengthwise in the Bucky drawer.	☐	☐	☐	☐	☐	☐
45. Instructs the patient to flex his or her hips and knees up to a comfortable position.	☐	☐	☐	☐	☐	☐
46. Supports the patient's waist so that the spine is parallel, places a support between the knees, and supports the patient's head to avoid rotation.	☐	☐	☐	☐	☐	☐
47. Adjusts the patient's arms so that they are at right angles to the body.	☐	☐	☐	☐	☐	☐
48. Directs the central ray to the center of the spine.	☐	☐	☐	☐	☐	☐
49. Centers the central ray perpendicularly to T6 (or if the spine is not supported, the central ray should be angled cephalad until it is perpendicular to the spine, usually 10°–15°).	☐	☐	☐	☐	☐	☐
50. Places a lead blocker behind the patient.	☐	☐	☐	☐	☐	☐

(continued)

Lumbar Spine
Anteroposterior
The student:

	Procedure		Repeat		Competency	
	Yes	No	Yes	No	Yes	No
51. Places the patient in the supine position on the radiographic table, without rotation.	☐	☐	☐	☐	☐	☐
52. Selects the appropriate receptor or places the cassette lengthwise. For conventional cassettes, the flash must be at the bottom and away from any anatomy.	☐	☐	☐	☐	☐	☐
53. Instructs the patient to flex his or her hips and knees slightly.	☐	☐	☐	☐	☐	☐
54. Centers the central ray to the midsagittal plane of the body.	☐	☐	☐	☐	☐	☐
55. Directs the central ray perpendicularly at the level of the iliac crest.	☐	☐	☐	☐	☐	☐

Lateral
The student:

	Procedure		Repeat		Competency	
	Yes	No	Yes	No	Yes	No
56. Places the patient in the left lateral position on the radiographic table, without rotation.	☐	☐	☐	☐	☐	☐
57. Selects the appropriate receptor or places the cassette lengthwise. For conventional cassettes, the flash must be at the bottom and away from any anatomy.	☐	☐	☐	☐	☐	☐
58. Instructs the patient to flex his or her hips and knees up toward his or her chest.	☐	☐	☐	☐	☐	☐
59. Supports the patient's waist so that the spine is parallel, and places a support between the knees to avoid rotation.	☐	☐	☐	☐	☐	☐
60. Adjusts the patient's arms so that they are at right angles to the body.	☐	☐	☐	☐	☐	☐
61. Directs the central ray to the center of the spine (3 inches anteriorly from the spinous process).	☐	☐	☐	☐	☐	☐
62. Centers the central ray perpendicularly at the level of the iliac crest, or if the spine is not supported/parallel, the central ray is angled caudad until it is perpendicular to the spine, usually 5° for male patients and 8° for female patients.	☐	☐	☐	☐	☐	☐
63. Places a lead blocker behind the patient.	☐	☐	☐	☐	☐	☐

Pelvis
Anteroposterior
The student:

	Procedure		Repeat		Competency	
	Yes	No	Yes	No	Yes	No
64. Places the patient in the supine position on the radiographic table, without rotation.	☐	☐	☐	☐	☐	☐
65. Selects the appropriate receptor or places the cassette crosswise (CW) in the Bucky drawer, with the top of the cassette/receptor 1–2 inches above the iliac crest.	☐	☐	☐	☐	☐	☐
66. Rotates the legs internally (approximately 15°).	☐	☐	☐	☐	☐	☐
67. Centers the central ray to the midsagittal plane of the body.	☐	☐	☐	☐	☐	☐
68. Centers the central ray perpendicularly to the pelvis, midway between the crest and the symphysis pubis.	☐	☐	☐	☐	☐	☐

Humerus (If Possible, Including the Elbow)
Anteroposterior
The student:

	Procedure		Repeat		Competency	
	Yes	No	Yes	No	Yes	No
69. Places the patient in the supine position on the table or the erect position at the upright Bucky/receptor.	☐	☐	☐	☐	☐	☐

	Procedure		Repeat		Competency	
	Yes	No	Yes	No	Yes	No
70. Selects the appropriate receptor or places the cassette lengthwise to have a 1-inch margin from the top of the shoulder to the top of the cassette/receptor. For conventional cassettes, the flash must be away from any anatomy.	☐	☐	☐	☐	☐	☐
71. Supinates the hand to place the posterior surface of the humerus against the Bucky/receptor, with the epicondyles parallel to the cassette/receptor.	☐	☐	☐	☐	☐	☐
72. Centers the anatomy of interest to the center of the cassette/receptor, including both joints.	☐	☐	☐	☐	☐	☐
73. Centers the central ray perpendicularly to the midshaft of the humerus.	☐	☐	☐	☐	☐	☐

Femur (Including the Knee)
Anteroposterior
The student:

	Procedure		Repeat		Competency	
	Yes	No	Yes	No	Yes	No
74. Instructs the patient to extend the knee, and places the posterior surface of the leg on the appropriate area of the table.	☐	☐	☐	☐	☐	☐
75. Rotates the leg medially until the femoral epicondyles are parallel with the table.	☐	☐	☐	☐	☐	☐
76. Centers the anatomy of interest to the center of the cassette/receptor, including the knee joint.	☐	☐	☐	☐	☐	☐
77. Centers the central ray perpendicularly to the midfemur area (the center of the cassette/receptor).	☐	☐	☐	☐	☐	☐

Ribs
Anteroposterior
The student:

	Procedure		Repeat		Competency	
	Yes	No	Yes	No	Yes	No
78. Places the patient's back against the upright Bucky/receptor.	☐	☐	☐	☐	☐	☐
79. Selects the appropriate receptor or places the cassette lengthwise. For conventional cassettes, the flash must be at the top and away from any anatomy.	☐	☐	☐	☐	☐	☐
80. Centers the central ray to the midsagittal plane of the body.	☐	☐	☐	☐	☐	☐
81. Directs the central ray perpendicularly at the level of T6.	☐	☐	☐	☐	☐	☐

Both RPO and LPO
The student:

	Procedure		Repeat		Competency	
	Yes	No	Yes	No	Yes	No
82. Places the patient in the oblique position, at a 45° angle, against the upright Bucky/receptor.	☐	☐	☐	☐	☐	☐
83. Selects the appropriate receptor or places the cassette lengthwise. For conventional cassettes, the flash must be at the top and away from any anatomy.	☐	☐	☐	☐	☐	☐
84. Directs the central ray halfway between the spinous processes and the lateral rib margin of the side of interest (side down).	☐	☐	☐	☐	☐	☐
85. Centers the central ray perpendicularly at the level of T6.	☐	☐	☐	☐	☐	☐

Comments:

_____

_____

(continued)

IMPORTANT DETAILS
The student:

	Procedure		Repeat		Competency	
	Yes	No	Yes	No	Yes	No
86. Instills confidence in the patient by exhibiting self-confidence throughout the examination.	☐	☐	☐	☐	☐	☐
87. Places a lead marker in the appropriate area of the cassette/receptor (top/bottom/anteriorly/laterally), where they will be visualized, on the proper anatomical side (right/left), and in the appropriate position (face up/face down), depending on the patient's position.	☐	☐	☐	☐	☐	☐
88. Provides radiation protection (shield) for the patient (when appropriate), self, and others (closes doors).	☐	☐	☐	☐	☐	☐
89. Applies proper collimation and makes adjustments as necessary.	☐	☐	☐	☐	☐	☐
90. Properly measures the patient along the course of the central ray.	☐	☐	☐	☐	☐	☐
91. Sets the proper exposure technique:	☐	☐	☐	☐	☐	☐

Conventional systems
- Sets the proper kVp, mA, and time and makes adjustments as necessary.

or

CR or DR systems
- Identifies the patient on the work-list (or manually types the patient information into the system).
- Selects appropriate body region, specific body part, and accurate view/projection.
- Double-checks preset parameters:
  —Adult vs. pediatric patients
  ○ Small, medium, or large
  —Bucky/receptor (upright vs. table) or non-Bucky
  —AEC vs. fixed
  ○ If AEC, checks ion chambers
  ○ Density setting
  —kVp and mA; adjusts if necessary
  —Focal spot/filament size

	Procedure		Repeat		Competency	
92. Exposes the cassette/receptor after telling the patient to hold still and after giving him or her proper breathing instructions (as necessary) *for each projection.*	☐	☐	☐	☐	☐	☐
93. Provides each radiograph with the proper identification (flash) and/or processes each cassette (image) without difficulty (regardless of technology: film, CR, or DR).	▣	▣	▣	▣	☐	☐
94. Properly completes the examination by filling out all necessary paperwork, entering the examination in the computer, having images checked by the appropriate staff members, providing postprocedural instructions and answering last-minute questions, and informing the patient that he or she is finished. Provides proper post-exam instructions as required.	▣	▣	▣	▣	☐	☐
95. Exhibits the ability to adapt to new and difficult situations if and when necessary.	▣	▣	▣	▣	☐	☐
96. Accepts constructive criticism and uses it to his or her advantage.	☐	☐	☐	☐	☐	☐
97. Leaves the radiographic room neat and clean for the next examination.	▣	▣	▣	▣	☐	☐
98. Completes the examination within a reasonable time frame.	☐	☐	☐	☐	☐	☐

Comments:

_____

_____

RADIOGRAPHIC IMAGE QUALITY

The student is able to critique his or her radiographs as to whether they demonstrate:

	Procedure		Repeat		Competency	
	Yes	No	Yes	No	Yes	No
99. Proper technique/optimal density	☐	☐	☐	☐	☐	☐
100. Enhanced detail, without evidence of motion and without any visible artifacts	☐	☐	☐	☐	☐	☐
101. Proper positioning (all anatomy included, evidence of proper centering/alignment, etc.)	☐	☐	☐	☐	☐	☐
102. Proper marker placement						
103. Evidence of proper collimation and radiation protection	☐	☐	☐	☐	☐	☐
104. Long vs. short scale of contrast	☐	☐	☐	☐	☐	☐

Comments:

_____

_____

SKELETAL/BONE SURVEY ANATOMY

Skull
The student is able to identify:

	Procedure		Repeat		Competency	
	Yes	No	Yes	No	Yes	No
105. Frontal bone	☐	☐	☐	☐	☐	☐
106. Parietal bones	☐	☐	☐	☐	☐	☐
107. Sella turcica	☐	☐	☐	☐	☐	☐
108. Sphenoid sinus	☐	☐	☐	☐	☐	☐

Cervical
The student is able to identify:

	Procedure		Repeat		Competency	
	Yes	No	Yes	No	Yes	No
109. Cervical body	☐	☐	☐	☐	☐	☐
110. Cervical transverse process	☐	☐	☐	☐	☐	☐
111. Spinous process	☐	☐	☐	☐	☐	☐
112. Cervical disk space	☐	☐	☐	☐	☐	☐

Thoracic
The student is able to identify:

	Procedure		Repeat		Competency	
	Yes	No	Yes	No	Yes	No
113. Thoracic body	☐	☐	☐	☐	☐	☐
114. Thoracic transverse process	☐	☐	☐	☐	☐	☐
115. Thoracic spinous process	☐	☐	☐	☐	☐	☐
116. Thoracic disk space	☐	☐	☐	☐	☐	☐

Lumbar
The student is able to identify:

	Procedure		Repeat		Competency	
	Yes	No	Yes	No	Yes	No
117. Lumbar body	☐	☐	☐	☐	☐	☐
118. Lumbar intervertebral foramen	☐	☐	☐	☐	☐	☐
119. L5–S1 articulation	☐	☐	☐	☐	☐	☐

Pelvis
The student is able to identify:

	Procedure		Repeat		Competency	
	Yes	No	Yes	No	Yes	No
120. Iliac crest	☐	☐	☐	☐	☐	☐
121. Acetabulum	☐	☐	☐	☐	☐	☐
122. Symphysis pubis	☐	☐	☐	☐	☐	☐

(continued)

Humerus
The student is able to identify:

	Procedure		Repeat		Competency	
	Yes	No	Yes	No	Yes	No
123. Humeral head and glenoid fossa	▣	▣	▣	▣	☐	☐
124. Capitellum	▣	▣	▣	▣	☐	☐
125. Trochlea	▣	▣	▣	▣	☐	☐

Femur
The student is able to identify:

	Procedure		Repeat		Competency	
	Yes	No	Yes	No	Yes	No
126. Femoral epicondyles vs. condyles	▣	▣	▣	▣	☐	☐
127. Femoral head and neck	▣	▣	▣	▣	☐	☐
128. Greater and lesser trochanters	▣	▣	▣	▣	☐	☐

Ribs
The student is able to identify:

	Procedure		Repeat		Competency	
	Yes	No	Yes	No	Yes	No
129. Rib head and tubercle	▣	▣	▣	▣	☐	☐
130. Rib angle	▣	▣	▣	▣	☐	☐
131. Obvious pathology	▣	▣	▣	▣	☐	☐

Comments:

_____

_____

Procedure Evaluator Signature	Repeat Evaluator Signature	Competency Evaluator Signature

Date	Date	Date

END SKELETAL/BONE SURVEY EVALUATION

Student Name:_____

	Procedure Grade	Repeat Grade	Competency Grade

PATIENT INFORMATION OR SIMULATED PROCEDURE *(circle if simulated)*

	Procedure	Repeat	Competency
Age			
Medical Record No.			
Ability to Cooperate			
Condition/Pathology			
Technical Factors Used			
Exposure Index			

FACILITY PREPARATION
The student:

	Procedure Yes	Procedure No	Repeat Yes	Repeat No	Competency Yes	Competency No
1. Examines the radiographic room and cleans/straightens it before escorting the patient in.	☐	☐	☐	☐	☐	☐
2. Has all equipment and supplies (patient gown, shield, markers, tape, cassettes, etc.) readily available before escorting the patient in.	☐	☐	☐	☐	☐	☐
3. Is able to manipulate all radiographic equipment with ease, and centers the central ray to the cassette/receptor *for all projections.*	☐	☐	☐	☐	☐	☐
4. Adjusts the tube to the proper SID.	☐	☐	☐	☐	☐	☐
5. Selects the appropriate receptor or cassettes of the appropriate sizes *for all projections,* according to the patient's size and examination.	☐	☐	☐	☐	☐	☐

Comments:

_____

_____

PATIENT PREPARATION
The student:

	Procedure Yes	Procedure No	Repeat Yes	Repeat No	Competency Yes	Competency No
6. Identifies the correct patient and examination according to the requisition while establishing a good rapport with him or her.	☐	☐	☐	☐	☐	☐
7. Obtains and documents the patient's history before the examination.	▣	▣	▣	▣	☐	☐
8. Asks female patients of childbearing age the date of their last menstrual period and documents this; inquires about the possibility of pregnancy and has them sign pregnancy consent forms	☐	☐	☐	☐	☐	☐
9. Explains the examination in terms the patient fully understands, and properly communicates with the patient throughout the examination.	☐	☐	☐	☐	☐	☐
10. Removes all obscuring objects (snaps, zippers, jewelry, etc.) so as *not* to produce radiographic artifacts.	☐	☐	☐	☐	☐	☐

(continued)

	Procedure		Repeat		Competency	
	Yes	No	Yes	No	Yes	No
11. Respects the patient's modesty and provides ample comfort for the patient while positioning him or her to begin the examination.	☐	☐	☐	☐	☐	☐

Comments:

_____

_____

PATIENT POSITIONING FOR A BONE AGE (PA HAND AND WRIST)
The student:

	Procedure		Repeat		Competency	
	Yes	No	Yes	No	Yes	No
12. Places the left hand and wrist palm down on the appropriate area of the cassette/receptor.	☐	☐	☐	☐	☐	☐
13. Slightly separates the fingers, ensuring that the thumb forms a 30° angle with the rest of the hand.	☐	☐	☐	☐	☐	☐
14. Centers the anatomy of interest to the center of the cassette/receptor.	☐	☐	☐	☐	☐	☐
15. Directs the central ray perpendicularly to the head of the third metacarpal.	☐	☐	☐	☐	☐	☐

Comments:

_____

_____

IMPORTANT DETAILS
The student:

	Procedure		Repeat		Competency	
	Yes	No	Yes	No	Yes	No
16. Instills confidence in the patient by exhibiting self-confidence throughout the examination.	☐	☐	☐	☐	☐	☐
17. Places a lead marker in the appropriate area of the cassette/receptor (top/bottom/anteriorly/laterally), where they will be visualized, on the proper anatomical side (right/left), and in the appropriate position (face up/face down), depending on the patient's position.	☐	☐	☐	☐	☐	☐
18. Provides radiation protection (shield) for the patient (when appropriate), self, and others (closes doors).	☐	☐	☐	☐	☐	☐
19. Applies proper collimation and makes adjustments as necessary.	☐	☐	☐	☐	☐	☐
20. Properly measures the patient along the course of the central ray.	☐	☐	☐	☐	☐	☐
21. Sets the proper exposure technique:	☐	☐	☐	☐	☐	☐

Conventional systems
- Sets the proper kVp, mA, and time and makes adjustments as necessary.

or

CR or DR systems
- Identifies the patient on the work-list (or manually types the patient information into the system).
- Selects appropriate body region, specific body part, and accurate view/projection.
- Double-checks preset parameters:
  —Adult vs. pediatric patients
  　○ Small, medium, or large
  —Bucky/receptor (upright vs. table) or non-Bucky
  —AEC vs. fixed
  　○ If AEC, checks ion chambers
  　○ Density setting
  —kVp and mA; adjusts if necessary
  —Focal spot/filament size

	Procedure		Repeat		Competency	
	Yes	No	Yes	No	Yes	No
22. Exposes the cassette/receptor after telling the patient to hold still *for each projection.*	☐	☐	☐	☐	☐	☐
23. Provides each radiograph with the proper identification (flash) and/or processes each cassette (image) without difficulty (regardless of technology: film, CR, or DR).	▣	▣	▣	▣	☐	☐
24. Properly completes the examination by filling out all necessary paperwork, entering the examination in the computer, having images checked by the appropriate staff members, providing postprocedural instructions and answering last-minute questions, and informing the patient that he or she is finished. Provides proper post-exam instructions as required.	▣	▣	▣	▣	☐	☐
25. Exhibits the ability to adapt to new and difficult situations if and when necessary.	▣	▣	▣	▣	☐	☐
26. Accepts constructive criticism and uses it to his or her advantage.	☐	☐	☐	☐	☐	☐
27. Leaves the radiographic room neat and clean for the next examination.	▣	▣	▣	▣	☐	☐
28. Completes the examination within a reasonable time frame.	▣	▣	▣	▣	☐	☐

Comments:

_____

_____

RADIOGRAPHIC IMAGE QUALITY
The student is able to critique his or her radiographs as to whether they demonstrate:

	Procedure		Repeat		Competency	
	Yes	No	Yes	No	Yes	No
29. Proper technique/optimal density	▣	▣	▣	▣	☐	☐
30. Enhanced detail, without evidence of motion and without any visible artifacts	▣	▣	▣	▣	☐	☐
31. Proper positioning (all anatomy included, evidence of proper centering/alignment, etc.)	▣	▣	▣	▣	☐	☐
32. Proper marker placement						
33. Evidence of proper collimation and radiation protection	▣	▣	▣	▣	☐	☐
34. Long vs. short scale of contrast	▣	▣	▣	▣	☐	☐

Comments:

_____

BONE AGE ANATOMY
The student is able to identify:

	Procedure		Repeat		Competency	
	Yes	No	Yes	No	Yes	No
35. Distal phalanges	▣	▣	▣	▣	☐	☐
36. Middle phalanges	▣	▣	▣	▣	☐	☐
37. Proximal phalanges	▣	▣	▣	▣	☐	☐
38. Distal interphalangeal joints	▣	▣	▣	▣	☐	☐
39. Proximal interphalangeal joints	▣	▣	▣	▣	☐	☐
40. Metacarpophalangeal joints	▣	▣	▣	▣	☐	☐
41. Metacarpals	▣	▣	▣	▣	☐	☐
42. Carpometacarpal joints	▣	▣	▣	▣	☐	☐
43. Carpals	▣	▣	▣	▣	☐	☐
44. Radius	▣	▣	▣	▣	☐	☐

(continued)

	Procedure		Repeat		Competency	
	Yes	No	Yes	No	Yes	No
45. Ulna	☐	☐	☐	☐	☐	☐
46. Obvious pathology	☐	☐	☐	☐	☐	☐

Comments:

_____

_____

_____   _____   _____
Procedure Evaluator Signature   Repeat Evaluator Signature   Competency Evaluator Signature

_____   _____   _____
Date   Date   Date

END BONE AGE EVALUATION

Student Name:_____

Procedure Grade	Repeat Grade	Competency Grade

PATIENT INFORMATION OR SIMULATED PROCEDURE *(circle if simulated)*

	Procedure	Repeat	Competency
Age			
Medical Record No.			
Ability to Cooperate			
Condition/Pathology			
Technical Factors Used			
Exposure Index			

FACILITY PREPARATION
The student:

	Procedure Yes No	Repeat Yes No	Competency Yes No
1. Examines the radiographic room and cleans/straightens it before escorting the patient in.	☐ ☐	☐ ☐	☐ ☐
2. Has all equipment and supplies (patient gown, shield, markers, tape, cassettes, etc.) readily available before escorting the patient in.	☐ ☐	☐ ☐	☐ ☐
3. Is able to manipulate all radiographic equipment with ease, and centers the central ray to the cassette/receptor *for all projections.*	☐ ☐	☐ ☐	☐ ☐
4. Adjusts the tube to the proper SID.	☐ ☐	☐ ☐	☐ ☐
5. Selects the appropriate receptor or cassettes of the appropriate sizes *for all projections,* according to the patient's size and examination.	☐ ☐	☐ ☐	☐ ☐

Comments:

_____

_____

PATIENT PREPARATION
The student:

	Procedure Yes No	Repeat Yes No	Competency Yes No
6. Identifies the correct patient and examination according to the requisition while establishing a good rapport with him or her.	☐ ☐	☐ ☐	☐ ☐
7. Obtains and documents the patient's history before the examination.	▪ ▪	▪ ▪	☐ ☐
8. Explains the examination in terms the patient fully understands, and properly communicates with the patient throughout the examination.	☐ ☐	☐ ☐	☐ ☐
9. Asks female patients of childbearing age the date of their last menstrual period and documents this; inquires about the possibility of pregnancy and has them sign pregnancy consent forms	☐ ☐	☐ ☐	☐ ☐
10. Removes all obscuring objects (snaps, zippers, jewelry, etc.) so as *not* to produce radiographic artifacts.	☐ ☐	☐ ☐	☐ ☐

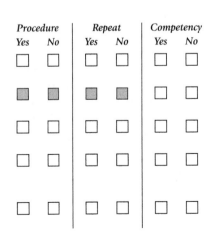

(continued)

	Procedure		Repeat		Competency	
	Yes	No	Yes	No	Yes	No
11. Respects the patient's modesty and provides ample comfort for the patient while positioning him or her to begin the examination.	☐	☐	☐	☐	☐	☐

Comments:

_____

_____

PATIENT POSITIONING FOR A LONG BONE MEASUREMENT/SCANOGRAM
AP Hips
The student:

	Procedure		Repeat		Competency	
	Yes	No	Yes	No	Yes	No
12. Places the patient in the supine position on the radiographic table.	☐	☐	☐	☐	☐	☐
13. Places the special metal ruler beneath the limbs and examines both sides simultaneously for comparison.	☐	☐	☐	☐	☐	☐
14. Localizes the hip joints and centers the hips to the top third of the cassette/receptor, imagining the line from the anterior superior iliac spine to the pubic symphysis and centering 2–3 cm laterally and distally from the midpoint of that line.	☐	☐	☐	☐	☐	☐
15. Directs the central ray perpendicularly midway between the two hips (midsagittal plane).	☐	☐	☐	☐	☐	☐
16. Does not remove the cassette or move the patient, but moves the central ray and cassette/receptor to the next centering point.	☐	☐	☐	☐	☐	☐

AP Knees
The student:

	Procedure		Repeat		Competency	
	Yes	No	Yes	No	Yes	No
17. Leaves the patient in the supine position on the radiographic table.	☐	☐	☐	☐	☐	☐
18. Does not adjust the special ruler beneath the limbs, and examines both sides simultaneously for comparison.	☐	☐	☐	☐	☐	☐
19. Localizes the knee joints and centers the knees, just below the apex of the patella at the level of the depression between the femoral and tibial condyles, to the middle third of the cassette/receptor.	☐	☐	☐	☐	☐	☐
20. Directs the central ray perpendicularly, midway between the two knees (midsagittal plane).	☐	☐	☐	☐	☐	☐
21. Does not remove the cassette or move the patient, but moves the central ray and cassette/receptor to the next centering point.	☐	☐	☐	☐	☐	☐

AP Ankles
The student:

	Procedure		Repeat		Competency	
	Yes	No	Yes	No	Yes	No
22. Leaves the patient in the supine position on the radiographic table.	☐	☐	☐	☐	☐	☐
23. Does not adjust the special ruler beneath the limbs, and examines both sides simultaneously for comparison.	☐	☐	☐	☐	☐	☐
24. Localizes the ankle joints and centers the ankles (midway between the malleoli) to the bottom third of the cassette/receptor.	☐	☐	☐	☐	☐	☐
25. Directs the central ray perpendicularly, midway between the two ankles (midsagittal plane).	☐	☐	☐	☐	☐	☐

Comments:

_____

_____

IMPORTANT DETAILS
The student:

	Procedure		Repeat		Competency	
	Yes	No	Yes	No	Yes	No
26. Instills confidence in the patient by exhibiting self-confidence throughout the examination.	☐	☐	☐	☐	☐	☐
27. Places a lead marker in the appropriate area of the cassette/receptor (top/bottom/anteriorly/laterally), where they will be visualized, on the proper anatomical side (right/left), and in the appropriate position (face up/face down), depending on the patient's position.	☐	☐	☐	☐	☐	☐
28. Provides radiation protection (shield) for the patient (when appropriate), self, and others (closes doors).	☐	☐	☐	☐	☐	☐
29. Applies *tight* collimation and makes adjustments as necessary.	☐	☐	☐	☐	☐	☐
30. Properly measures the patient along the course of the central ray.	☐	☐	☐	☐	☐	☐
31. Sets the proper exposure technique:	☐	☐	☐	☐	☐	☐

Conventional systems
- Sets the proper kVp, mA, and time and makes adjustments as necessary.

or

CR or DR systems
- Identifies the patient on the work-list (or manually types the patient information into the system).
- Selects appropriate body region, specific body part, and accurate view/projection.
- Double-checks preset parameters:
  —Adult vs. pediatric patients
    ○ Small, medium, or large
  —Bucky/receptor (upright vs. table) or non-Bucky
  —AEC vs. fixed
    ○ If AEC, checks ion chambers
    ○ Density setting
  —kVp and mA; adjusts if necessary
  —Focal spot/filament size

	Procedure		Repeat		Competency	
32. Exposes the cassette/receptor after telling the patient to hold still and after giving him or her proper breathing instructions (as necessary) *for each projection.*	☐	☐	☐	☐	☐	☐
33. Provides each radiograph with the proper identification (flash) and/or processes each cassette (image) without difficulty (regardless of technology: film, CR, or DR).	▧	▧	▧	▧	☐	☐
34. Properly completes the examination by filling out all necessary paperwork, entering the examination in the computer, having images checked by the appropriate staff members, providing postprocedural instructions and answering last-minute questions, and informing the patient that he or she is finished. Provides proper post-exam instructions as required.	▧	▧	▧	▧	☐	☐
35. Exhibits the ability to adapt to new and difficult situations if and when necessary.	▧	▧	▧	▧	☐	☐
36. Accepts constructive criticism and uses it to his or her advantage.	☐	☐	☐	☐	☐	☐
37. Leaves the radiographic room neat and clean for the next examination.	▧	▧	▧	▧	☐	☐
38. Completes the examination within a reasonable time frame.	☐	☐	☐	☐	☐	☐

Comments:

_____

_____

(continued)

RADIOGRAPHIC IMAGE QUALITY
The student is able to critique his or her radiographs as to whether they demonstrate:

	Procedure		Repeat		Competency	
	Yes	No	Yes	No	Yes	No
39. Proper technique/optimal density	☐	☐	☐	☐	☐	☐
40. Enhanced detail, without evidence of motion and without any visible artifacts	☐	☐	☐	☐	☐	☐
41. Proper positioning (all anatomy included, evidence of proper centering/alignment, etc.)	☐	☐	☐	☐	☐	☐
42. Proper marker placement						
43. Evidence of proper collimation and radiation protection	☐	☐	☐	☐	☐	☐
44. Long vs. short scale of contrast	☐	☐	☐	☐	☐	☐

Comments:

_____

_____

LONG BONE MEASUREMENT/SCANOGRAM ANATOMY
The student is able to identify:

	Procedure		Repeat		Competency	
	Yes	No	Yes	No	Yes	No
45. Acetabulum	☐	☐	☐	☐	☐	☐
46. Femoral head	☐	☐	☐	☐	☐	☐
47. Greater and lesser trochanters	☐	☐	☐	☐	☐	☐
48. Femoral neck	☐	☐	☐	☐	☐	☐
49. Medial and lateral femoral condyles	☐	☐	☐	☐	☐	☐
50. Medial and lateral femoral epicondyles	☐	☐	☐	☐	☐	☐
51. Fibula	☐	☐	☐	☐	☐	☐
52. Tibia	☐	☐	☐	☐	☐	☐
53. Medial and lateral tibial condyles	☐	☐	☐	☐	☐	☐
54. Medial and lateral malleoli	☐	☐	☐	☐	☐	☐
55. Talus	☐	☐	☐	☐	☐	☐
56. Obvious pathology	☐	☐	☐	☐	☐	☐

Comments:

_____

_____

_____	_____	_____
Procedure Evaluator Signature	Repeat Evaluator Signature	Competency Evaluator Signature

_____	_____	_____
Date	Date	Date

END LONG BONE MEASUREMENT/SCANOGRAM EVALUATION

Bibliography

Ballinger, PW. Merrill's Atlas of Radiographic Positions and Radiologic Procedures, 6th ed, Vols 1-3. St Louis: Mosby, 1986.

Ballinger, PW, Frank, ED. Merrill's Atlas of Radiographic Positions and Radiologic Procedures, 9th ed, Vols 1-3. St Louis: Mosby, 1999.

Ballinger, PW, Frank, ED. Merrill's Atlas of Radiographic Positions and Radiologic Procedures, 10th ed, Vols 1-3. St Louis: Mosby, 2003.

Kiser, D. The Competency-Based Rad Tech Workbook. Philadelphia: W.B. Saunders, 1991.

Index